T0309998

Atlas of Dermatopathology: Tumors, Nevi, and Cysts

Atlas of Dermatopathology
Tumors, Nevi, and Cysts

Günter Burg MD

Department of Dermatology
University of Zurich
Switzerland

Heinz Kutzner MD

Department of Dermatology
Institute of Dermatopathology
Friedrichshafen
Germany

Werner Kempf MD

Department of Dermatopathology
University of Zurich
Switzerland

Josef Feit MD, PhD

Department of Pathology
University of Ostrava
Czech Republic

Bruce R. Smoller MD

University of Rochester Medical Center
School of Medicine and Dentistry
Rochester
USA

WILEY Blackwell

The right of Günter Burg, Heinz Kutzner, Werner Kempf, Josef Feit, Bruce R. Smoller to be identified as the authors of editorial material in this work has been asserted in accordance with law.

Registered Office(s)
John Wiley & Sons, Inc., 111 River Street, Hoboken, NJ 07030, USA
John Wiley & Sons Ltd, The Atrium, Southern Gate, Chichester, West Sussex, PO19 8SQ, UK

Editorial Office
9600 Garsington Road, Oxford, OX4 2DQ, UK

For details of our global editorial offices, customer services, and more information about Wiley products visit us at www.wiley.com.

Wiley also publishes its books in a variety of electronic formats and by print-on-demand. Some content that appears in standard print versions of this book may not be available in other formats.

Library of Congress Cataloging-in-Publication Data

Names: Burg, Günter, author. | Kutzner, Heinz, author. | Kempf, Werner, author. | Feit, Josef, author. | Smoller, Bruce R., author.
Title: Atlas of dermatopathology: Tumors, nevi, and cysts / Günter Burg, Heinz Kutzner, Werner Kempf, Josef Feit, Bruce R. Smoller.
Description: Hoboken, NJ : Wiley-Blackwell, [2018] | Includes bibliographical references and index. |
Identifiers: LCCN 2018023723 (print) | LCCN 2018024979 (ebook) | ISBN 9781119371557 (Adobe PDF) | ISBN 9781119371564 (ePub) | ISBN 9781119371540 (hardcover)
Subjects: | MESH: Skin Neoplasms–diagnosis | Skin Neoplasms–pathology | Cutaneous Cyst–diagnosis | Cutaneous Cyst–pathology | Diagnosis, Differential | Atlases
Classification: LCC RC280.S5 (ebook) | LCC RC280.S5 (print) | NLM WR 17 | DDC 616.99/477–dc23
LC record available at https://lccn.loc.gov/2018023723

Cover Design: Wiley
Cover Image: All images courtesy of Günter Burg

Set in 8.5/12pt Meridien by SPi Global, Pondicherry, India
Printed and bound in Singapore by Markono Print Media Pte Ltd

10 9 8 7 6 5 4 3 2 1

To our families and teachers, who have supported and guided us

Contents

Preface

In tumorous processes, the typical cytomorphology and growth pattern assessed by histological examination are the major hallmarks of correct diagnosis. Therefore, this text-atlas, in 13 well-illustrated chapters, presents the major cytomorphological elements of the skin, and describes the histological characteristics of epidermal and organoid nevi, hamartomas and tumors of the epidermis, adnexal structures, melanocytic lesions, and tumors of connective tissue, vessels, fat, muscles, nerves, mast cells, histiocytes, and hematopoietic cells, i.e. lymphomas and leukemias. In addition to the histology, the clinical features and differential diagnoses (DD:) are presented for each entity. As cysts may be clinically misdiagnosed as tumorous lesions, a chapter on cysts has been added for differential diagnostic purposes.

The text of the clinical features (Cl:) is given in prose form, whereas the description of the histological features (Hi:) follows the approved bullet point style in order to keep the information as compact and concise as possible.

Some of the diagnoses listed lack clinical or histological pictures.

Even though we have tried to cover most common diagnoses, the book is far from being comprehensive. Many variants of tumors described in the literature are waiting to be included in the next edition and may be studied in special books dealing with distinct adnexal, vascular, soft tissue, hematopoietic or other neoplasias.

Günter Burg, Heinz Kutzner, Werner Kempf,
Josef Feit, Bruce R. Smoller
2018

Acknowledgments

Computational resources for the atlases were provided by the CESNET LM2015042 and CERIT Scientific Cloud LM2015085 large research and development programs.

We appreciate the support of the Wiley Publishing Group and its co-workers, especially of Mrs Yogalakshmi Mohanakrishnan and Mrs Monisha Swaminathan from the Health Science Office in India.

CHAPTER 1

Epidermis

Atlas of Dermatopathology: Tumors, Nevi, and Cysts, First Edition. Günter Burg, Heinz Kutzner,
Werner Kempf, Josef Feit, and Bruce R. Smoller.
© 2019 John Wiley & Sons Ltd. Published 2019 by John Wiley & Sons Ltd.

Nevi

Epidermal Nevus

Hyperkeratotic streaks or plaques

Psoriasiform hyperkeratosis, acanthosis and papillomatosis

Mild hypergranulosis

Cl: Epidermal nevi are the most common manifestations of cutaneous mosaicism. They are autosomal dominant segmental hyperkeratotic verrucous or papular lesions present at birth. They present as brown or gray isolated, linear, zosteriform, or whorled patches or follow Blaschko lines.

Hi: Psoriasiform acanthosis, papillomatosis, orthohyperkeratosis.

Reference

Chi, C.C., Wang, S.H., and Lin, P.Y. (2009) Combined epidermal-connective tissue nevus of proteoglycan (a type of mucinous nevus): a case report and literature review. *J Cutan Pathol* **36**(7): 808–11.

DD: Seborrheic keratosis; epidermolytic hyperkeratosis.

Variant: Inflammatory Linear Verrucous Epidermal Nevus (ILVEN)

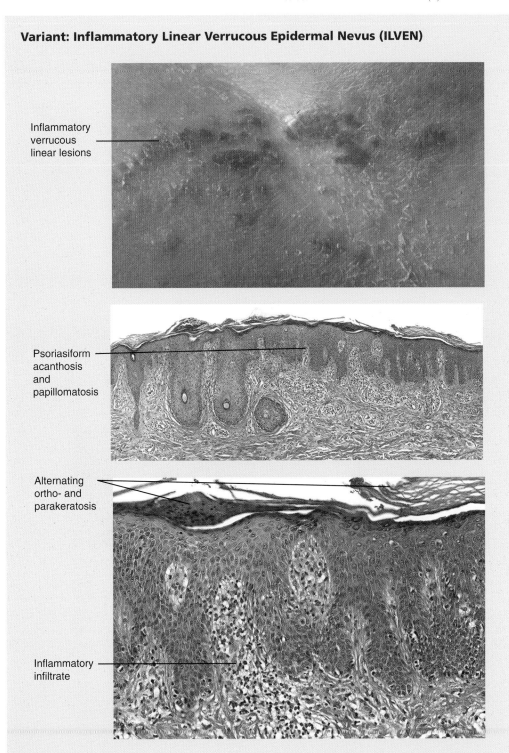

Inflammatory verrucous linear lesions

Psoriasiform acanthosis and papillomatosis

Alternating ortho- and parakeratosis

Inflammatory infiltrate

SEBORRHEIC KERATOSIS AND VARIANTS

Cl: ILVEN is considered a variant of epidermal nevus. It shows linear verrucous streaks with inflammatory erythema, scaling, and pruritus.
Hi:
- Psoriasiform acanthosis and papillomatosis
- Alternating areas of ortho- and parakeratosis
- Decreased to absent granular layer
- Prominent acantholysis in some cases
- Inflammatory infiltrate in the papillary dermis

Keratoses

Seborrheic Keratosis (SK) and Variants

Most common epidermal tumor. Synonyms: Senile keratosis, seborrheic wart. Even though resembling common warts, there is no association with human papilloma virus (HPV). They are benign but cosmetically disturbing, sometimes irritated, and occasionally are confused with pigmented tumors like malignant melanoma or pigmented basal cell carcinoma.
Cl: Seborrheic keratosis may present various clinical features. The most common variants are *acanthotic seborrheic keratoses*, which occur as multiple elevated light or dark brown lesions of various sizes preferentially on the trunk, head, and neck of elderly people, sparing palms and soles. *Flat seborrheic keratoses* are referred to as solar lentigo in sun-exposed areas. Others are *papillomatous* and hyperkeratotic with a ceribriform surface. They may be inflamed (*irritated* or "activated"). *Melanoacanthoma* is a dark pigmented seborrheic keratosis in elderly people, which may be confused with malignant melanoma. *Dermatosis papulosa nigra*, preferentially occurring in the suborbital and temporal region of black and dark-skinned individuals, presents as tiny pigmented papules. *Reticulated adenoid* (pigmented) and *clonal* (intraepidermal, Borst–Jadassohn) seborrheic keratosis or SK with "*monster cells*" are distinct histological features without special clinical presentation. Hyperkeratotic SK (*stucco keratoses*) appear as tiny multiple whitish hyperkeratotic lesions like gypsum splatters on the dorsum of hands, feet, and lower legs.
DD: Verruca vulgaris; acrokeratosis verruciformis (Hopf).

Variant: Acanthotic Seborrheic Keratosis

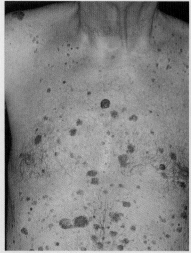

Multiple seborrheic keratoses on the trunk

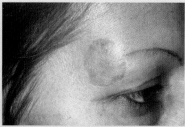
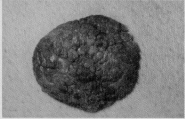

Flat (above) and papillomatous (below) seborrheic keratoses

SEBORRHEIC KERATOSIS AND VARIANTS

Variant: Acanthotic Seborrheic Keratosis

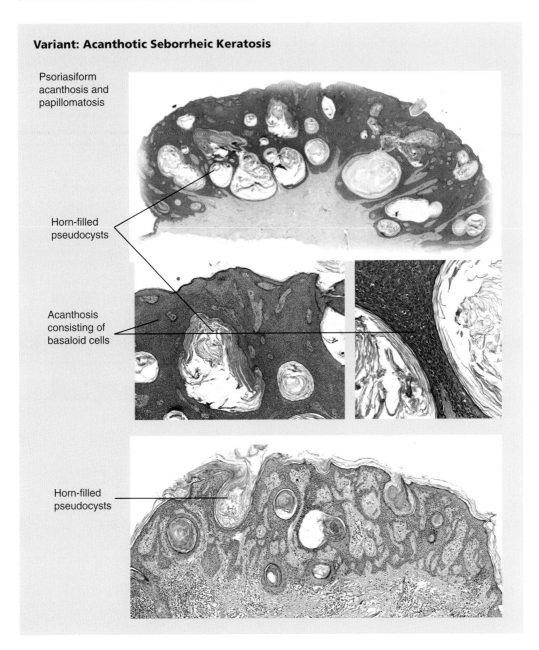

Psoriasiform acanthosis and papillomatosis

Horn-filled pseudocysts

Acanthosis consisting of basaloid cells

Horn-filled pseudocysts

Hi: Broad acanthotic epidermis composed of basaloid cells. Anastomosing horny pseudocysts filled with keratin.

SEBORRHEIC KERATOSIS AND VARIANTS

Variant: Reticulated, Pigmented Seborrheic Keratosis

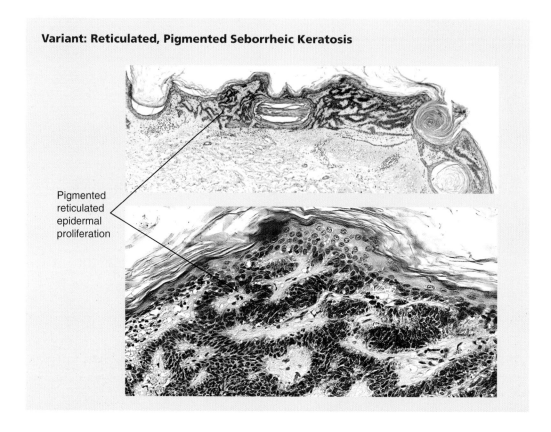

Pigmented
reticulated
epidermal
proliferation

Hi: Anastomosing small epithelial cords mostly with basal pigmentation forming a reticular net.

Variant: Flat Seborrheic Keratosis

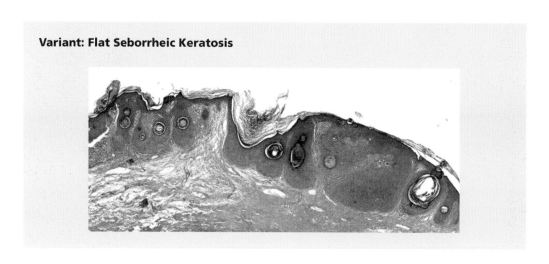

Hi: Flat plump acanthosis with keratin-filled horny pseudocysts.

SEBORRHEIC KERATOSIS AND VARIANTS

Variant: Papillomatous Seborrheic Keratosis

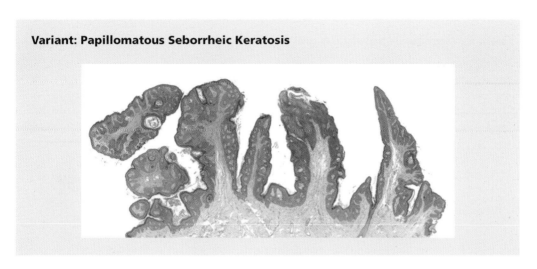

Hi:
- Church spire-like proliferations
- Papillomatosis
- Ortho- and parakeratosis

Variant: Activated (Irritated) Seborrheic Keratosis

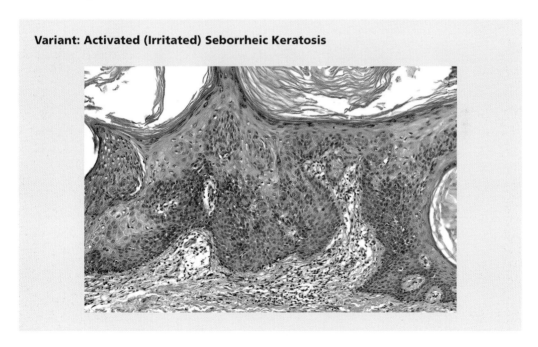

Hi: Mixed cellular inflammatory infiltrate in the upper dermis and between rete ridges.

Variant: Dermatosis Papulosa Nigra
Cl: Multiple tiny black papules in almost 50% of black-skinned individuals, commonly located on the cheeks and periorbital region. They resemble small seborrheic keratosis.

Hi: Corresponds to flat or reticulated pigmented seborrheic keratosis.

DD: Small seborrheic keratosis; fibromas.

Reference

Grimes, P.E., Arora, S., Minus, H.R., and Kenney, J.A. Jr (1983) Dermatosis papulosa nigra. *Cutis* **32**(4)L 385–6, 392.

SEBORRHEIC KERATOSIS AND VARIANTS

Variant: Dermatosis Papulosa Nigra

Variant: Melanoacanthoma (Pigmented Seborrheic Keratosis)

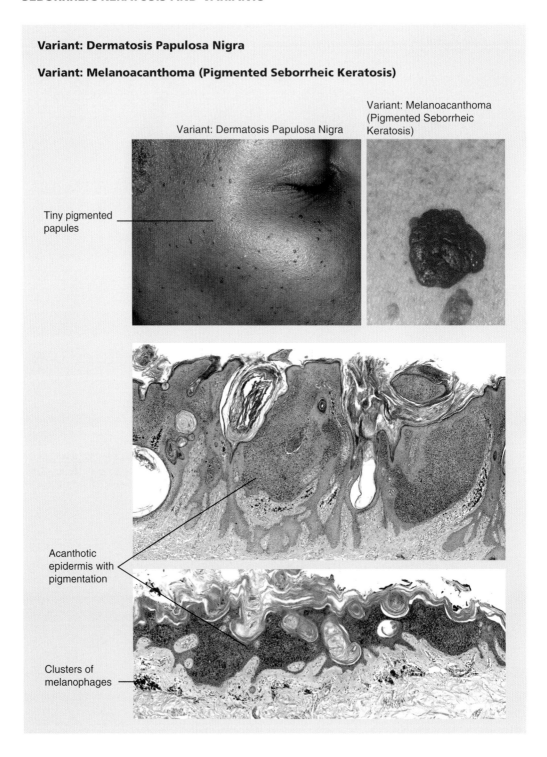

Variant: Dermatosis Papulosa Nigra

Variant: Melanoacanthoma (Pigmented Seborrheic Keratosis)

Tiny pigmented papules

Acanthotic epidermis with pigmentation

Clusters of melanophages

Hi: Deeply pigmented variant of acanthotic seborrheic keratosis, consisting of a mixture of pigmented keratinocytes and dendritic melanocytes.

SEBORRHEIC KERATOSIS AND VARIANTS

Variant: Clonal (Intraepidermal) Seborrheic Keratosis (Borst–Jadassohn)

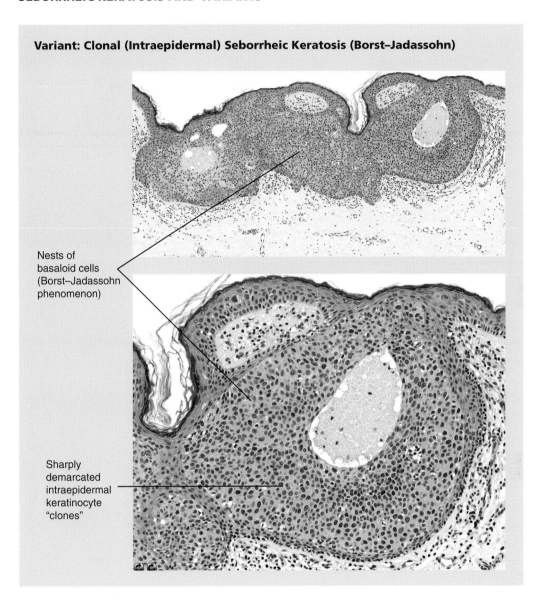

Nests of basaloid cells (Borst–Jadassohn phenomenon)

Sharply demarcated intraepidermal keratinocyte "clones"

Hi: Intraepidermal clonal accumulation of epidermal cells, sometimes demarcated by stronger pigmentation.

DD: Hidroacanthoma simplex (eccrine poroma); clonal Bowen disease; intraepidermal squamous cell carcinoma.

Reference

Lora, V., Chouvet, B., and Kanitakis, J. (2011) The "intraepidermal epithelioma" revisited: immunohistochemical study of the Borst-Jadassohn phenomenon. *Am J Dermatopathol* **33**(5): 492–497.

SEBORRHEIC KERATOSIS AND VARIANTS

Variant: Seborrheic Keratosis with Monster Cells (Bowenoid)

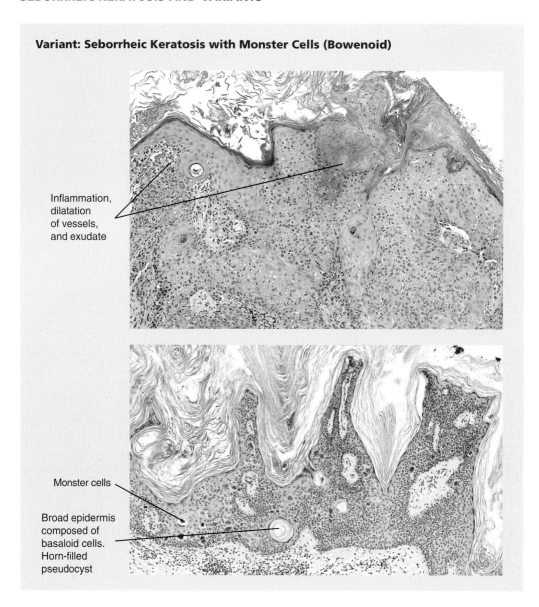

Inflammation, dilatation of vessels, and exudate

Monster cells

Broad epidermis composed of basaloid cells. Horn-filled pseudocyst

Hi: Morphological variant of SK with scattered large, haloed cells.

SEBORRHEIC KERATOSIS AND VARIANTS

Variant: Hyperkeratotic Seborrheic Keratosis (Stucco Keratosis)

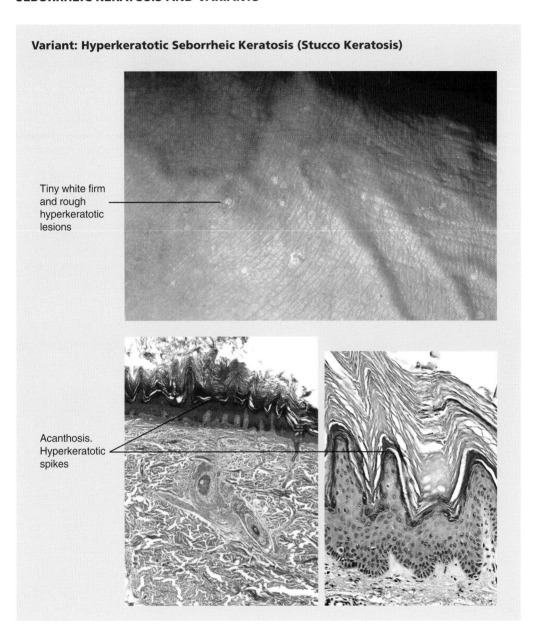

Tiny white firm and rough hyperkeratotic lesions

Acanthosis. Hyperkeratotic spikes

Hi: Acanthosis and orthohyperkeratotic spikes.

Confluent and Reticulate Papillomatosis (Gougerot and Carteaud)

Confluent and
reticulated brownish
patches resembling
pityriasis versicolor

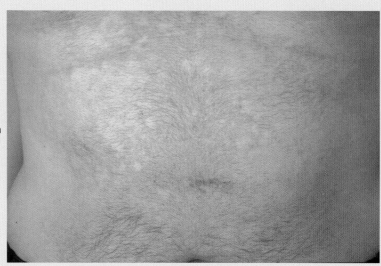

Hyperkeratosis and
slight acanthosis;
no inflammation

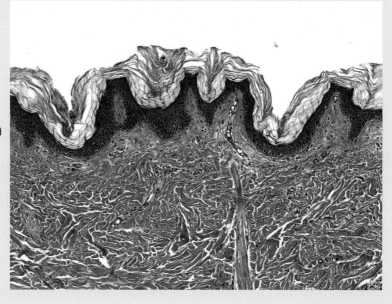

Cl: Gray-brown tiny asymptomatic papules, similar to seborrheic keratosis, coalescing to larger plaques or reticular net, resembling pityriasis versicolor or acanthosis nigricans. Sternum and back are the favorite localisations.

Hi: Slight papillomatosis and hyperkeratosis resembling acanthosis nigricans. Often colonization with *Pityrosporon (Malassezia) orbiculare* (PAS stain).

Reticulate Pigmented Anomaly of the Flexures (Dowling–Degos Disease)

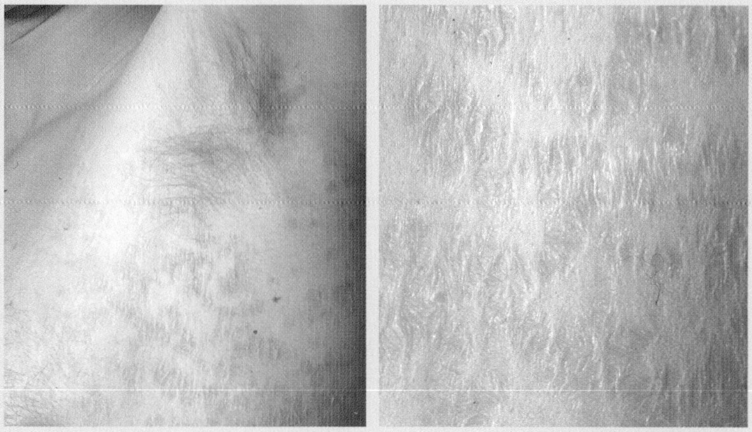

Reticulate hyper-pigmentation on the lateral side of the chest

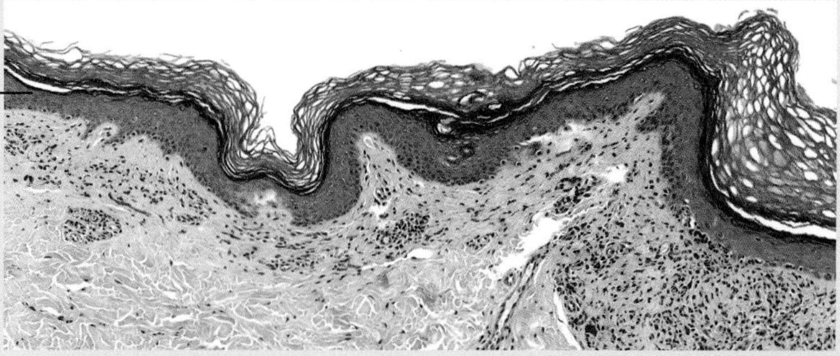

Slight atrophy

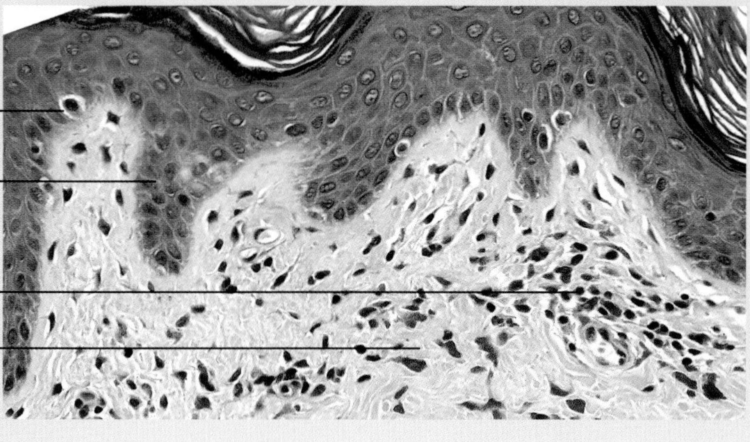

Melanocyte

Downward projection of rete ridges

Slight inflammation

Melanophages loaded with pigment

Cl: Congenital, autosomal dominant inherited disease (mutation in the keratin 5-gene *KRT5*), manifesting mostly in adults. Symmetrical small brown macules, resulting in reticular hyperpigmentation of flexural areas (cubital and popliteal fossae, axillae, lateral aspects of the neck, groins).

Hi: Similar to flat seborrheic keratosis with basal hyperpigmentation; normal number of melanocytes. Downward projection of the epidermal rete ridges.

Acanthosis Nigricans

Gray-brown verruciform papules and crests

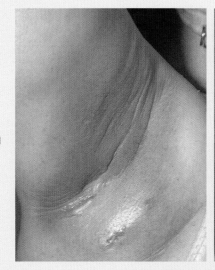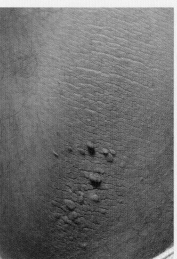

Alternate ortho- and parahyperkeratosis, acanthosis, papillomatosis (left)

Morphological variant with marked hypergranulosis (right)

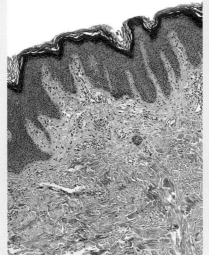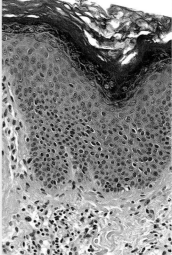

Cl: Gray-brown verruciform papules in major intertriginous and flexural areas or neck. The skin shows a velvety surface with crests. It may be associated with a variety of underlying disorders, including obesity (pseudo-acanthosis nigricans benigna), congenital syndromes, hormonal disorders, or malignancies as a paraneoplastic process (acanthosis nigricans maligna).

Hi:
- Alternate ortho- and parahyperkeratosis
- Acanthosis
- Papillomatosis
- Little or no basal layer hyperpigmentation

DD: Acrochordon; small seborrheic keratosis; epidermal nevus.

Solar (Actinic) Keratosis

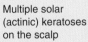

Multiple solar (actinic) keratoses on the scalp

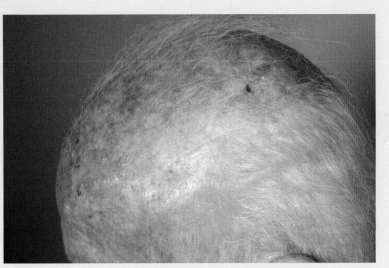

Cl: Actinic keratoses are considered by some to be squamous cell carcinomas *in situ*. However, from a prognostic point of view, they are nosologically different. They are induced by chronic (sunlight) UV exposure and therefore the most common locations are the face, especially nose and ears, and back of the hands and the scalp of bald-headed men. Several variants exist: hypertrophic, bowenoid, atrophic, lichenoid, pigmented. The development of a cutaneous horn, bleeding with hemorrhagic crust, may simulate squamous cell carcinoma or should raise suspicion of malignant transition into squamous cell carcinoma.

Hi:
- Many different histological patterns may be seen, reflecting the great clinical variability
- Focal areas of orthohyperkeratosis (pink) alternating with parakeratosis (blue)
- Abnormal keratinocytes, especially in the lower third of the epidermis and the basal layer
- Pseudopod-like proliferations of the epidermis
- In some cases, acantholysis (acantholytic variant) is present in the lower part of the epidermis
- The dysplastic epithelium usually expands downward into the epithelium of the hair follicles
- In the upper dermis, there are solar elastosis and a sparse inflammatory infiltrate and telangiectases

Variant: Acantholytic Solar Keratosis

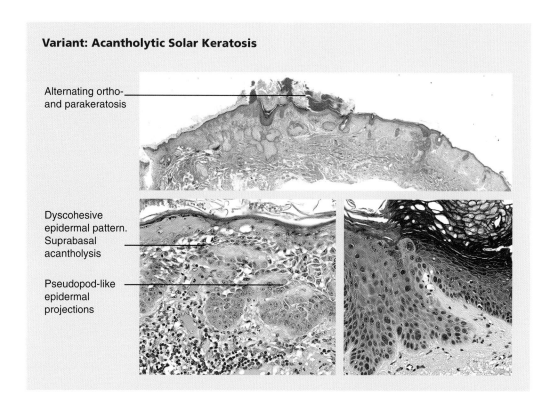

Alternating ortho- and parakeratosis

Dyscohesive epidermal pattern. Suprabasal acantholysis

Pseudopod-like epidermal projections

Hi: Suprabasal acantholysis and split formation.

Variant: Atrophic Solar Keratosis

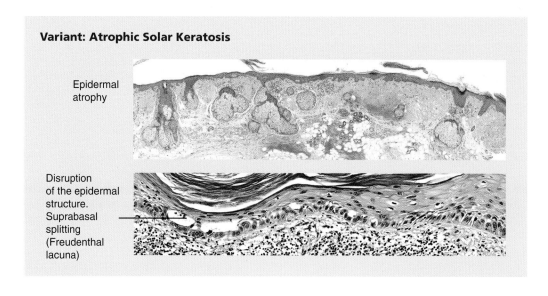

Epidermal atrophy

Disruption of the epidermal structure. Suprabasal splitting (Freudenthal lacuna)

Hi: Atrophy of the epidermis.

Variant: Lichen Planus-Like Solar Keratosis

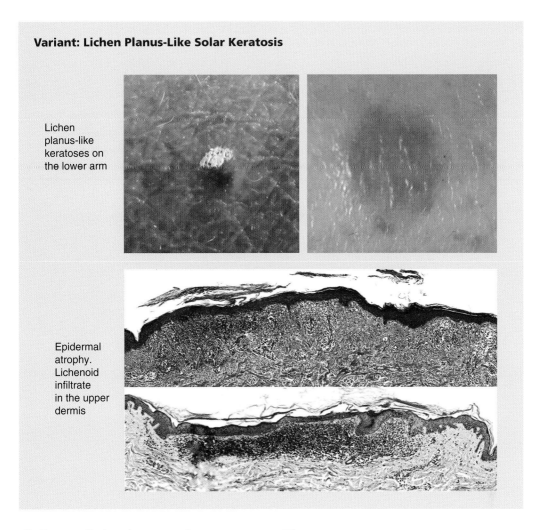

Lichen planus-like keratoses on the lower arm

Epidermal atrophy. Lichenoid infiltrate in the upper dermis

Cl: Circumscribed erythematous plaque, not necessarily hyperkeratotic.

Hi:
- Alternating para- and orthohyperkeratosis
- Acanthosis
- Lichenoid infiltrate in the upper dermis

Variant: Hypertrophic (Bowenoid) Solar Keratosis

Hyperkeratosis, acanthosis, papillomatosis, atypical keratinocytes in all levels of the epidermis featuring a bowenoid pattern

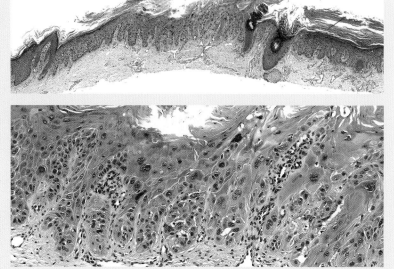

Hi:

• Hypertrophic epidermis
• Bowenoid features with atypical cells in mid and lower levels of the epidermis

Cornu Cutaneum

Keratotic horn on actinic keratoses (left)

Spike-like apposition of horny masses on top of a hypertrophic actinic keratosis (right)

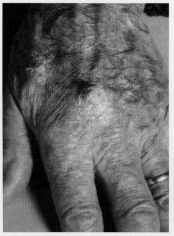 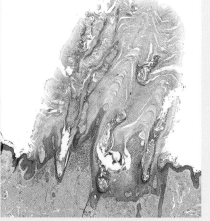

This clinical term describes the apposition of horny material forming a horn. It may be seen in association with various underlying disorders, including actinic keratosis, lupus erythematosus, radiation-induced scars, keratoacanthoma, squamous cell carcinoma, and several other conditions.

Cl: Horn-like hyperkeratosis.

Hi:
- Massive apposition of ortho- or parakeratotic horny masses
- Specific changes of the respective underlying disorder

Acanthomas, Non-Viral

Solar Lentigo

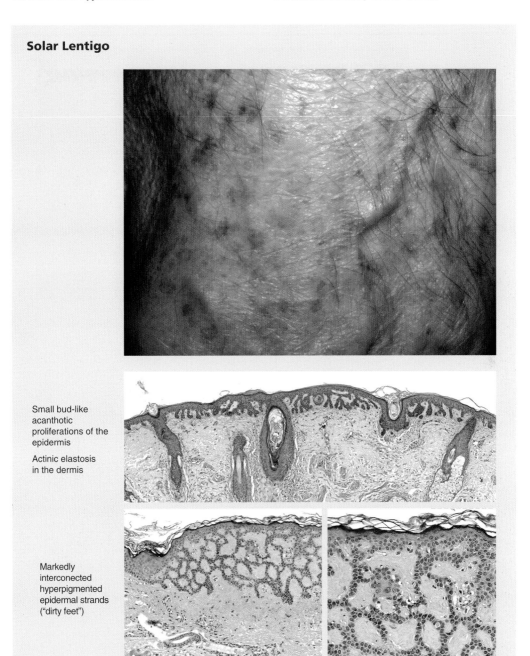

Small bud-like acanthotic proliferations of the epidermis

Actinic elastosis in the dermis

Markedly interconected hyperpigmented epidermal strands ("dirty feet")

Cl: Multiple brown pigmented macules in sun-exposed locations in elderly individuals.

Hi:

- Small, bud-like acanthotic proliferations
- Anastomosing network in some cases
- Hyperpigmentation of the basal layer

- Variable increase of melanocytes
- Solar elastosis in the upper dermis

DD: Pigmented actinic (solar) keratosis and flat seborrheic keratosis.

Callus, Factitial Acanthoma

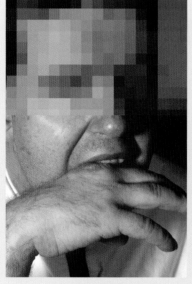 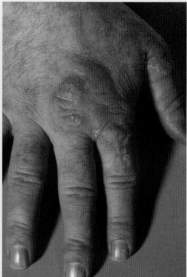

Factitial acantoma from chewing

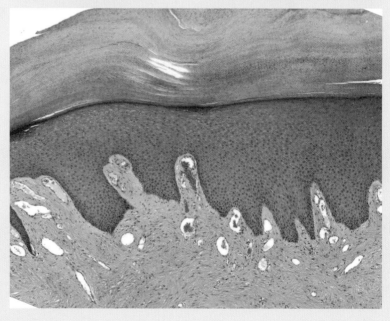

Alternating stratified ortho- and parakeratosis

Marked acanthosis with plump rete ridges

Cl: Corns typically develop in response to pressure and show compact apposition of horny material, sometimes surrounded by faint erythema.

Hi:

- Alternating stratified ortho- and parahyperkeratosis
- Acanthosis of the epidermis without koilocytes

- Pseudopod-like rete ridges
- Granular layer normal or prominent
- Fibrosis and telangiectases

Knuckle Pads (Chewing Pads)

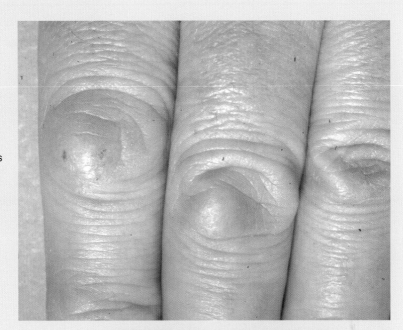

Knuckle pads in typical location

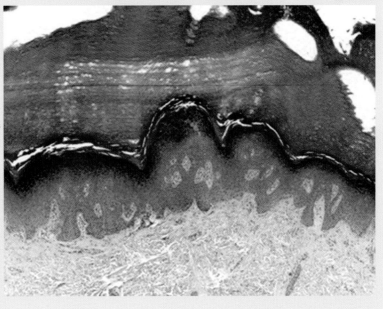

Hyperorthokeratosis with hypergranulosis and marked acanthosis

Cl: Knuckle pads, usually located at the dorsal aspect of the joints of the finger, are considered a subtype of callus.

Hi: See above (callus).

Pale (Clear) Cell Acanthoma

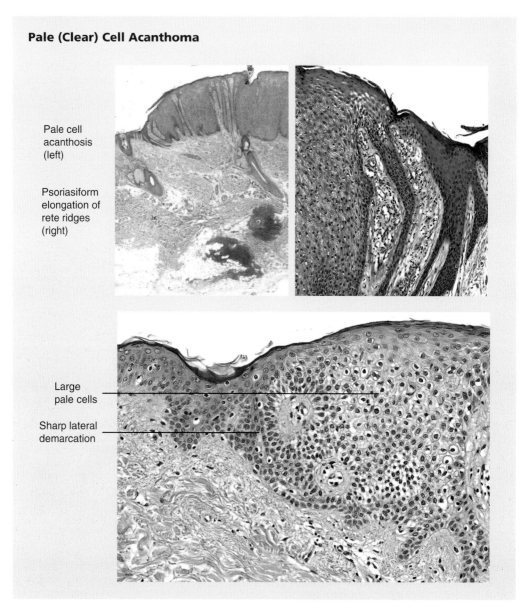

Pale cell acanthosis (left)

Psoriasiform elongation of rete ridges (right)

Large pale cells

Sharp lateral demarcation

Cl: This uncommon, benign, slowly exophytic growing and slightly hyperkeratotic tumor usually presents as a solitary sharply bordered lesion on the leg of elderly individuals.

Hi:
• Slight hyperkeratosis

• Acanthotic epidermis, dominated by large pale cells which replace all but the basal layer
• Sharp demarcation against the adjacent normal epidermis
• Large cells are rich in glycogen (PAS)
• Psoriasiform elongation of rete ridges

References

Garcia-Gavin, J., Gonzalez-Vilas, D., Montero, I., Rodriguez-Pazos, L., Pereiro, M.M., and Toribio, J. (2011) Disseminated eruptive clear cell acanthoma with spontaneous regression: further evidence of an inflammatory origin? *Am J Dermatopathol* **33**(6): 599–602.

Lin, C.Y., Lee, L.Y., and Kuo, T.T. (2016) Malignant clear cell acanthoma: report of a rare case of clear cell acanthoma-like tumor with malignant features. *Am J Dermatopathol* **38**(7): 553–6.

Shalin, S.C., Rinaldi, C., and Horn, T.D. (2013) Clear cell acanthoma with changes of eccrine syringofibroadenoma: reactive change or clue to etiology? *J Cutan Pathol* **40**(12): 1021–6.

Large Cell Acanthoma

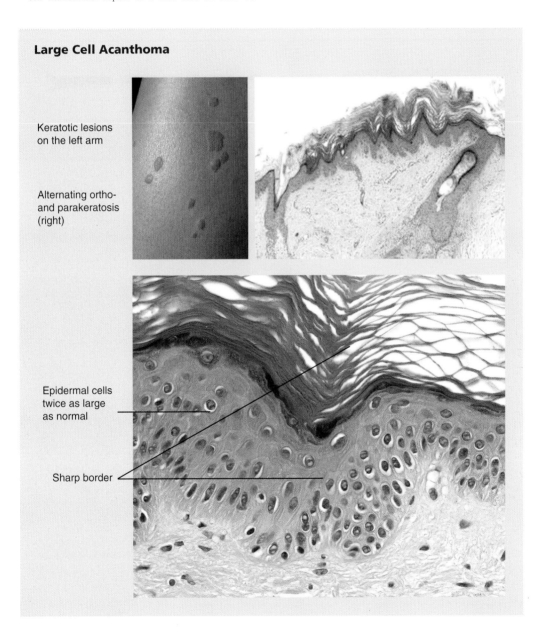

Keratotic lesions on the left arm

Alternating ortho- and parakeratosis (right)

Epidermal cells twice as large as normal

Sharp border

Cl: This pale flat benign tumor with sharp borders in sun-exposed areas is considered to be a variant of solar keratosis and is a histological rather than a clinical diagnosis.

Hi:

- Hyperkeratosis
- Keratinocytes are twice as large as in normal epidermis
- Sharp demarcation from adjacent normal epidermis

Reference

Fraga, G.R., and Amin, S.M. (2014) Large cell acanthoma: a variant of solar lentigo with cellular hypertrophy. *J Cutan Pathol* **41**(9): 733–739.

Differential Diagnosis: Epidermolytic Acanthoma

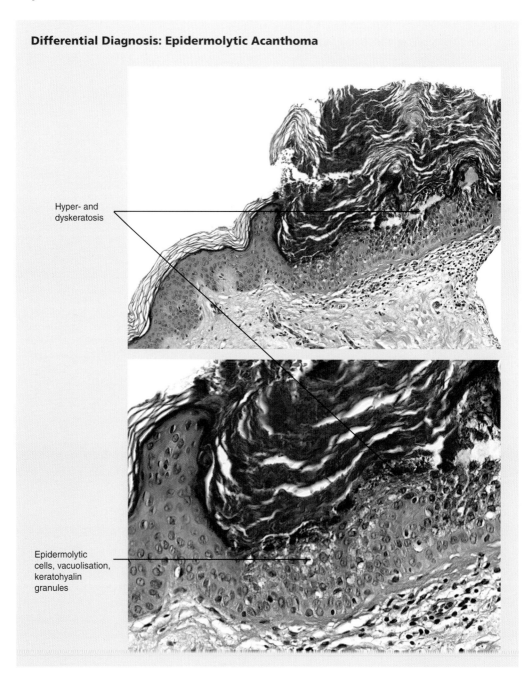

Hyper- and dyskeratosis

Epidermolytic cells, vacuolisation, keratohyalin granules

Cl: Epidermolytic acanthoma are uncommon solitary or disseminated benign tumors on the trunk or in the anogenital region presenting as wart-like lesions.

Hi:

- Hyper- and dyskeratosis
- Vacuolisation in the spinous and granular layer
- Keratohyaline granules
- Suprabasal epidermolytic cells in the upper two-thirds of the epidermis
- Suprabasilar vesiculation may occur

DD: Epidermolytic hyperkeratosis as seen in congenital ichthyosiform erythroderma, incidental finding in other lesions such as actinic keratosis, transient acantholytic dermatosis (Grover's), dyskeratosis follicularis (Darier's).

References

Egozi-Reinman, E., Avitan-Hersh, E., Barzilai, A., Indelman, M., and Bergman, R. (2016) Epidermolytic acanthoma of the genitalia does not show mutations in KRT1 or KRT10. *Am J Dermatopathol* **38**(2): 164–5.

Kazlouskaya, V., Lambe, J., and Elston, D. (2013) Solitary epidermolytic acanthoma. *J Cutan Pathol* **40**(8): 701–707.

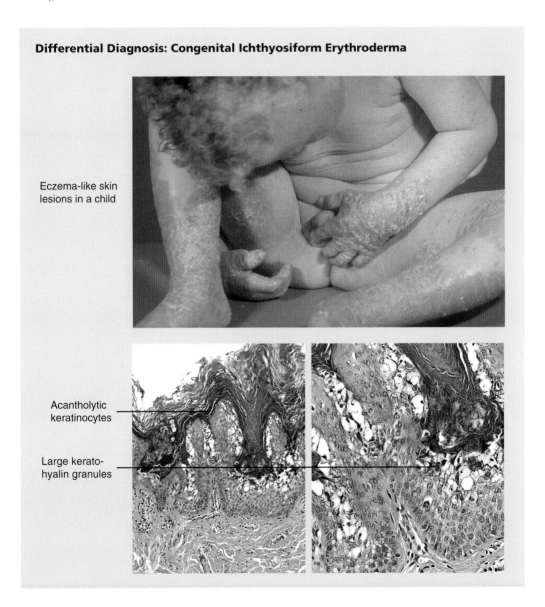

Differential Diagnosis: Congenital Ichthyosiform Erythroderma

Eczema-like skin lesions in a child

Acantholytic keratinocytes

Large kerato-hyalin granules

Inborn keratinization disorder with widespread skin lesions at birth or early in life.

Cl: Widespread erythroderma with blistering transforming to warty plaques, preferentially located in big flexural skinfolds.

Hi:
- Thick epidermis
- Acanthokeratolysis
- Clumps of keratin tonofilaments

Acantholytic Acanthoma

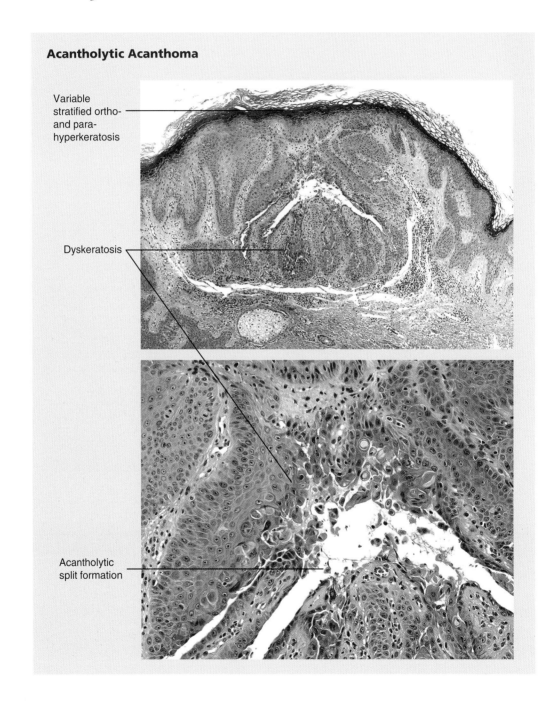

Variable stratified ortho- and para-hyperkeratosis

Dyskeratosis

Acantholytic split formation

Cl: Solitary or multiple papules most commonly found on the trunk, anogenital or mucosal areas, resembling verruca vulgaris or seborrheic keratosis. Immunosuppression may be an underlying pathogenetic factor.

Hi:

- Variable hyperkeratosis
- Symmetrical, well-circumscribed downward proliferation of keratinocytes without atypia
- Dyskeratosis
- Prominent acantholysis throughout all epidermal layers is the hallmark of the lesions

DD: Resembles Hailey–Hailey, Grover's or pemphigus, but the process is localized.

References

Brownstein, M.H. (1988) Acantholytic acanthoma. *J Am Acad Dermatol* **19**(1): 783–6.

Megahed, M., and Scharffetter-Kochanek, K. (1993) Acantholytic acanthoma. *Am J Dermatopathol* **15**(3): 283–5.

Warty Dyskeratoma

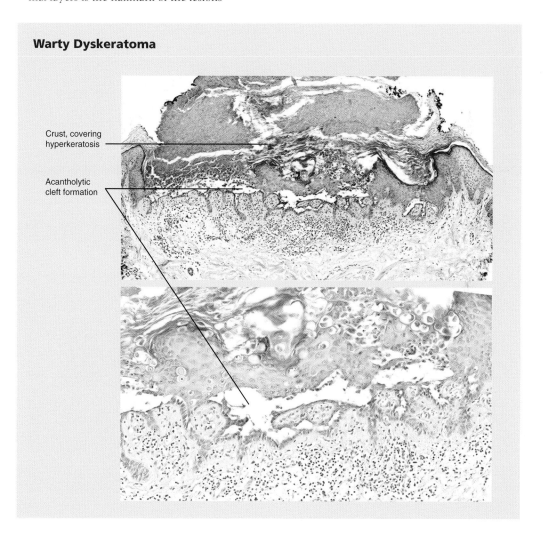

Crust, covering hyperkeratosis

Acantholytic cleft formation

Warty Dyskeratoma

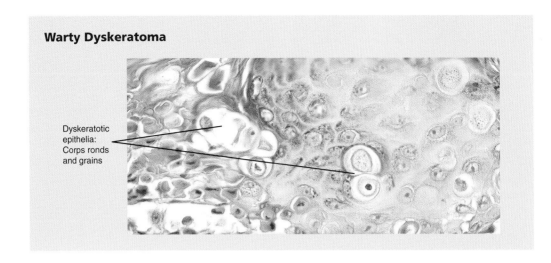

Dyskeratotic epithelia: Corps ronds and grains

Cl: Solitary verrucous papule, sometimes crusted when traumatized.

Hi: Warty dyskeratoma simulates the histological features of Darier's disease and has been considered to be a localized variant of that disease.

- Papular or verrucous lesion
- Focal parakeratosis
- Irregular acanthosis with acantholysis
- Dyskeratotic corps ronds and grains
- Frequent association with pilosebaceous structures

DD: Dyskeratosis follicularis (Darier's disease; see Volume I, page 65), pemphigus benignus familiaris (Hailey–Hailey; see Volume I, page 64), transient acantholytic dermatosis (Grover's disease; see Volume I, page 67).

DD: Dyskeratosis Follicularis (Darier)

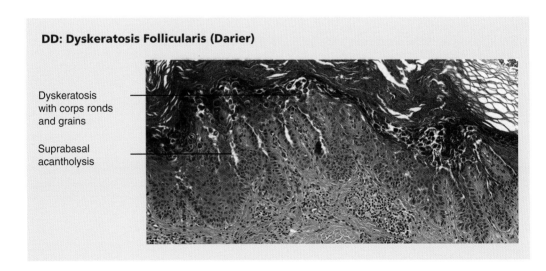

Dyskeratosis with corps ronds and grains

Suprabasal acantholysis

DD: Pemphigus Benignus Familiaris (Hailey-Hailey)

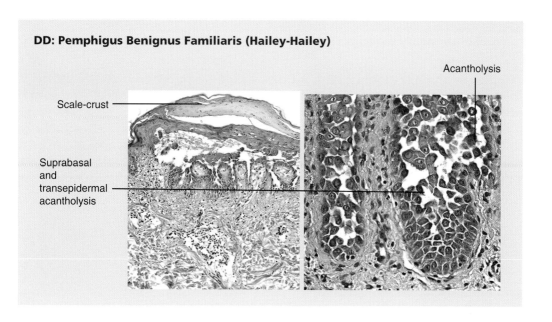

Acantholysis

Scale-crust

Suprabasal and transepidermal acantholysis

DD: Transient Acantholytic Dermatosis (Grover's Disease)

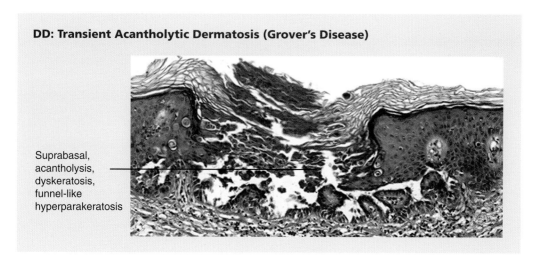

Suprabasal, acantholysis, dyskeratosis, funnel-like hyperparakeratosis

References

Lora, V., Scarabello, A., and Cota, C. (2015) Warty dyskeratoma as a cutaneous horn of the mons pubis. *Am J Dermatopathol* **37**(10): 802–4.

Martorell-Calatayud, A., Sanmartin-Jimenez, O., Traves, V., and Guillen, C. (2012) Numerous umbilicated papules on the trunk: multiple warty dyskeratoma. *Am J Dermatopathol* **34**(6): 674–5.

Porokeratoma (Porokeratosis Mibelli)

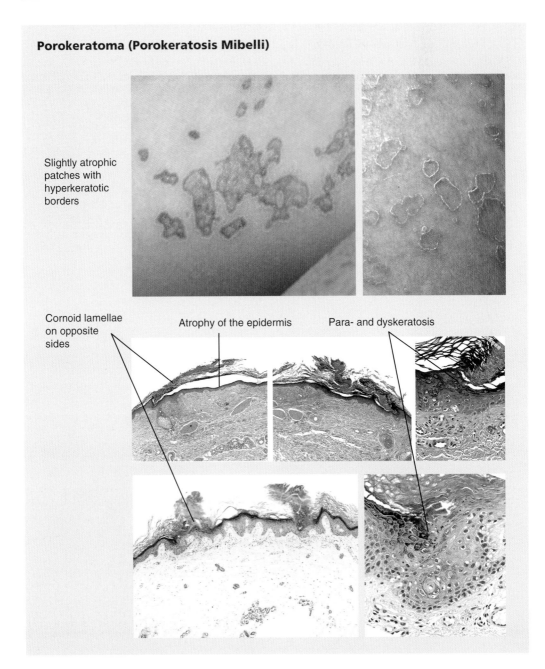

Slightly atrophic patches with hyperkeratotic borders

Cornoid lamellae on opposite sides

Atrophy of the epidermis

Para- and dyskeratosis

This group of autosomal dominant inherited keratinization disorders is defined histologically by the presence of a cornoid lamella, which is seen best when the biopsy is taken perpendicular to the border of the lesion.

Cl: The lesions may appear at any age and occur more often in men. The extremities are the favored sites of manifestation, but other parts of the body may also be affected. The initial lesion starts as a small red papule with a central keratotic spine which spreads peripherally, forming a slightly atrophic patch with irregular hyperkeratotic borders. Linear porokeratosis and giant porokeratosis are variants. There is an increased risk for the development of squamous cell carcinoma.

Hi:

- No relationship to sweat pores, as suggested by the name
- Narrow ridge of hyperkeratosis with parakeratosis (cornoid lamella)
- Cornoid lamella (with PAS-positive grains) amidst parakeratotically layered corneocytes
- Dyskeratotic cells are almost always found beneath the cornoid lamella
- Focal absence of stratum granulosum
- Central atrophy of the epidermis – imitating atrophic lupus erythematosus
- Underlying lichenoid infiltrate
- Advanced stages may show epithelial dysplasia in the center

References

Biswas, A. (2015) Cornoid lamellation revisited: apropos of porokeratosis with emphasis on unusual clinicopathological variants. *Am J Dermatopathol* **37**(2): 145–55.

Tallon, B., and Emanuel, P. (2017) Follicular porokeratosis, a porokeratosis variant. *Am J Dermatopathol* **39**: e1-7–e109.

Tan, T.S., and Tallon, B. (2016) Pigmented porokeratosis. A further variant? *Am J Dermatopathol* **38**(3): 218–21.

Acanthomas, Viral

Verruca Vulgaris

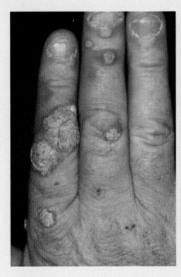
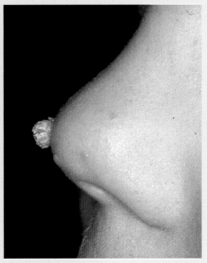

Hyperkeratotic verrucae on fingers and nose

Verruca Vulgaris

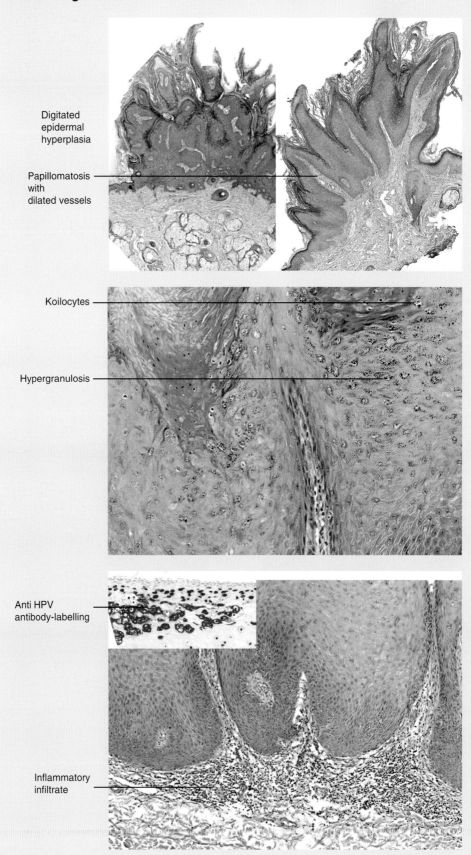

Digitated epidermal hyperplasia

Papillomatosis with dilated vessels

Koilocytes

Hypergranulosis

Anti HPV antibody-labelling

Inflammatory infiltrate

HUMAN PAPILLOMA VIRUS (HPV)

Cl: Solitary or grouped papules showing massive hyperkeratosis and sometimes significant inflammation.

Hi:

- Epidermal hyperplasia with a "multiple raised fingers" silhouette
- Hyperkeratosis with focal parakeratosis
- Intracorneal inclusions of hemorrhagic exudate (capillary thrombi)
- Hypergranulosis with enlarged keratohyalin granules
- Koilocytes (bird's eye cells) in the granular layer and upper stratum spinosum
- Dilated vessels in the papillary dermis
- Inflammatory infiltrate in the upper dermis

Variant: Verruca Plana

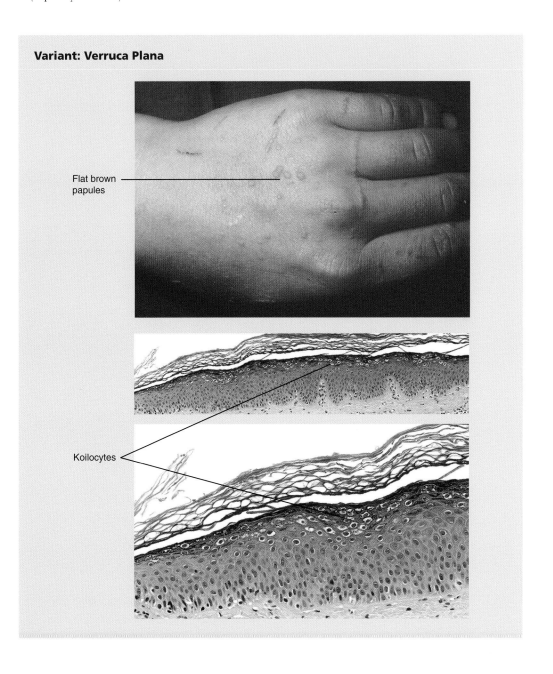

Flat brown papules

Koilocytes

HUMAN PAPILLOMA VIRUS (HPV)

Cl: Flat hyperkeratotic (verruciform) papules.

Hi:
- Hyperkeratosis
- Slight acanthosis

- No papillomatosis
- Confluent band of koilocytes (bird's eye cells) in the granular layer

Variant: Condyloma Acuminatum

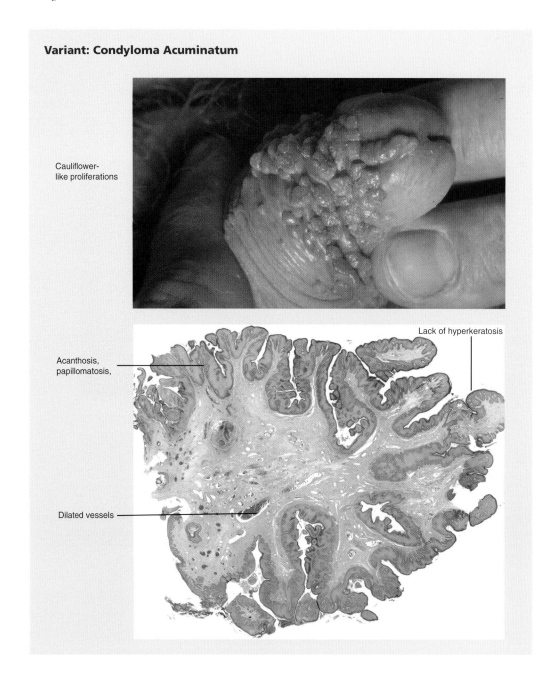

Cauliflower-like proliferations

Lack of hyperkeratosis

Acanthosis, papillomatosis,

Dilated vessels

Cl: Papular and verruciform lesions in anogenital or oral localisation.

Hi: Acanthopapilloma with focal hyperparakeratosis and lack of pseudocysts ("naked seborrheic keratosis"). Presence of koilocytes, even sometimes sparse.

HUMAN PAPILLOMA VIRUS (HPV)

Bowenoid Papulosis

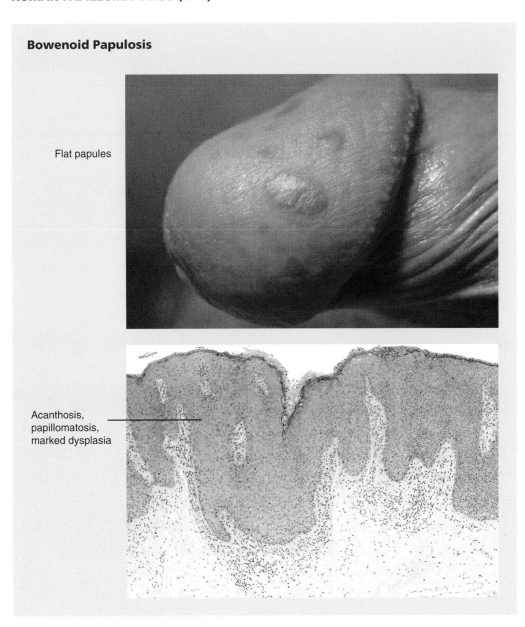

Flat papules

Acanthosis,
papillomatosis,
marked dysplasia

HUMAN PAPILLOMA VIRUS (HPV)

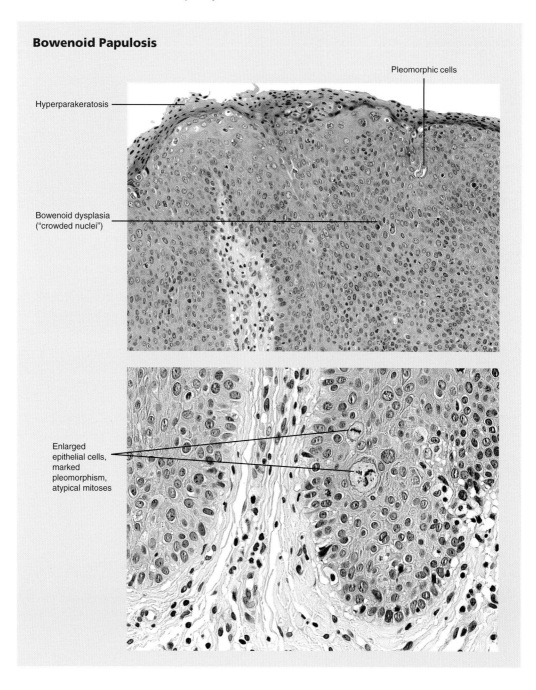

Bowenoid Papulosis

Pleomorphic cells

Hyperparakeratosis

Bowenoid dysplasia ("crowded nuclei")

Enlarged epithelial cells, marked pleomorphism, atypical mitoses

Cl: Solitary or confluent flat papular eruptions in anogenital localisation, often associated with onco-genic HPV infection (HPV16, HPV18).

Hi: Atypical epithelial cells with nuclear pleo-morphism and mitotic activity, identical with Bowen's disease.

HUMAN PAPILLOMA VIRUS (HPV)

Acrokeratosis Verruciformis (Hopf)

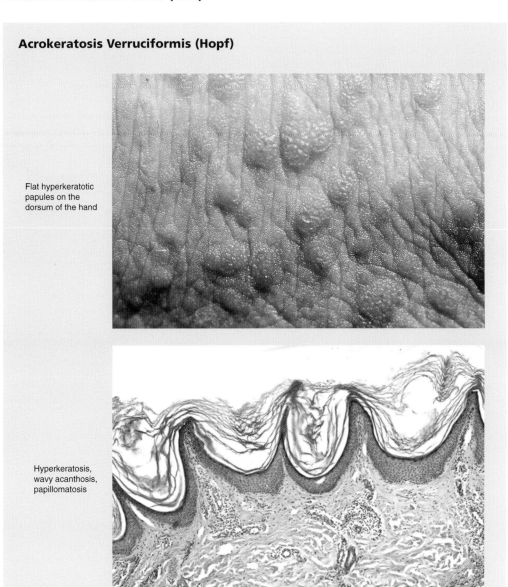

Flat hyperkeratotic papules on the dorsum of the hand

Hyperkeratosis, wavy acanthosis, papillomatosis

Considered to be associated with HIV infection by some and to be an autosomal dominant inherited disorder by others. There is close relationship to Darier's disease and to epidermodysplasia verruciformis.

Cl: Multiple flat hyperkeratotic papules in distal parts of the extremities (dorsa of the hands, feet, forearms).

Hi:
- Orthohyperkeratosis
- Wavy acanthosis
- Papillomatosis
- Thin papillae

MOLLUSCUM POXVIRUS

References

Bergman, R., Sezin, T., Indelman, M., Helou, W.A., and Avitan-Hersh, E. (2012) Acrokeratosis verruciformis of Hopf showing P602L mutation in ATP2A2 and overlapping histopathological features with Darier disease. *Am J Dermatopathol* **34**(6): 597–601.

Matsumoto, A., Gregory, N., Rady, P.L., Tyring, S.K., and Carlson, J.A. (2017) Brief Report: HPV-17 infection in Darier disease with acrokeratosis verrucosis of Hopf. *Am J Dermatopathol* **39**(5): 370–3.

Molluscum Contagiosum

Grouped umbilicated papules

Crateriform symmetric tumor with Molluscum bodies

Molluscum bodies (basophilic virus capsid – Molluscum poxvirus)

MOLLUSCUM POXVIRUS

Cl: Molluscum poxvirus is the causative agent. Typically children and immunocompromised patients are affected. Lesions are mostly multiple, sometimes extensive and eczematous. Characteristic features are elevated papules with a central dell.

Hi:
- Epidermal hyperplasia
- Central invagination, corresponding to the clinically visible dell
- Dell filled with necrotic keratinocytes, containing large, prominent, basophilic intracytoplasmic inclusions (molluscum bodies) that stain positive with Melan A
- Massive inflammatory reaction when ruptured

Molluscum Contagiosum, Inflamed

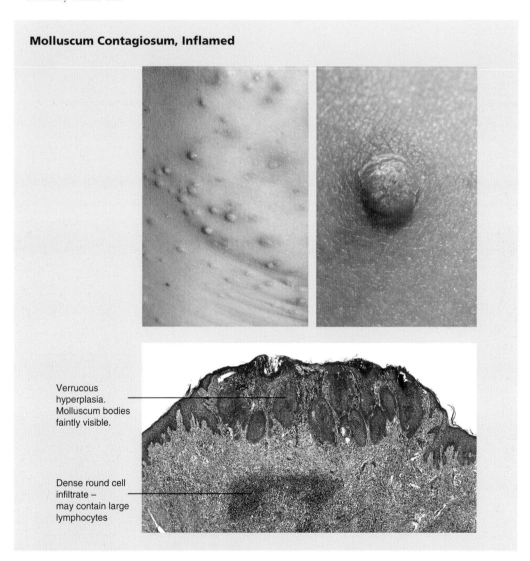

Verrucous hyperplasia. Molluscum bodies faintly visible.

Dense round cell infiltrate – may contain large lymphocytes

Reference

Ishikawa, M.K., Arps, D.P., Chow, C., Hocker, T.L., and Fullen, D.R. (2015) Histopathological features of molluscum contagiosum other than molluscum bodies. *Histopathology* **67**(6): 836–42.

"Pseudocarcinomas" and Neoplasms with Intermediate Malignant Potential

Keratoacanthoma, epithelioma cuniculatum, papillomatosis cutis carcinoides, Buschke–Löwenstein giant condyloma, and florid oral papillomatosis form a group of disorders which are biologically benign, do not metastasize and histologically simulate large warts or well-differentiated squamous cell carcinoma.

Keratoacanthoma (KA)

Hyperkeratotic craterifom tumor on the nose (left)

Nodule with central keratotic horn (right)

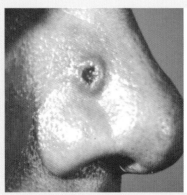
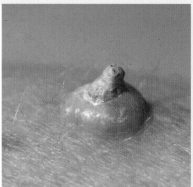

Cl: Most KAs develop in sun-exposed areas. They are biologically benign and develop within weeks, in contrast to squamous cell carcinoma which develops over months. Multiple KAs are encountered in conjunction with hereditary cancer syndromes (Muir–Torre) or as specific clinical variants (e.g. Grzybowski, Ferguson–Smith). The typical lesion is a dome-shaped keratotic nodule with a central dell filled by a keratotic plug. KA centrifugum marginatum is a centrifugal spreading variant, which most commonly occurs on the extremities.

Variant: Keratoacanthoma Centrifugum Marginatum

Centrifugally growing flat hyperkeratotic tumors on hand (left) and lower limb (right)

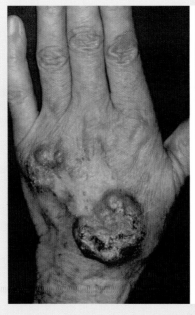
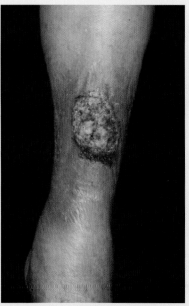

Variants of Keratoacanthoma

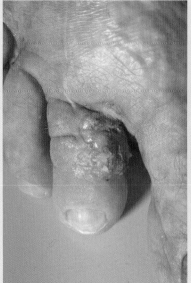

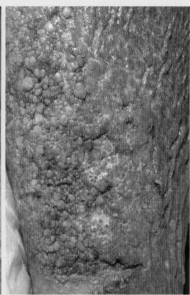

Verrucous carcinoma
(epithelioma cuniculatum)

Papillomatosis cutis carcinoides
(pseudocarcinomatous hyperplasia)

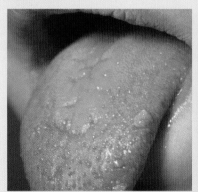

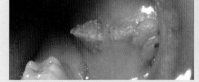

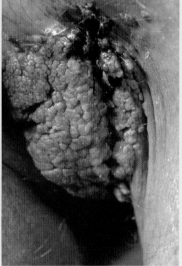

Florid oral papillomatosis

Giant condyloma
(Buschke–Löwenstein)

Keratoacanthoma

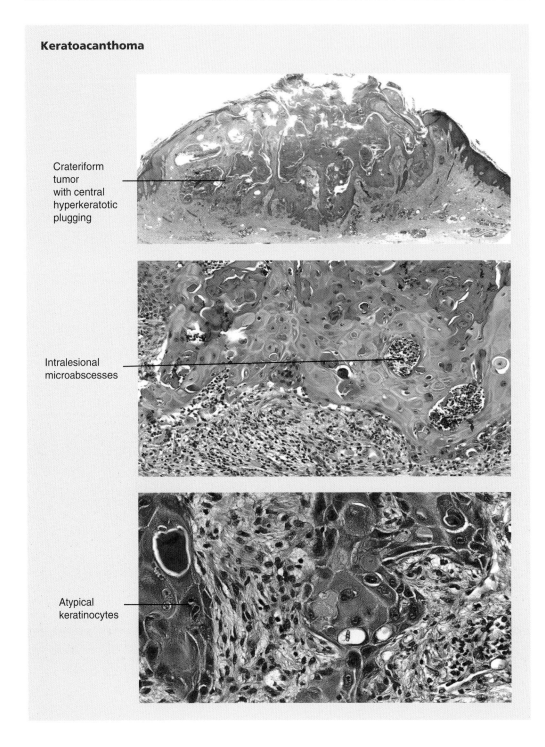

Crateriform tumor with central hyperkeratotic plugging

Intralesional microabscesses

Atypical keratinocytes

Keratoacanthoma

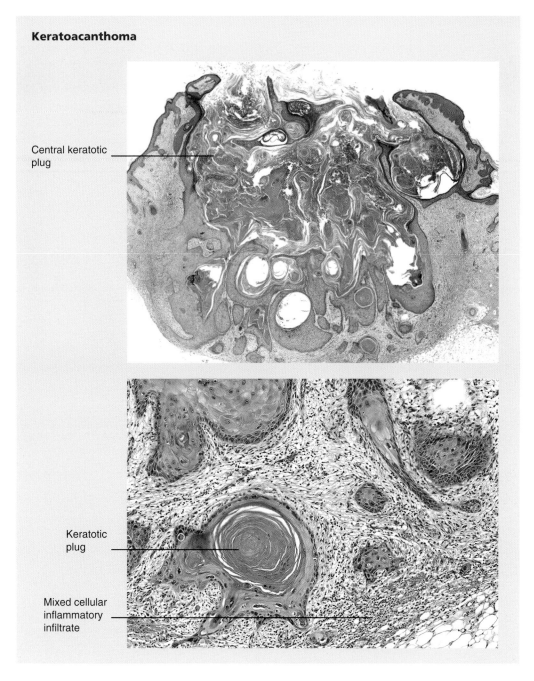

Central keratotic plug

Keratotic plug

Mixed cellular inflammatory infiltrate

Hi:
- Symmetrical cup-shaped tumor, filled with cornified debris and with smooth outer margins
- Central keratotic plug with massive acanthosis and papillomatosis
- Bilateral epithelial lip formation of adjacent rete ridges
- Proliferation of atypical keratinocytes and mitoses
- Parakeratosis
- Intraepidermal formation of microabscesses, filled with mixed inflammatory cells and debris
- Mixed cellular infiltrate in the dermis

References

Kluger, N. (2010) Issues with keratoacanthoma, pseudoepitheliomatous hyperplasia and squamous cell carcinoma within tattoos: a clinical point of view. *J Cutan Pathol* **37**(7): 812–13.

Misago, N., Takai, T., Toda, S., and Narisawa, Y. (2014) The histopathologic changes in keratoacanthoma depend on its stage. *J Cutan Pathol* **41**(7): 617–19.

Resnik, K.S. and Kutzner, H. (2010) Of lymphocytes and cutaneous epithelium: keratoacanthomatous hyperplasia in CD30+ lymphoproliferative disorders and CD30+ cells associated with keratoacanthoma. *Am J Dermatopathol* **32**(3): 314–15.

Savage, J.A. and Maize, J.C. Sr (2014) Keratoacanthoma clinical behavior: a systematic review. *Am J Dermatopathol* **36**(5): 422–9.

Epithelioma Cuniculatum (Verrucous Carcinoma) (EC/VC)

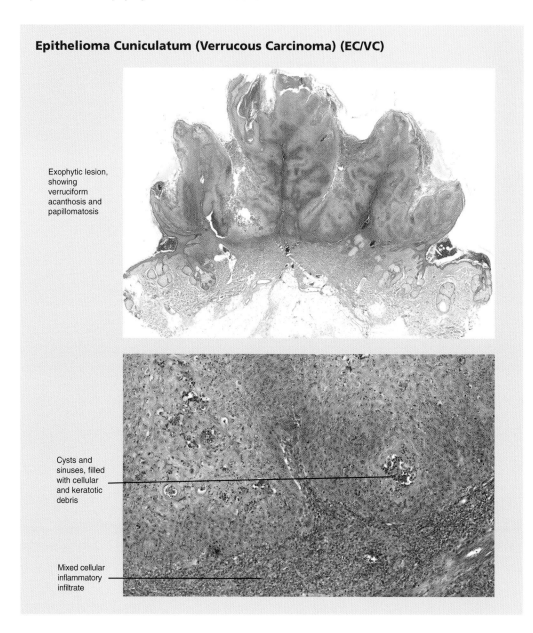

Exophytic lesion, showing verruciform acanthosis and papillomatosis

Cysts and sinuses, filled with cellular and keratotic debris

Mixed cellular inflammatory infiltrate

Cl: Both exo- and endophytic verrucous lesions, mostly of the soles or perigenital area. Association with HPV infection has been reported.

Hi:

- Exo- or endophytic verrucous hyperkeratosis
- Irregular papillomatosis and acanthosis
- Adjacent epidermis normal
- Well-differentiated keratinocytes
- Low proliferative activity, minimal epithelial dysplasia
- Cysts and sinuses ("fox's burrow"-like), allowing discharge of pus, blood, or cornified debris

DD: Large warts; well-differentiated squamous cell carcinoma.

Comment: Epithelioma cuniculatum/verrucous carcinoma is a genuine carcinoma, albeit lacking the classic histopathological squamous cell carcinoma features, e.g. massive epithelial dysplasia and high proliferative activity. EC/VC is a unique carcinomatous tumor growing by lack of apoptosis rather than by increased proliferation rate. Pathologists should be aware that behind the silhouette of an exo-endophytic epithelial hyperplasia with minimal cytological atypia and scant mitoses, there is a genuine carcinoma.

References

Kubik, M.J. and Rhatigan, R.M. (2012) Carcinoma cuniculatum: not a verrucous carcinoma. *J Cutan Pathol* **39**(12): 1083–7.

Nakamura, Y., Kashiwagi, K., Nakamura, A., and Muto, M. (2015) Verrucous carcinoma of the foot diagnosed using p53 and Ki-67 immunostaining in a patient with diabetic neuropathy. *Am J Dermatopathol* **37**(3): 257–9.

Odar, K., Bostjancic, E., Gale, N., Glavac, D., and Zidar, N. (2012) Differential expression of microRNAs miR-21, miR-31, miR-203, miR-125a-5p and miR-125b and proteins PTEN and p63 in verrucous carcinoma of the head and neck. *Histopathology* **61**(2): 257–65.

Zidar, N., Langner, C., Odar, K., et al. (2017) Anal verrucous carcinoma is not related to infection with human papillomaviruses and should be distinguished from giant condyloma (Buschke–Lowenstein tumour). *Histopathology* **70**(6): 938–45.

Papillomatosis Cutis Carcinoides

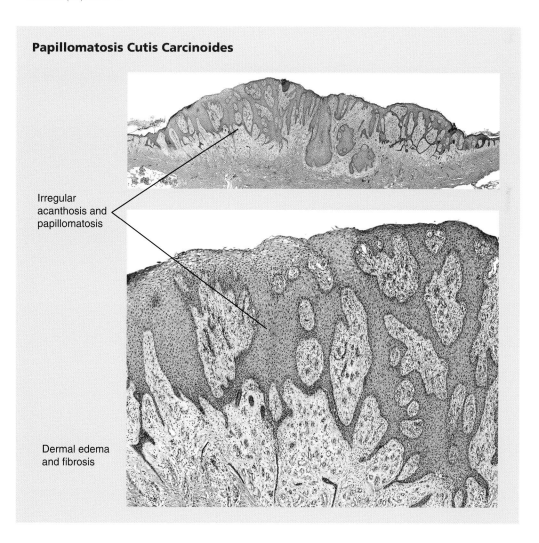

Irregular acanthosis and papillomatosis

Dermal edema and fibrosis

Cl: Large, cauliflower-like reactive hyperkeratotic process around chronic inflammatory processes, ulceration or tumor, preferentially on the shins or dorsal aspect of the feet, resembling squamous cell carcinoma.

Hi:

- Irregular acanthosis of pale epithelium with elongation of rete ridges
- Irregular papillomatosis
- Normal keratinocytes
- Edema and fibrosis in the upper dermis
- Variable chronic inflammatory changes of the surrounding tissue

DD: Blastomycosis-like pyoderma.

References

Allerga, F., Manifredi, G., Colli, V., Magnanini, M., and Manfredi, M. (1975) [An uncommon pseudo tumoral skin disease; the so-called Papillomatosis cutis carcinoides. A review (author's transl)]. *Ateneo Parmense Acta Biomed* **46**(6): 649–63.

Balda, B.R. and Wilhelm, K. (1970) [Verruca vulgaris gigantea with the aspect of papillomatosis cutis carcinoides]. *Hautarzt* **21**(12): 550–2.

Baldauf, K., Strohbach, F., and Laslop, M. (1982) [Malignant transformation of papillomatosis cutis carcinoides Cottron]. *Z Arztl Fortbild (Jena)* **76**(1–2): 69–71.

Bues, M., Muller, K.M., and Schwering, H. (1983) [Pseudocancer of the skin following lower leg amputation. Rare case of Gottron's papillomatosis cutis carcinoides]. *Zentralbl Chir* **108**(14): 895–9.

Cajkovac, V., Trbuljak, M., and Petricic, B. (1970) [Papillomatosis cutis carcinoides Gottron]. *Rad Med Fak Zagrebu* **18**(1): 81–7.

Rathjens, B. (1953). [Papillomatosis cutis carcinoides Gottron]. *Dermatol Wochenschr* **127**(14): 313–17.

Ruppe, J.P. Jr (1981) Verrucous carcinoma. Papillomatosis cutis carcinoides. *Arch Dermatol* **117**(3): 184–5.

Stevanovic, D.V. (1963) Papillomatosis cutis carcinoides (Gottron). *Oncologia* **16**: 116–22.

Vilanova, X. and Cabre, J. (1964) [Pseudoepithelioma (J. De Az'ua) Papillomatosis Cutis Carcinoides (Grottron)]. *Actas Dermosifiliogr* **55**: 753–62.

Florid Papillomatosis of the Oral Cavity (Oral Verrucous Carcinoma)

Cl: Whitish cobblestone-like plaques and papules of the buccal mucosa. Lesions may progress to cauliflower-like exophytic neoplasms.

Hi:

- Hyperplastic epithelial layer
- Focal granulosis and slight parakeratosis
- No significant proliferative activity

DD: Hairy leukoplakia occurs mostly in immunocompromised patients, preferentially at the lateral margins of the tongue, presenting with poorly circumscribed whitish plaques similar to hyperplastic leukoplakia. Histopathologically, there is a typical zonation or "tricolore" pattern with superficial eosinophilic parakeratosis in conjunction with a verrucous surface, a midepithelial pale zone of ballooned keratinocytes, and a basal zone of eosinophilic banal epithelia. EBER *in situ* hybridization shows Epstein–Barr virus in the superficial layer. There may be HPV co-infection.

References

Collangettes, D., Chollet, P., and Fonck, Y. (1993) Oral florid papillomatosis. *Eur J Cancer B Oral Oncol* **29B**(1): 81–2.

Grillo, E., Miguel-Morrondo, A., Vano-Galvan, S., and Jaen-Olasolo, P. (2012) [Oral florid papillomatosis]. *Rev Clin Esp* **212**(11): e93.

Perez-Belmonte, L.M., Gomez-Moyano, E., Herrero-Lifona, L., and Jimenez-Onate, F. (2015) [Verrocous mass on the tongue: oral florid papillomatosis]. *Enferm Infecc Microbiol Clin* **33**(2): 135–6.

Buschke–Löwenstein Tumor (Giant Condyloma)

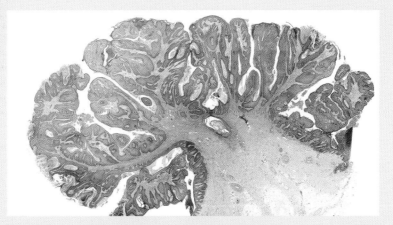

Exophytic lesion, showing verruciform acanthosis and papillomatosis

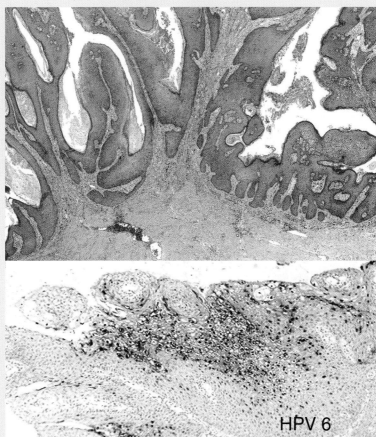

HPV6
In-situ
hybridization

BOWEN'S DISEASE

Cl: Large, almost cerebriform, foul-smelling papillomatous tumor, evolving from recurring and progressing small genital or perianal lesions.
Hi: Large condyloma, epithelial proliferation and dysplasia.

Reference

Zidar, N., Langner, C., Odar, K., et al. (2017) Anal verrucous carcinoma is not related to infection with human papillomaviruses and should be distinguished from giant condyloma (Buschke–Lowenstein tumour). *Histopathology* **70**(6): 938–45.

Malignant Epidermal Neoplasms

Bowen's Disease (Carcinoma *in situ*)

Psoriasiform and keratotic plaque on the trunk (left) and finger (right) respectively

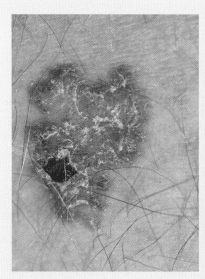
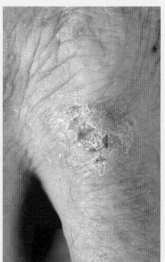

Erythroplasia (Queyrat)

Sharply demarcated irregular plaque on the glans penis

Plaque in the perianal region without sharp demarcation (circle)

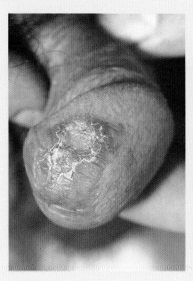
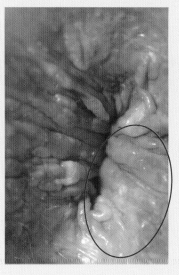

BOWEN'S DISEASE

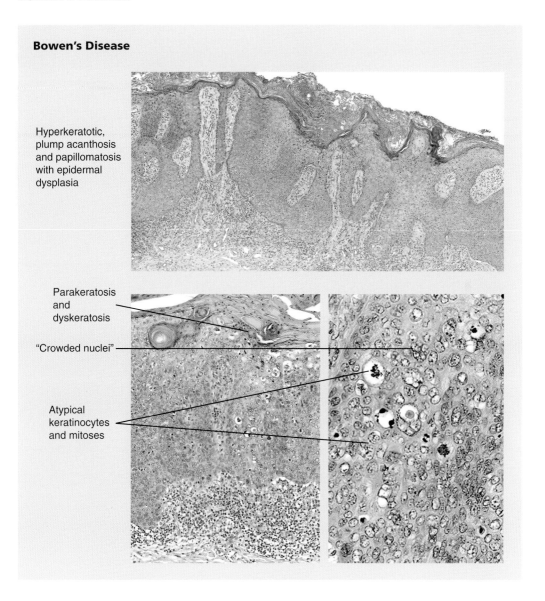

Bowen's Disease

Hyperkeratotic, plump acanthosis and papillomatosis with epidermal dysplasia

Parakeratosis and dyskeratosis

"Crowded nuclei"

Atypical keratinocytes and mitoses

Cl: Flat, slowly expanding, psoriasiform, sharply bordered red or pink patch or plaque most frequently located on the trunk, but also at any other site of the body. Variants are erythroplasia of Queyrat at the male genitalia or pigmented Bowen's disease, preferentially in the anogenital region; the latter is often associated with HPV16/18 infection. Bowen's disease of the nailbed may be easily misdiagnosed.

Hi:
- Parahyperkeratosis and plump acanthosis
- The hallmarks are large, atypical, occasionally dyskeratotic multinucleated keratinocytes and many atypical mitotic figures, disseminated over all levels of the epidermis
- "Crowded nuclei"
- Preservation of a regular basal layer
- The tumor is *in situ* and does not cross the basement membrane. Invasive variants correspond to Bowen's carcinoma
- Tumor invasion into the epithelium of hair follicles and sweat glands may occur
- Clear cell type of Bowen's disease with multiple PAS-positive tumor cells may simulate Paget's disease

DD: Bowenoid actinic keratosis; bowenoid papulosis; superficial spreading melanoma; clonal seborrheic keratosis; pigmented Paget's disease of the mamilla.

BOWEN'S DISEASE

References

Elbendary, A., Xue, R., Valdebran, M., et al. (2017) Diagnostic criteria in intraepithelial pagetoid neoplasms: a histopathologic study and evaluation of select features in paget disease, bowen disease, and melanoma in situ. *Am J Dermatopathol* **39**(6): 419–27.

Idriss, M.H., Misri, R., and Boer-Auer, A. (2016) Orthokeratotic Bowen disease: a histopathologic, immunohistochemical and molecular study. *J Cutan Pathol* **43**(1): 24–31.

Kalegowda, I.Y. and Boer-Auer, A. (2017) Clonal seborrheic keratosis versus pagetoid bowen disease: histopathology and role of adjunctive markers. *Am J Dermatopathol* **39**(6): 433–9.

Kogut, M., Toberer, F., Enk, A.H., and Hassel, J.C. (2016) Limitations of Ber-EP4 for distinction of Bowen disease from basal cell carcinoma. *J Cutan Pathol* **43**(4): 367–71.

Svajdler, M. Jr, Mezencev, R., Kaspirkova, J., et al. (2016) Human papillomavirus infection and p16 expression in extragenital/extraungual bowen disease in immunocompromised patients. *Am J Dermatopathol* **38**(10): 751–7.

Takayama, R., Ishiwata, T., Ansai, S., et al. (2013) Lumican as a novel marker for differential diagnosis of Bowen disease and actinic keratosis. *Am J Dermatopathol* **35**(8): 827–32.

Variant: Clear Cell Bowen's Disease

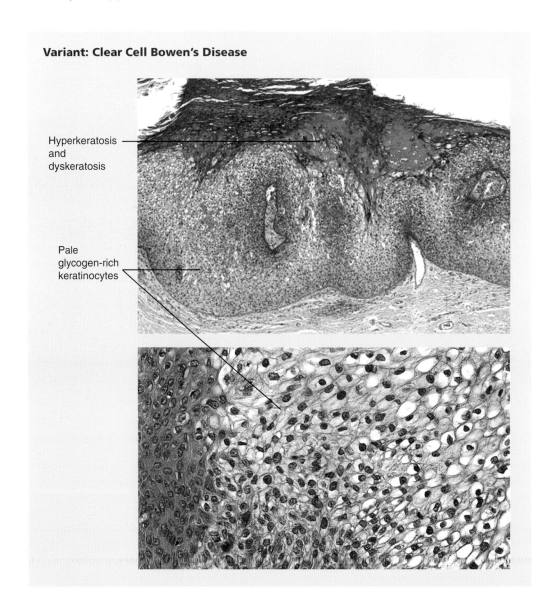

Hyperkeratosis and dyskeratosis

Pale glycogen-rich keratinocytes

BOWEN'S DISEASE

Hi: Pale keratinocytes with PAS-positive glycogen-rich cytoplasm.

Variant: Cutaneous Horn (Cornu Cutaneum) on Bowen's Disease

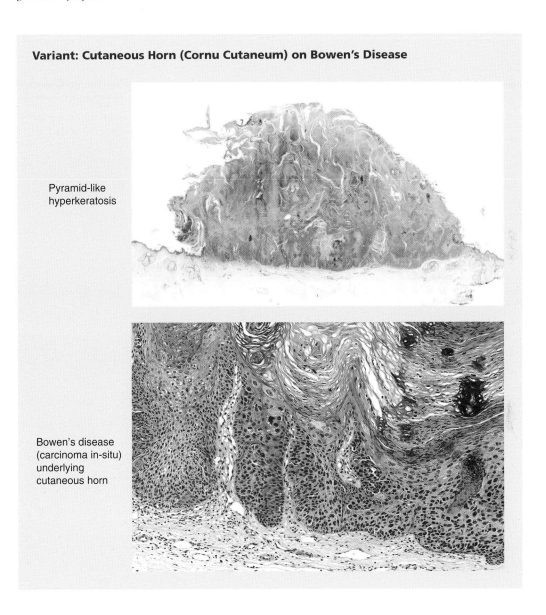

Pyramid-like hyperkeratosis

Bowen's disease (carcinoma in-situ) underlying cutaneous horn

Cl: Morphological term, describing a keratotic exophytic tumorous lesion, originating from various conditions, including Bowen's disease, actinic keratosis, squamous cell carcinoma.

Hi:
• Pyramid-shaped hyperkeratosis
• At the base histological features of Bowen's disease

DD: Cutaneous horn on actinic keratosis; warty dyskeratoma; squamous cell carcinoma; lupus erythematosus.

BOWEN'S DISEASE

Reference

Lora, V., Scarabello, A., and Cota, C. (2015) Warty dyskeratoma as a cutaneous horn of the mons pubis. *Am J Dermatopathol* **37**(10): 802–4.

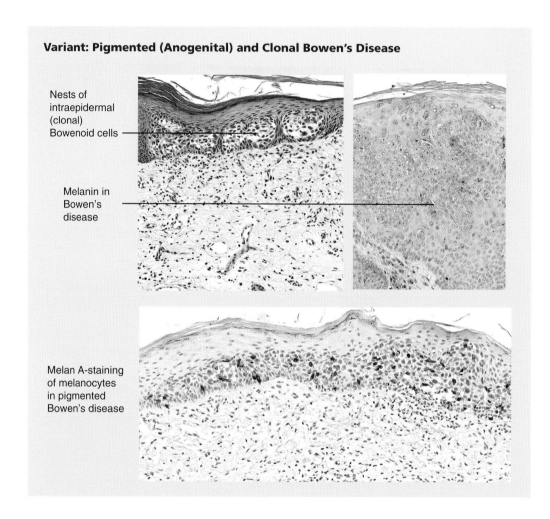

Variant: Pigmented (Anogenital) and Clonal Bowen's Disease

Nests of intraepidermal (clonal) Bowenoid cells

Melanin in Bowen's disease

Melan A-staining of melanocytes in pigmented Bowen's disease

Cl: Bowen's disease in the anogenital region frequently is pigmented, especially in dark-skinned individuals. Most cases are associated with oncogenic HPV infection (HPV16, HPV18).

Hi:
- Hyperpigmented bowenoid keratinocytes
- Atypical keratinocytes are AE1/AE3 positive but CK7 negative
- Slightly increased number of Melan A-positive melanocytes

BOWEN'S DISEASE

Variant: Erythroplasia of Queyrat and Vulvar Intraepithelial Neoplasia

Glans penis

Acanthosis,
bowenoid cells
in all levels of
the epidermis

Inflammatory
infiltrate,
containing many
plasma cells

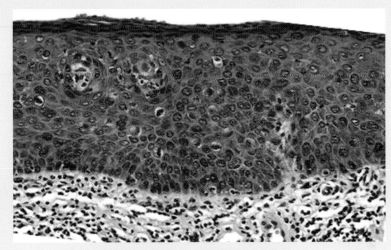

Vulva

Acanthosis,
papillomatosis

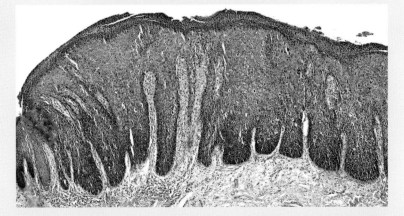

Bowenoid cells
with marked
pleomorphism
and mitoses

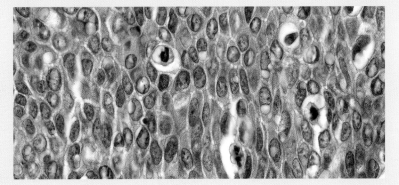

BASAL CELL CARCINOMA

Cl: Red, velvety, sharply bordered irregular patch or plaque on the glans penis. Similar lesions can be found in anogenital localisations and oral mucosa of both sexes. By some authors, Queyrat's disease is considered to be a separate entity with a worse prognosis rather than a variant of Bowen's disease.
Hi:
- Superficial erosion
- Slight acanthosis and/or papillomatosis

- Minimal dyskeratosis
- Atypical "bowenoid" keratinocytes in all levels of the epidermis
- Inflammatory infiltrate on the basis of the lesion, containing many plasma cells

Basal Cell Carcinoma (BCC)
Many variants exist.

Variant: Nodular BCC

Pearly, waxy tumor with elevated border and telangiectases

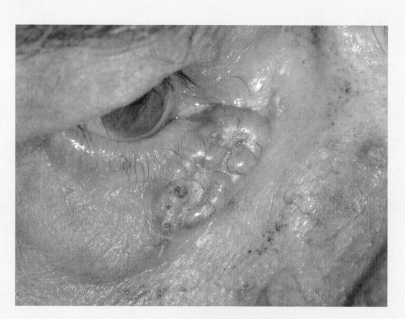

Exophytic proliferation of basaloid cells

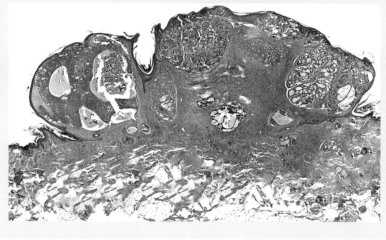

Variant: Nodular BCC

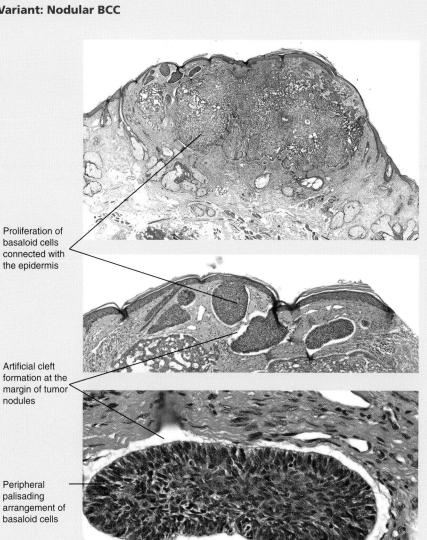

Proliferation of basaloid cells connected with the epidermis

Artificial cleft formation at the margin of tumor nodules

Peripheral palisading arrangement of basaloid cells

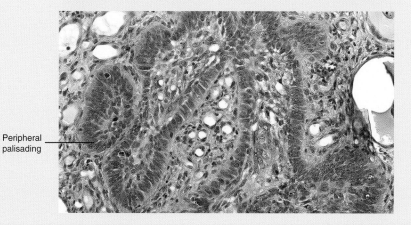

Peripheral palisading

BASAL CELL CARCINOMA

Cl: Pink or red well-circumscribed nodule, preferentially localized in sun-exposed skin. Pearly or waxy elevated border, telangiectases. Often central superficial erosion and crust formation.

Hi:
- Basophilic roundish and oval-shaped epithelial cells

- Peripheral band-like palisading arrangement
- Connection between tumor and epidermis or adnexa
- Prominent shrinkage clefts between tumor and surrounding stroma
- Immunohistochemical expression of BerEP4

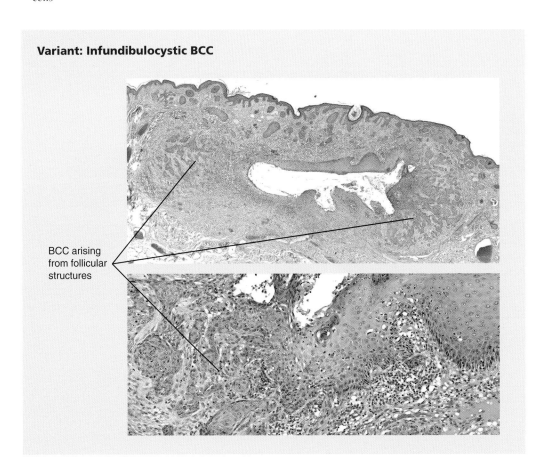

Variant: Infundibulocystic BCC

BCC arising from follicular structures

Cl: No specific clinical appearance.

Hi: Proliferation of basaloid cells, originating from follicular structures.

BASAL CELL CARCINOMA

Variants of BCC With Ductal, Matrical or Sebaceous Differentiation

Variant: BCC with Ductal Differentiation

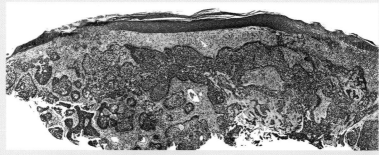

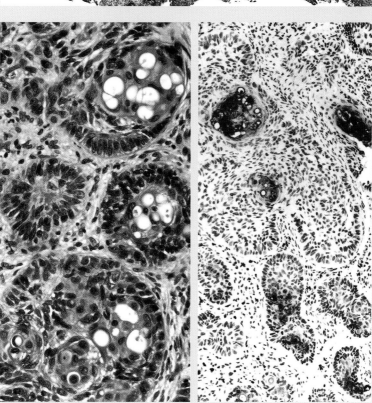

BCC with ductal
structures;
CEA-positive

Courtesy of Luis Requena, Madrid

BASAL CELL CARCINOMA

Variant: BCC with Matrical Differentiation

BCC with matrical
differentiation;
beta-catenin
(right)

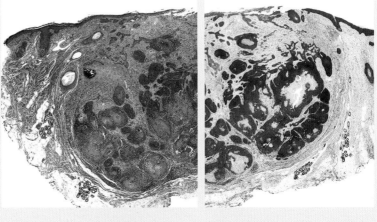

Nests of basaloid
cells; shadow
cells (right)

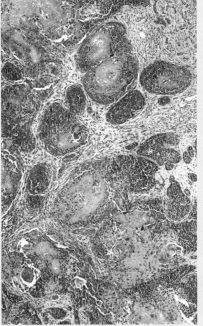
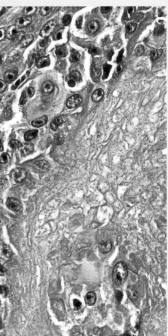

Courtesy of Luis Requena, Madrid

BASAL CELL CARCINOMA

Variant: BCC with Sebaceous Differentiation

BCC with strong fibrous stroma reaction

Nests of basaloid cells with sebaceous differentiation

Courtesy of Luis Requena, Madrid

Comment: Distinct differentiation towards various structures may be seen in some BCC, which sometimes leads to diagnostic pitfalls.

References

Ambrojo, P., Aguilar, A., Simon, P., Requena, L., and Sanchez Yus, E. (1992) Basal cell carcinoma with matrical differentiation. *Am J Dermatopathol* **14**(4): 293–7.

Del Sordo, R., Cavaliere, A., and Sidoni, A. (2007) Basal cell carcinoma with matrical differentiation: expression of beta-catenin [corrected] and osteopontin. *Am J Dermatopathol* **29**(5): 470–4.

BASAL CELL CARCINOMA

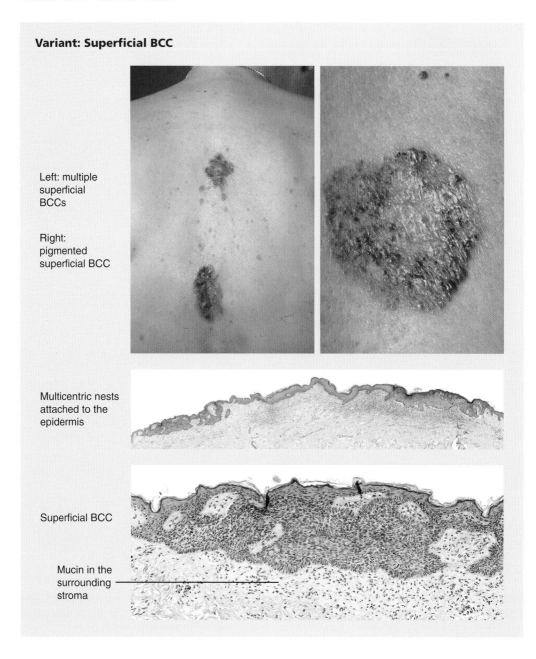

Variant: Superficial BCC

Left: multiple superficial BCCs

Right: pigmented superficial BCC

Multicentric nests attached to the epidermis

Superficial BCC

Mucin in the surrounding stroma

Cl: Solitary or multiple plaques; mostly located on the trunk.

Hi:

- Solitary or confluent superficial nests of basaloid epithelial cells
- Connection with the epidermis or with adnexal structures
- Peripheral palisading
- Distinct shrinkage clefts
- Adjacent tumor stroma containing mucin
- Fibrosis and inflammatory infiltrate in the upper dermis

BASAL CELL CARCINOMA

Variant: Pigmented BCC

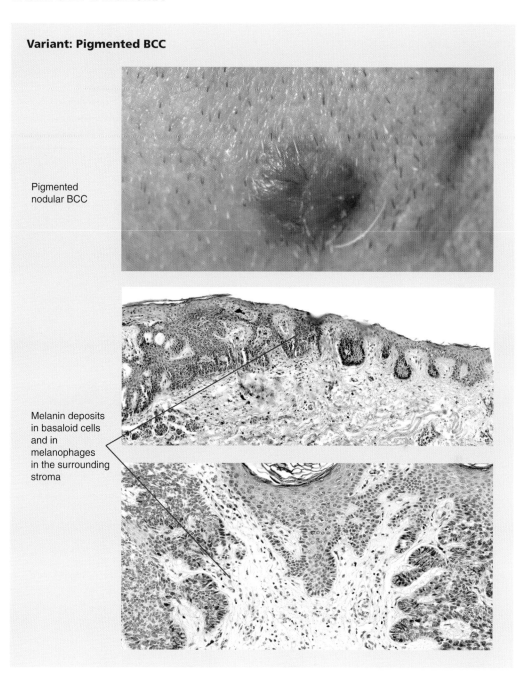

Pigmented
nodular BCC

Melanin deposits
in basaloid cells
and in
melanophages
in the surrounding
stroma

Cl: Nodular or superficial pigmented lesion.
Hi: Increased number of intratumoral melanocytes in scattered array.

BASAL CELL CARCINOMA

Variant: Adenoid-Cystic BCC

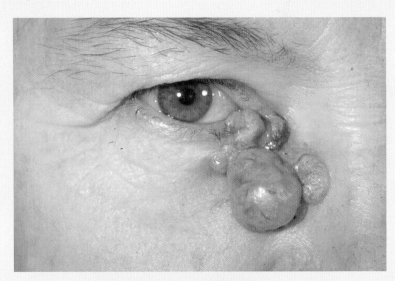

Adenoid-cystic BCC, originating from the lower eyelid

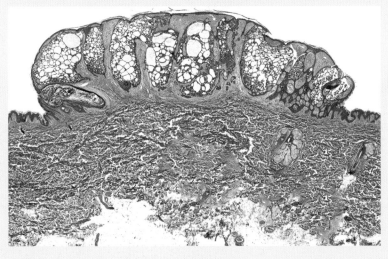

Tumor from the trunk. Fenestrated tumor pattern. Intralesional cystic spaces

Cl: Single or multiple confluent soft, translucent bluish-white nodules with discrete telangiectases. Preferential localisation is the eyelids. Hidrocystoma is the most common differential diagnosis.

Hi: Solid nodules of basaloid cells and intratumoral mucin-filled cystic spaces.

DD: Mucinous eccrine carcinoma, showing slender strands of basaloid epithelial cells lying in "puddles of mucin." Endocrine mucin-producing tumor (as a variant of mucinous eccrine carcinoma) presenting with roundish basaloid tumor nests in a "cannonball"-like arrangement. Nests may contain intratumoral mucinous lakes. Characteristic immunophenotype with expression of chromogranin, synaptophysin, estrogen, and progesterone.

BASAL CELL CARCINOMA

Variant: Adenoid-Cystic BCC

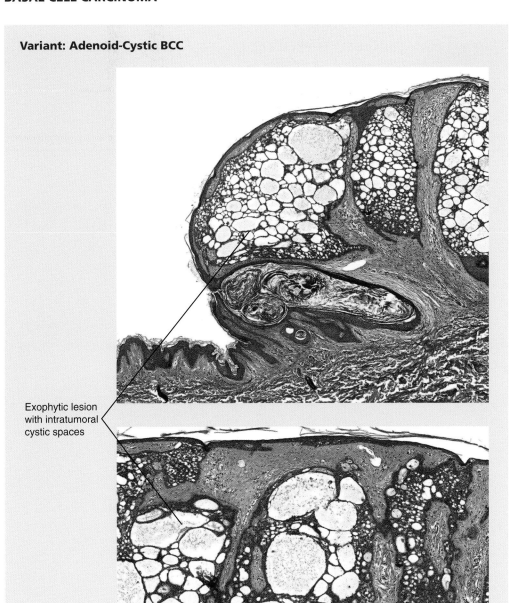

Exophytic lesion
with intratumoral
cystic spaces

BASAL CELL CARCINOMA

Variant: Sclerodermiform (Morpheaform) BCC

Slightly atrophic superficial lesions on the nose (left) and forehead (right)

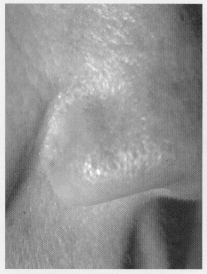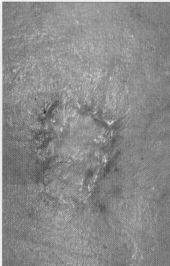

Delicate tumor strands within sclerotic stroma

Sclerosis between and underneath tumor islands

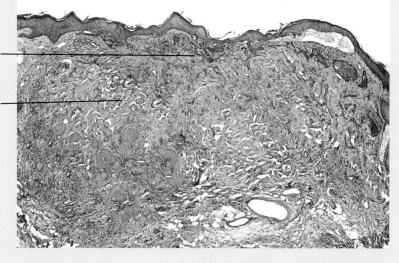

BASAL CELL CARCINOMA

Variant: Sclerodermiform (Morpheaform) BCC

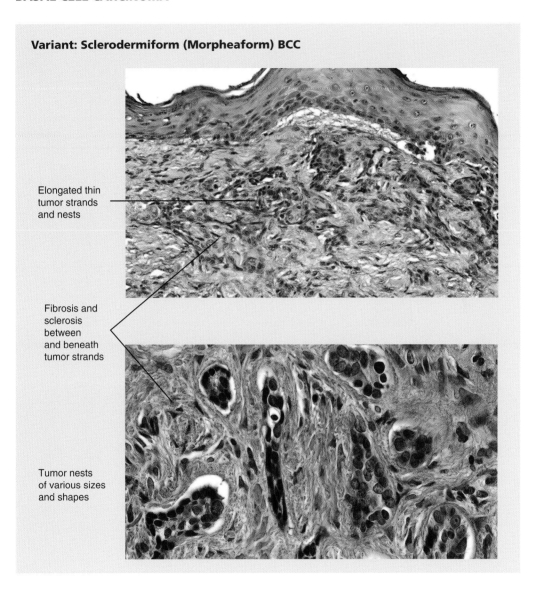

Elongated thin tumor strands and nests

Fibrosis and sclerosis between and beneath tumor strands

Tumor nests of various sizes and shapes

Cl: Poorly circumscribed indurated scar-like lesion. Spread beyond clinically recognizable borders. Aggressive course, especially in the nasolabial fold, where deeper structures may be involved. Ulceration is rare.

Hi:

- Small thin tumor islands and strands, proliferating between collagen bundles
- Absence of peripheral palisading
- Fibrosis of the surrounding dermis
- Cleft formation may occur, but is not typical
- Strong positivity for BerEP4

DD: Clinical differential diagnoses include traumatic scar, morphea, desmoplastic melanoma, desmoplastic trichoepithelioma, microcystic adnexal carcinoma.

BASAL CELL CARCINOMA

Clinical Variants: Ulcerating BCCs

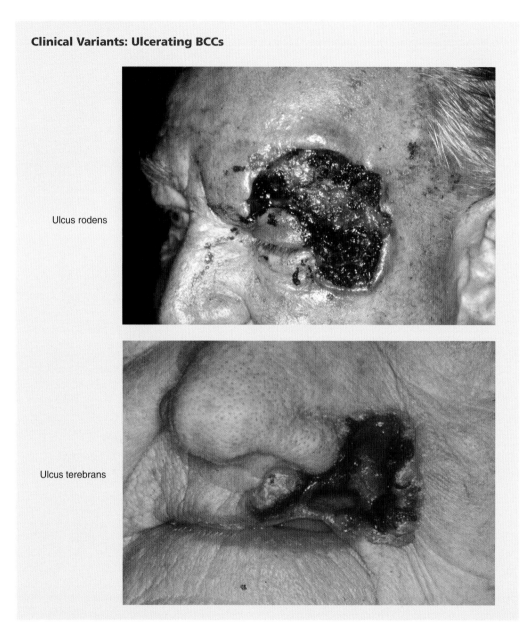

Ulcus rodens

Ulcus terebrans

Two types can be differentiated, both with an aggressive clinical course. Ulcus rodens ulcerates and spreads peripherally, whereas ulcus terebrans spreads into the depth, destroying underlying structures, including cartilage and bone.

BASAL CELL CARCINOMA

Histological Variants: Metatypic BCC with Squamoid Differentiation

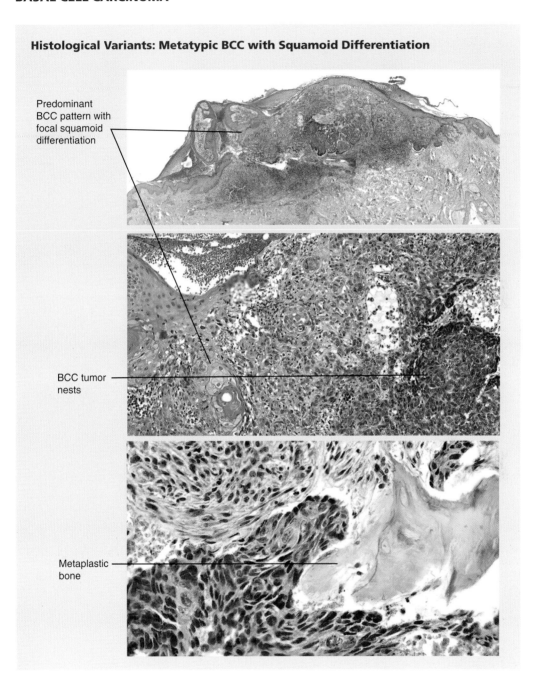

Predominant BCC pattern with focal squamoid differentiation

BCC tumor nests

Metaplastic bone

BASAL CELL CARCINOMA

Variant: Metatypic BCC with Squamoid Differentiation

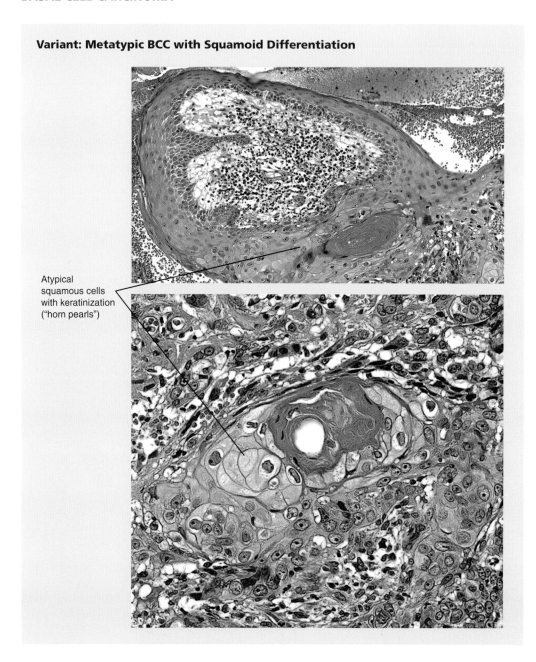

Atypical
squamous cells
with keratinization
("horn pearls")

Hi: Cytological features indeterminate between classic basal cell carcinoma and squamous cell carcinoma. Often with typical basaloid tumor formation blending into squamous cell carcinoma-like zones of differentiation.

Syndromatic BCC (Basal Cell Nevus Syndrome, Gorlin–Goltz)

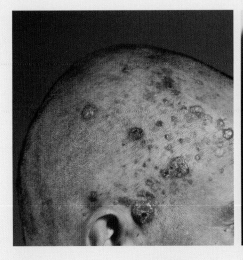
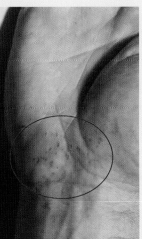

Multiple BCCs
on the scalp

Palmar pits
(circle)

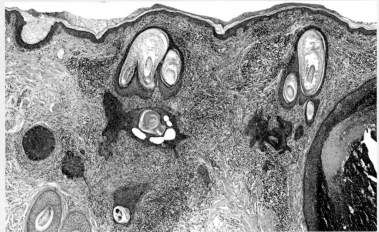

Proliferation
of basaloid cells
originating from
infundibulocystic
structures

Several syndromes are associated with increased risk of BCC: Bazex–Dupré–Christol syndrome, Rombo syndrome, multiple hereditary infundibulocystic basal cell carcinomas, basaloid follicular hamartoma.

Cl: Autosomal dominant inherited mutation of the PTCH gene, which is responsible for disorders affecting the skin, skeleton, and central nervous system. Patients develop multiple basal cell carcinomas disseminated over trunk, face, and extremities. Initially, BCC may resemble small melanocytic nevi, before developing into larger BCCs. As in non-syndromatic BCCs, UV light and x-rays are promoting factors. Additional clinical signs include palmar pits (tiny defects of the stratum corneum), mandibular cysts, kyphoscoliosis, and calcified falx cerebri.

Hi: Corresponds to sporadic BCC. Most commonly nodular or superficial subtype. Early lesions may show an infundibulocystic origin.

Fibroepithelioma of Pinkus

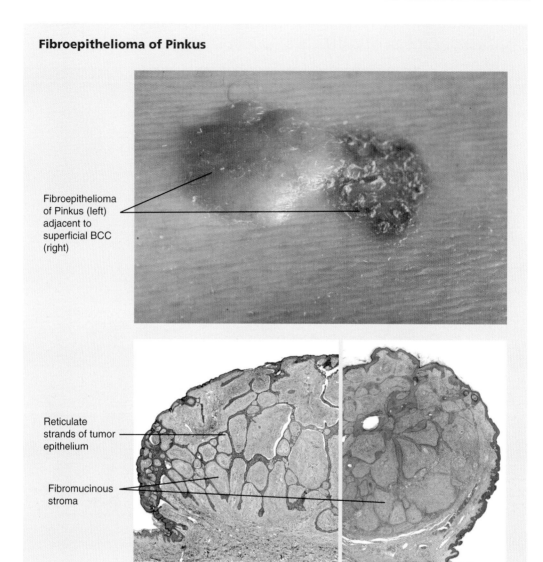

Fibroepithelioma of Pinkus (left) adjacent to superficial BCC (right)

Reticulate strands of tumor epithelium

Fibromucinous stroma

Fibroepithelioma of Pinkus

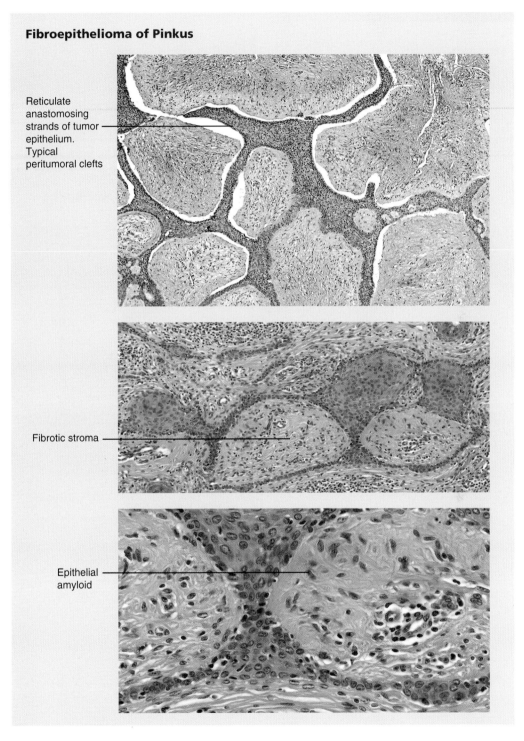

Reticulate anastomosing strands of tumor epithelium. Typical peritumoral clefts

Fibrotic stroma

Epithelial amyloid

Cl: Soft nodular, non-ulcerating lesion, preferentially in lumbosacral localisation.

Hi: Fibroepithelioma of Pinkus is considered to be a reticulated variant of BCC.

- Lacy strands of tumorous epithelium
- Connection with the epidermis
- Prominent fibromucinous stroma

- Peritumoral shrinkage clefts and peripheral palisading may be focally present
- At the tips of elongated tumor strands, there may be small, nub-like BerEP4-positive basaloid nests considered to be indicators of abortive hair bulb formation
- Focal positivity for PHLDA-1

SQUAMOUS CELL CARCINOMA

References

Bowen, A.R. and LeBoit, P.E. (2005) Fibroepithelioma of Pinkus is a fenestrated trichoblastoma. *Am J Dermatopathol* **27**(2): 149–54.

Katona, T.M., Ravis, S.M., Perkins, S.M., Moores, W.B., and Billings, S.D. (2007) Expression of androgen receptor by fibroepithelioma of Pinkus: evidence supporting classification as a basal cell carcinoma variant? *Am J Dermatopathol* **29**(1): 7–12.

Naeyaert, J.M., Pauwels, C., Geerts, M.L., and Verplancke, P. (2001) CD-34 and Ki-67 staining patterns of basaloid follicular hamartoma are different from those in fibroepithelioma of Pinkus and other variants of basal cell carcinoma. *J Cutan Pathol* **28**(10): 538–41.

Stern, J.B., Haupt, H.M., and Smith, R.R. (1994) Fibroepithelioma of Pinkus. Eccrine duct spread of basal cell carcinoma. *Am J Dermatopathol* **16**(6): 585–7.

Squamous Cell Carcinoma (SCC)

Variant: Well-Differentiated SCC

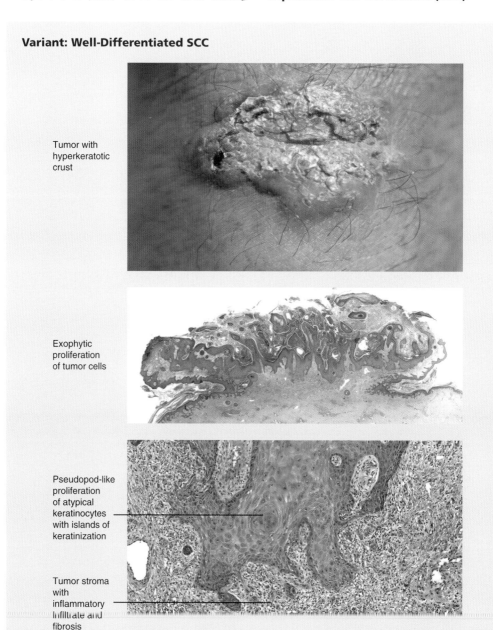

Tumor with hyperkeratotic crust

Exophytic proliferation of tumor cells

Pseudopod-like proliferation of atypical keratinocytes with islands of keratinization

Tumor stroma with inflammatory infiltrate and fibrosis

SQUAMOUS CELL CARCINOMA

Variant: Well-Differentiated SCC

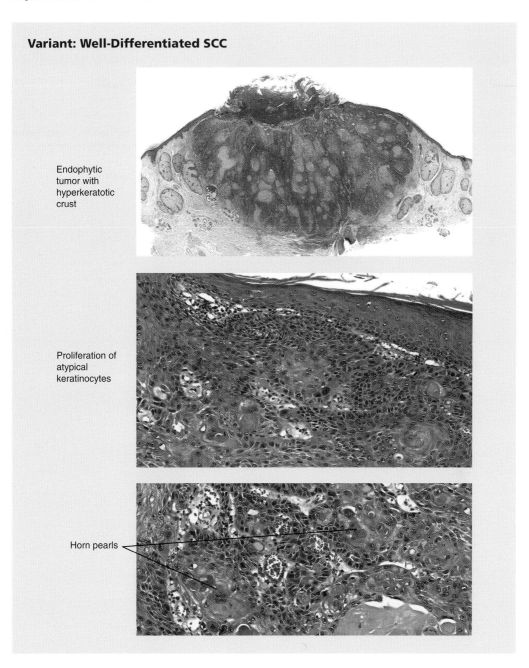

Endophytic tumor with hyperkeratotic crust

Proliferation of atypical keratinocytes

Horn pearls

Cl: SCCs usually arise on chronically damaged skin (UV or ionizing irradiation, scars from wounds, burning, chronic ulcers, fistulae, lupus erythematosus, lupus vulgaris). They can appear anywhere on the body, including lips, tongue, and anogenital region. The lower third of the face, lower lip, earlobe, and dorsa of the hands are favored sites. The firm, nodular plaques are usually covered with hyperkeratotic crusts. Well-differentiated, highly keratinizing SCCs have an intermediate malignant potential with a low tendency to metastasize.

Hi:
- Invasive epithelial tumor with asymmetry and poor circumscription
- Proliferation of pleomorphic epithelial tumor cells, corresponding to the keratinocytes of the spinous layer of the epidermis
- Eosinophilic cytoplasm

SQUAMOUS CELL CARCINOMA

- Intercellular bridges
- Focal keratinization and horn pearls
- Mitoses
- Focal necroses, not as pronounced as in keratoacanthoma

- Infiltrative growth
- Sometimes tumoral acantholysis may be present, simulating pattern of angiosarcoma

Variant: Acantholytic SCC (Epithelioma Spinocellulare Segregans of Delacretaz)

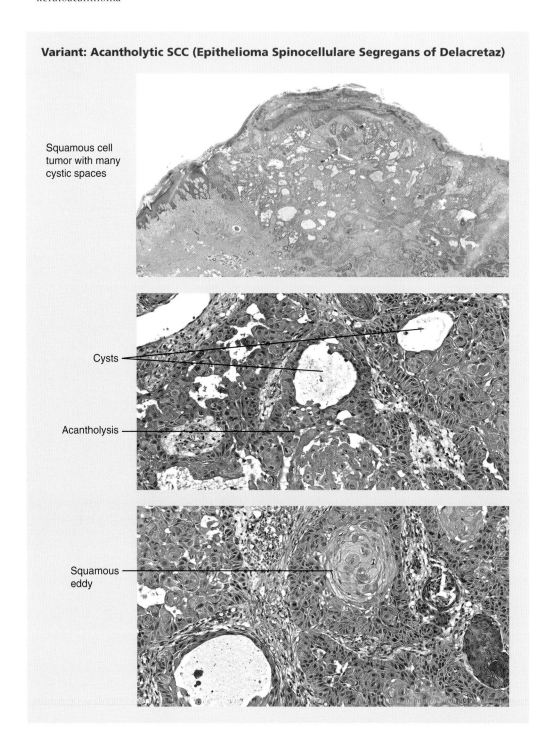

Squamous cell tumor with many cystic spaces

Cysts

Acantholysis

Squamous eddy

SQUAMOUS CELL CARCINOMA

Variant: Acantholytic SCC (Epithelioma Spinocellulare Segregans of Delacretaz)

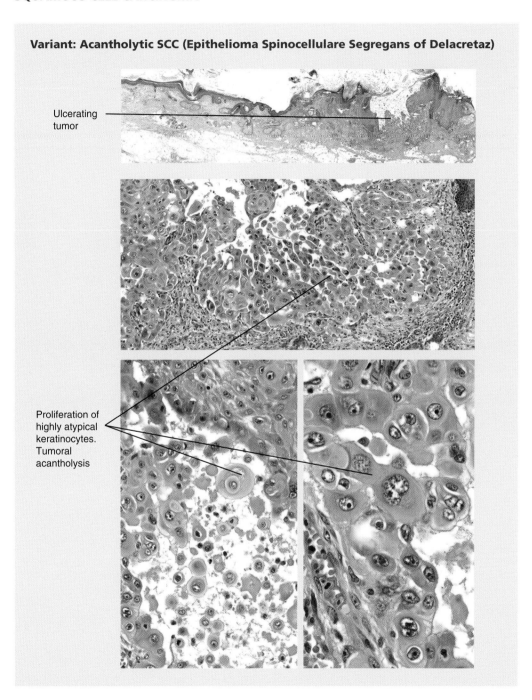

Ulcerating tumor

Proliferation of highly atypical keratinocytes. Tumoral acantholysis

This is not an entity in its own right but rather a poorly differentiated SCC variant with free-floating keratinocytes. Intercellular adhesion has been lost throughout the entire tumor, resulting in an angio-sarcoma-like tumor pattern (tumoral acantholysis). **Cl**: Minimal hyperkeratosis. Mostly ulcerated, bleeding or oozing, crust formation.

Hi:
- Pleomorphic and anaplastic keratinocytes
- Loss of intercellular bridges with acantholysis
- Inflammatory infiltrate, often containing many plasma cells

SQUAMOUS CELL CARCINOMA

Reference

Delacretaz, J., Madjedi, A.S., and Loretan, R.M. (1957)
[Epithelioma spinocellulare segregans; the so-called
adenoacanthoma of the sweat glands (Lever)].
Hautarzt **8**(11): 512–18.

Variant: Myxoid SCC

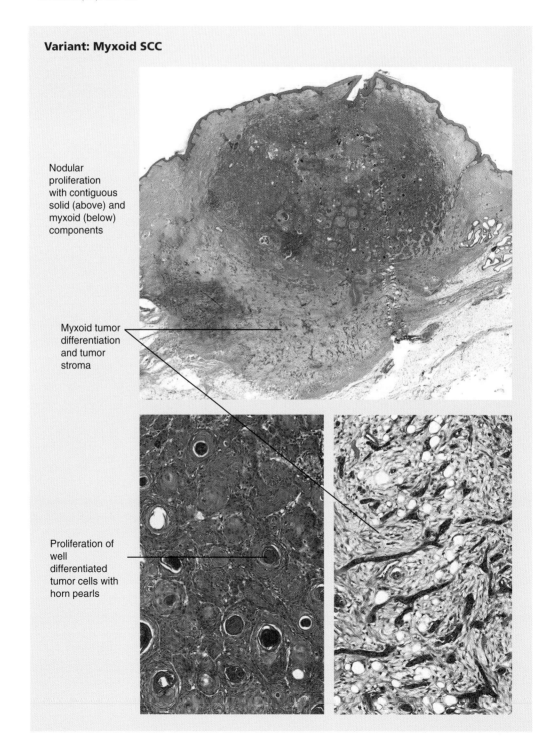

Nodular proliferation with contiguous solid (above) and myxoid (below) components

Myxoid tumor differentiation and tumor stroma

Proliferation of well differentiated tumor cells with horn pearls

SQUAMOUS CELL CARCINOMA

Cl: No specific clinical features.   **Hi**: Myxoid fibrous stroma.

Variant: Follicular (Infundibular) SCC

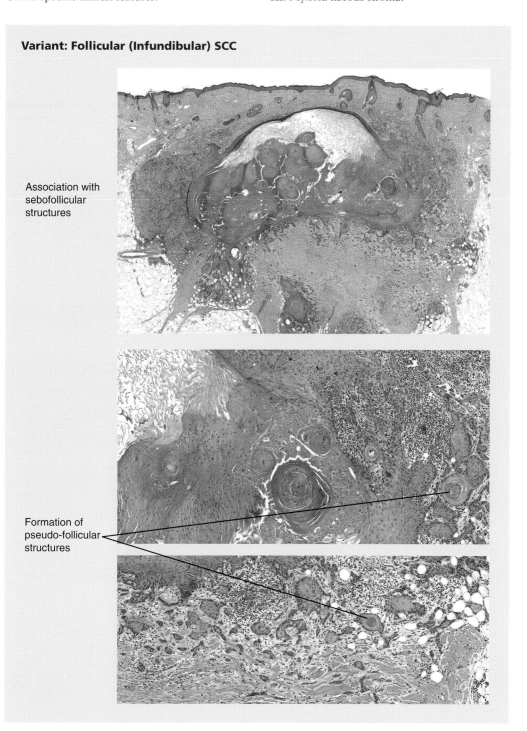

Association with sebofollicular structures

Formation of pseudo-follicular structures

SQUAMOUS CELL CARCINOMA

Some squamous cell carcinomas have follicular differentiation, arising from the infundibular portion of hair follicles. While they may overlap histologically with keratoacanthoma, clinically they are rarely confused with this entity.
Cl: Simulating keratoacanthoma.

Hi:
- Arising from the infundibular portion of the hair follicle
- Abortive follicular structures

Variant: Spindle Cell (Fusicellular) SCC

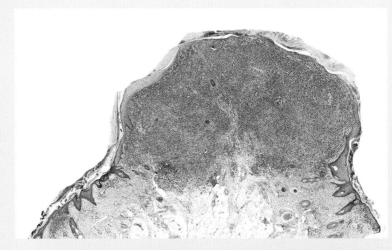

Exophytic epithelial tumor without keratinization

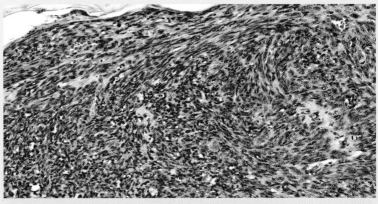

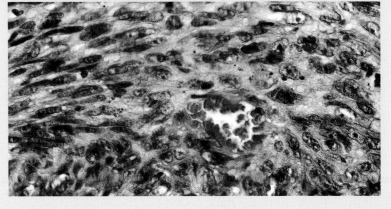

Epithelial spindle cells

SQUAMOUS CELL CARCINOMA

This variant presents with a tumor pattern that must be immunohistochemically separated from other epithelial and mesenchymal spindle cell tumors.

Cl: No specific clinical features.

Hi: Differentiation from other spindle cell tumors, especially from amelanotic melanoma, must be based on immunohistochemistry. Malignant melanoma reliably expresses S100 and SOX10, and is always negative for pancytokeratin. Spindled SCCs are frequently positive for vimentin, further adding to the confusion with mesenchymal neoplasms.

DD: Malignant (amelanotic) melanoma.

Squamous Cell Carcinomas in Special Sites

Cl: SCCs on ear, lip, penis, vulva, and tongue often are misdiagnosed at incipient stages of tumor evolution and may be mistaken for infectious disorders. However, due to the loss of differentiation, tumors at these sites often show a progressive course and tend to metastasize into the local lymph nodes.

Squamous Cell Carcinomas in Special Sites

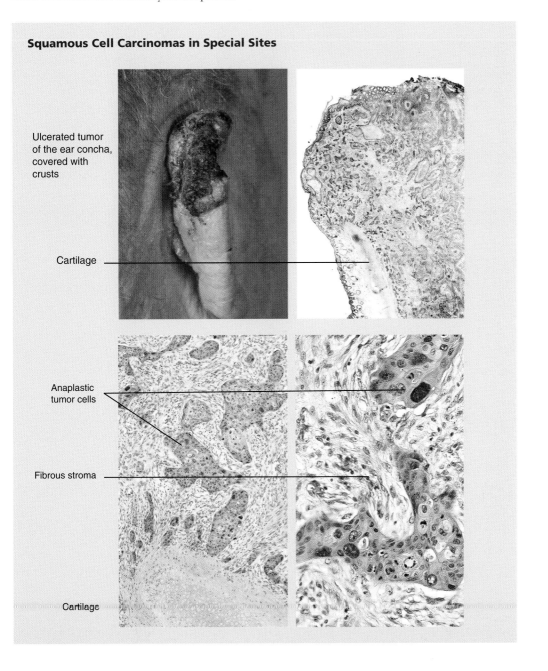

Ulcerated tumor of the ear concha, covered with crusts

Cartilage

Anaplastic tumor cells

Fibrous stroma

Cartilage

SQUAMOUS CELL CARCINOMA

Differential Diagnosis: Chondrodermatitis Nodularis Helicis of Winkler

Crateriform
lesion (left)

Endophytic crater
with epidermal
hyperplasia
and adjacent
granulation
tissue, overlying
eroded cartilage
(right)

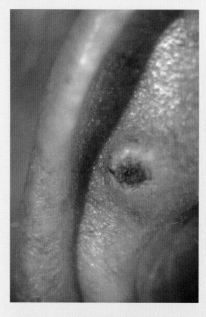 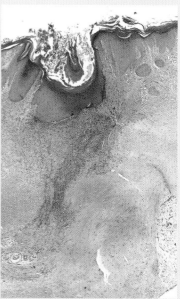

Epidermal
hyperplasia,
granulation
tissue, eroded
cartilage

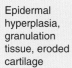 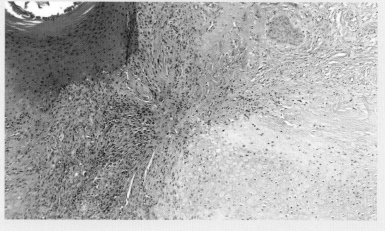

SQUAMOUS CELL CARCINOMA

Special Sites: SCC of the Lip

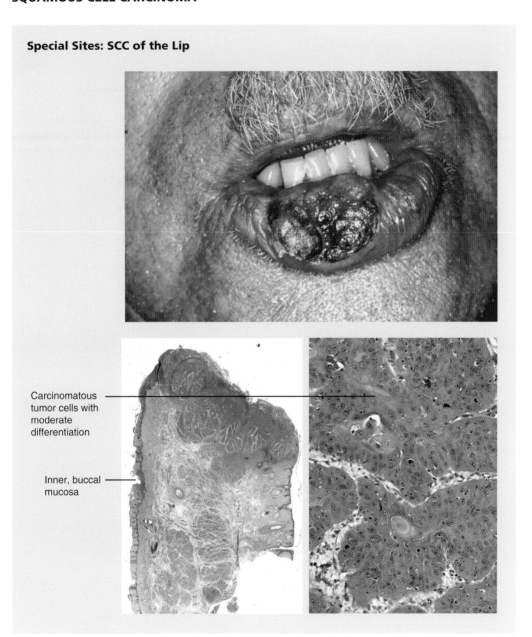

Carcinomatous tumor cells with moderate differentiation

Inner, buccal mucosa

SQUAMOUS CELL CARCINOMA

Special Sites: SCC of the Tongue

Ulcerated SCC
of the tongue

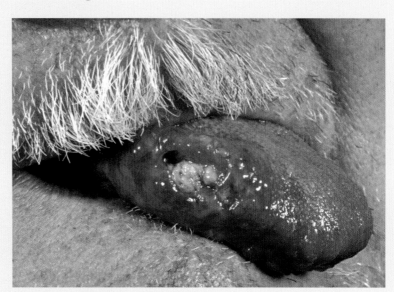

Invasive
carcinoma with
large, poorly
differentiated
squamous
epithelial cells

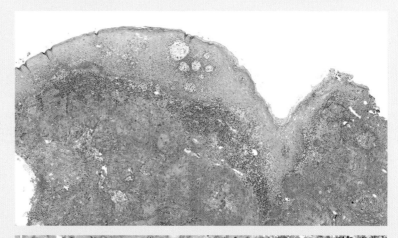

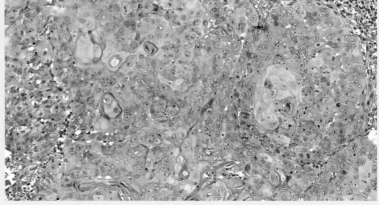

SQUAMOUS CELL CARCINOMA

Special Sites: SCC of the Penis

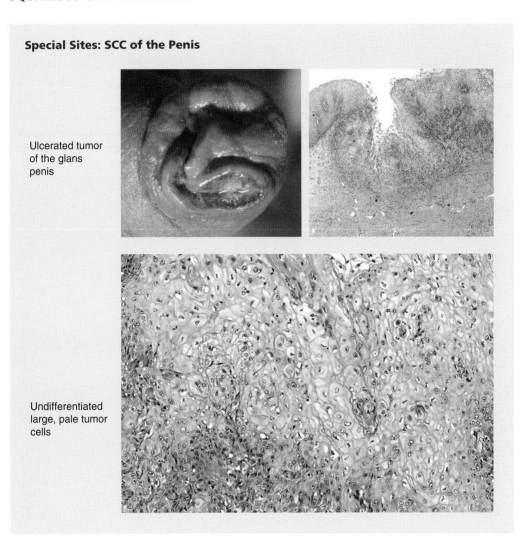

Ulcerated tumor of the glans penis

Undifferentiated large, pale tumor cells

Hi:
- Often ulcerated
- Undifferentiated cytomorphology with minimal keratinization
- Highly atypical, pale anaplastic epithelial tumor cells
- Many mitoses
- Inflammatory infiltrate, containing many plasma cells

DD (ear): Chondrodermatitis nodularis helicis of Winkler.

CHAPTER 2

Adnexal

Atlas of Dermatopathology: Tumors, Nevi, and Cysts, First Edition. Günter Burg, Heinz Kutzner,
Werner Kempf, Josef Feit, and Bruce R. Smoller.
© 2019 John Wiley & Sons Ltd. Published 2019 by John Wiley & Sons Ltd.

NEVI, HYPERPLASIAS, AND BENIGN ADNEXAL NEOPLASMS

Sweat Gland Differentiation

A clearcut differentiation between the preferential origin (eccrine or apocrine) of an adnexal neoplasm is often not possible, since both structural elements may be seen side by side in the same lesion. However, elongated ductal structures are a clue to an apocrine origin of the lesion.

Nevi, Hyperplasias, and Benign Adnexal Neoplasms (BAN)
Eccrine Differentiation

Sweat Gland Nevus

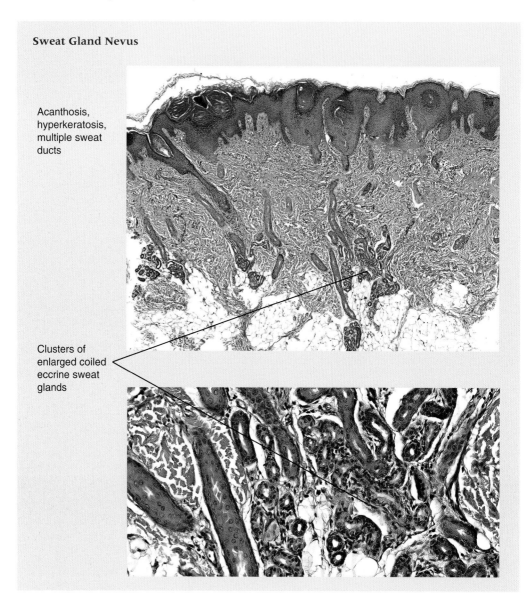

Acanthosis, hyperkeratosis, multiple sweat ducts

Clusters of enlarged coiled eccrine sweat glands

Cl: Plaque with localized hyperhidrosis. Very rare.
Hi:
- Densely packed clusters of normal or enlarged eccrine sweat glands, sometimes embedded in mucinous stroma
- Acanthosis and hyperkeratosis

DD: Epidermal nevus with eccrine differentiation.

References

Frouin, E., Riviere, B., Maillet, O., et al. (2016) Coccygeal polypoid eccrine nevus associated with imperforate anus and unilateral multicystic kidney dysplasia. *J Cutan Pathol* **43**(8), 697–701.

Luo, D.Q., Huang, C.Z., Xie, W.L., Xu, F.F., and Mo, L.Q. (2015) Hybrid eccrine gland and hair follicle

NEVI, HYPERPLASIAS, AND BENIGN ADNEXAL NEOPLASMS

hamartoma: a new entity of adnexal nevus. *Am J Dermatopathol* **37**(2): 167–70.

Martorell-Calatayud, A., Colmenero, I., Hernandez-Martin, A., Requena, L., and Torrelo, A. (2010) Porokeratotic eccrine and hair follicle nevus. *Am J Dermatopathol* **32**(5): 529–30.

Shaffer, H.C., Schosser, R., and Phillips, C. (2009) Acantholytic dyskeratotic epidermal nevus with eccrine differentiation: a case report and review of literature. *J Cutan Pathol* **36**(9): 1001–4.

Eccrine Syringofibroadenoma (Mascaro Tumor)

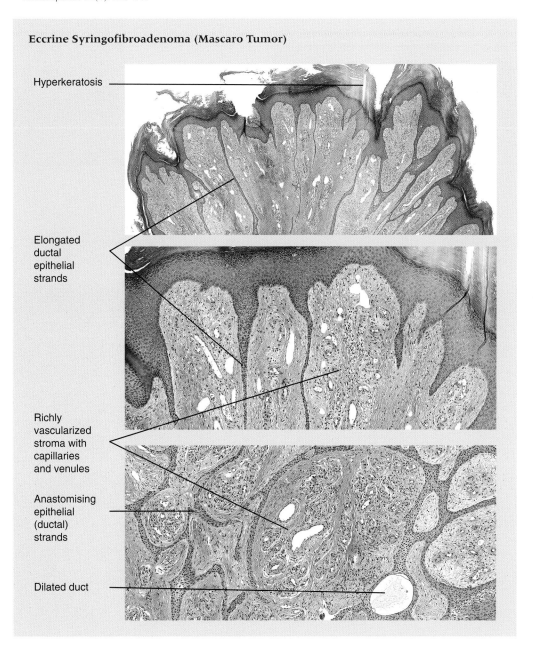

Hyperkeratosis

Elongated ductal epithelial strands

Richly vascularized stroma with capillaries and venules

Anastomising epithelial (ductal) strands

Dilated duct

Cl: Rare solitary, hyperkeratotic tumor, preferentially on the extremities. The tumor presents with a "tapioca pudding"-like surface. Considered to be a reactive change within chronic irritated skin; also designated as acrosyringial nevus.

Hi:
- Acanthosis with moderate hyperkeratosis
- Elongated rete ridges
- Small ductal structures within the epithelial strands
- Richly vascularized stroma

NEVI, HYPERPLASIAS, AND BENIGN ADNEXAL NEOPLASMS

DD: Fibroepithelioma of Pinkus; reticulate seborrheic keratosis; eccrine poroma.

References

Cota, C., Ferrara, G., Amantea, A., and Donati, P. (2011) Eccrine syringofibroadenoma and clear cell acanthoma: an association by chance? *Am J Dermatopathol* **33**(2): 195–8.

Shalin, S.C., Rinaldi, C., and Horn, T.D. (2013) Clear cell acanthoma with changes of eccrine syringofibroade-noma: reactive change or clue to etiology? *J Cutan Pathol* **40**(12): 1021–6.

Tan, T., Guitart, J., Liu, L.L., et al. (2017) Eccrine syringofibroadenoma in association with acquired epidermodysplasia verruciformis. *Am J Dermatopathol* **39**(7): 534–7.

Weedon, D. and Lewis, J. (1977) Acrosyringeal nevus. *J Cutan Pathol* **4**(3): 166–8.

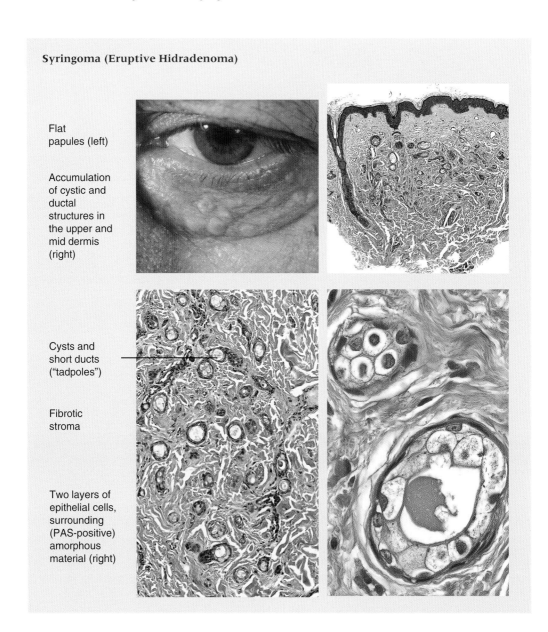

Syringoma (Eruptive Hidradenoma)

Flat papules (left)

Accumulation of cystic and ductal structures in the upper and mid dermis (right)

Cysts and short ducts ("tadpoles")

Fibrotic stroma

Two layers of epithelial cells, surrounding (PAS-positive) amorphous material (right)

NEVI, HYPERPLASIAS, AND BENIGN ADNEXAL NEOPLASMS

Cl: Most common, especially in young women, in the periorbital region but also occurs in other locations (vulva) in association with eccrine glands. Multiple tiny, smooth skin-colored or yellowish intradermal papules.

Hi:

- Involvement of the upper dermis
- Tiny tennis racket-like cystic and ductal structures ("tadpoles")
- Double layer of epithelial cells
- Fibrotic stroma
- PAS-positive clear cell variants (rare)

References

Alonso-Riano, M., Camara-Jurado, M., Garrido, M.C., and Rodriguez-Peralto, J.L. (2015) Papular clear cell hyperplasia of the eccrine duct: a precursor lesion of clear cell syringoma? *Am J Dermatopathol* **37**(9): 701–3.

Incel Uysal, P., Yalcin, B., Ozhamam, E., and Bozdogan, O. (2017) Coexistence of adult onset eruptive syringoma and bilateral renal cell carcinoma: a case report. *Am J Dermatopathol* **39**(1): 56–8.

Poroma

Three variants can be differentiated: common solid poroma, hidroacanthoma simplex, and dermal duct tumor.

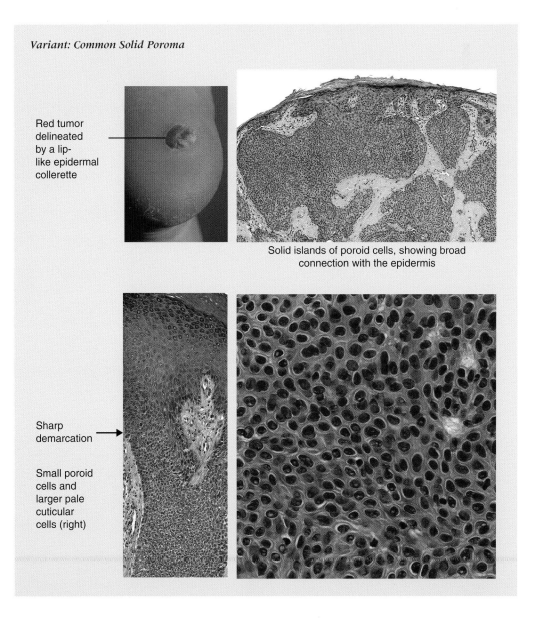

Variant: Common Solid Poroma

Red tumor delineated by a lip-like epidermal collerette

Solid islands of poroid cells, showing broad connection with the epidermis

Sharp demarcation

Small poroid cells and larger pale cuticular cells (right)

NEVI, HYPERPLASIAS, AND BENIGN ADNEXAL NEOPLASMS

Cl: Protuberant eroded painful (on pressure) benign, usually solitary, sharply circumscribed sweat gland tumor, preferentially on the foot. Multiple lesions may occur. Malignant poromas (porocarcinomas) are rare.

Hi:
- Solid invasive basaloid tumor, containing two morphologically different epithelial cell types:

  ○ Small poroid cells with eosinophilic basaloid roundish morphology
  ○ Larger, pale cuticular cells corresponding to the inner layer of sweat ducts
- Marked focal necrosis ("necrosis en masse")

DD: Eccrine acrospiroma; basal cell carcinoma; trichilemmoma.

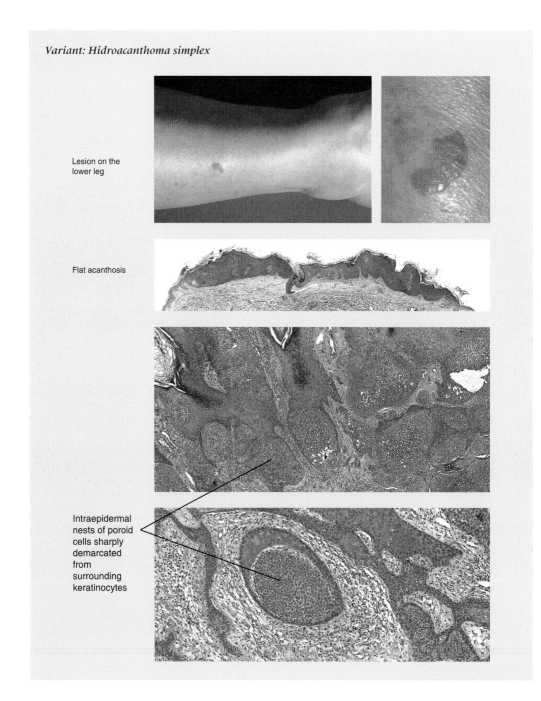

Variant: Hidroacanthoma simplex

Lesion on the lower leg

Flat acanthosis

Intraepidermal nests of poroid cells sharply demarcated from surrounding keratinocytes

NEVI, HYPERPLASIAS, AND BENIGN ADNEXAL NEOPLASMS

Cl: Circumscribed flat, brown, sometimes hyperkeratotic lesion, resembling flat seborrheic keratosis.

Hi:
- Acanthotic epidermis
- Clonal intraepidermal nests of poroid cells

- Prominent peripheral basaloid rimming by sharply demarcated regular keratinocytes

DD: Seborrheic keratosis with intraepidermal clonal proliferation (intraepidermal epithelioma of Borst–Jadassohn). Seborrheic keratoses do not appear on palms or soles.

Differential Diagnosis: Intraepidermal Epithelioma of Borst–Jadassohn (Seborrheic Keratosis)

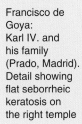

Francisco de Goya:
Karl IV. and his family (Prado, Madrid). Detail showing flat seborrheic keratosis on the right temple

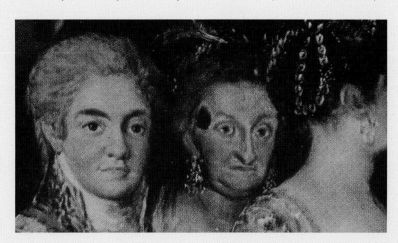

Intraepidermal clones of basaloid epidermal cells, surrounded by normal keratinocytes (mid and bottom)

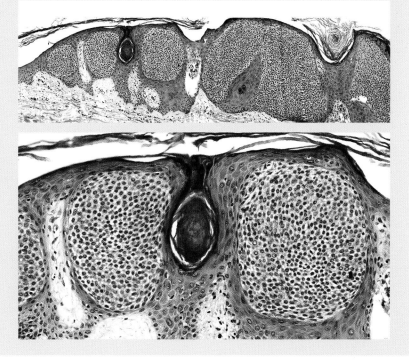

NEVI, HYPERPLASIAS, AND BENIGN ADNEXAL NEOPLASMS

Cl: Usually flat seborrheic keratosis, which does not occur on the planta or palma.
Hi: Acanthosis of the epidermis showing clonal nests of basaloid epidermal cells surrounded by regular keratinocytes. Nests are composed of irregularly arranged keratinocytes lacking cytological atypia.

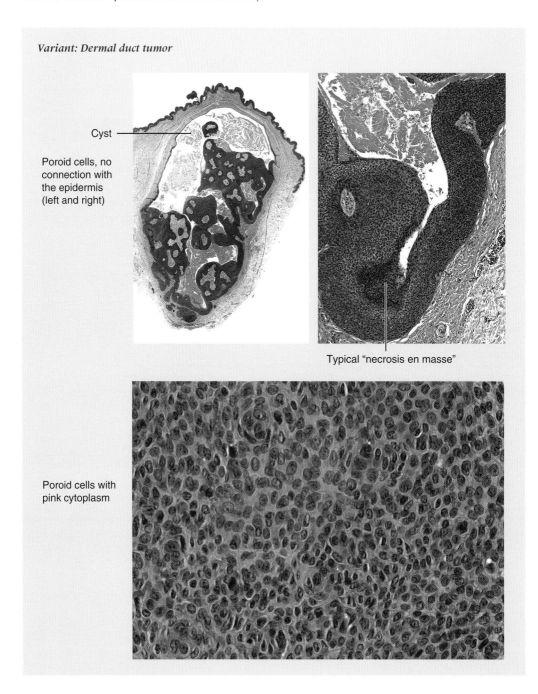

Variant: Dermal duct tumor

Cyst

Poroid cells, no connection with the epidermis (left and right)

Typical "necrosis en masse"

Poroid cells with pink cytoplasm

Cl: Inconspicuous papulonodular lesion.   **Hi**: No (broad) connection with the epidermis.

NEVI, HYPERPLASIAS, AND BENIGN ADNEXAL NEOPLASMS

Apocrine Differentiation

Apocrine Nevus

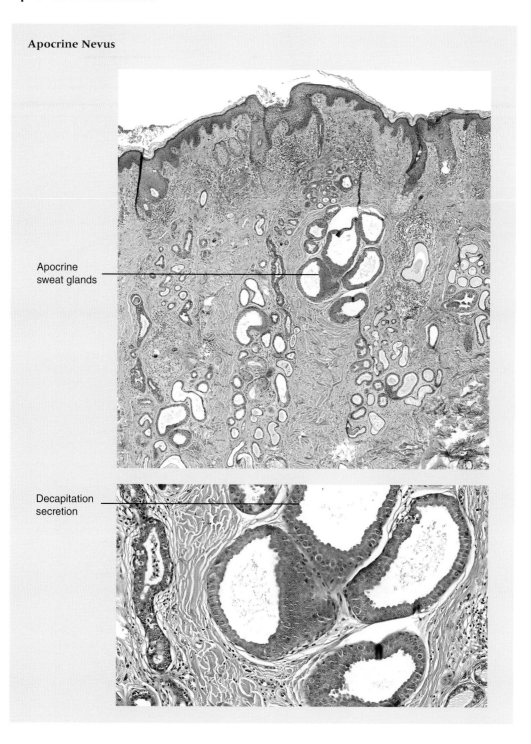

Apocrine
sweat glands

Decapitation
secretion

NEVI, HYPERPLASIAS, AND BENIGN ADNEXAL NEOPLASMS

Cl: Apocrine nevi are very rare and have no distinct clinical appearance.

Hi:

- Apocrine sweat gland structures
- Decapitation secretion
- Frequent association with proliferation of hair follicles or sebaceous glands

References

Ando, K., Hashikawa, Y., Nakashima, M., Nakayama, A., and Ohashi, M. (1991) Pure apocrine nevus. A study of light-microscopic and immunohistochemical features of a rare tumor. *Am J Dermatopathol* **13**(1): 71–6.

Cordero, S.C., Royer, M.C., Rush, W.L., Hallman, J.R., and Lupton, G.P. (2012) Pure apocrine nevus: a report of 4 cases. *Am J Dermatopathol* **34**(3): 305–9.

Kim, J.H., Hur, H., Lee, C.W., and Kim, Y.T. (1988) Apocrine nevus. *J Am Acad Dermatol* **18**(3): 579–81.

Neill, J.S. and Park, H.K. (1993) Apocrine nevus: light microscopic, immunohistochemical and ultrastructural studies of a case. *J Cutan Pathol* **20**(1): 79–83.

Mixed Tumor of the Skin (Chondroid Syringoma)

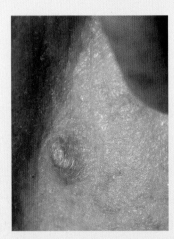

Nodule on the neck

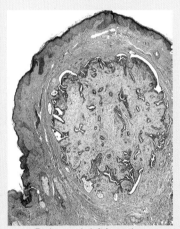

Peritumoral cleft formation (top and below)

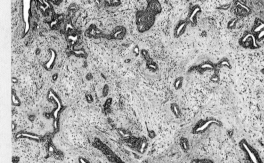

Branching tubular ducts within a mucinous stroma

NEVI, HYPERPLASIAS, AND BENIGN ADNEXAL NEOPLASMS

Cl: Small firm cutaneous or subcutaneous nodules, mostly located in the head and neck area. Usually benign, also considered to be a morphological variant of cutaneous myoepithelioma. Malignant mixed tumors of the skin exist.

Hi:

- Roundish sharply circumscribed tumor
- "Mixed" variety of structures: eccrine, apocrine, sebaceous, pilar, mucinous
- Branching tubules and clusters of epithelial cells with eccrine, apocrine, sebaceous or pilar differentiation
- All structures embedded in mucinous stroma
- Islands of chondroid (cartilage) differentiation and metaplastic ossification, especially in apocrine variant
- Clusters of large "plasmacytoid" epithelial cells (myoepithelial) with co-expression of S100 and alpha smooth muscle actin

- Eccrine variants present with a prominent chondroid stroma and embedded monomorphic tubular strands that strongly express S100

References

Headington, J.T. (1961) Mixed tumors of skin: eccrine and apocrine types. *Arch Dermatol* **84**: 989–96.

Jun, H.J., Cho, E., Cho, S.H., and Lee, J.D. (2012) Chondroid syringoma with marked calcification. *Am J Dermatopathol* **34**(8): e125–7.

Nguyen, C.M. and Cassarino, D.S. (2017) Local recurrence of cutaneous mixed tumor (chondroid syringoma) as malignant mixed tumor of the thumb 20 years after initial diagnosis. *J Cutan Pathol* **44**(3): 292–5.

Requena, C., Brotons, S., Sanmartin, O., et al. (2013) Malignant chondroid syringoma of the face with bone invasion. *Am J Dermatopathol* **35**(3): 395–8.

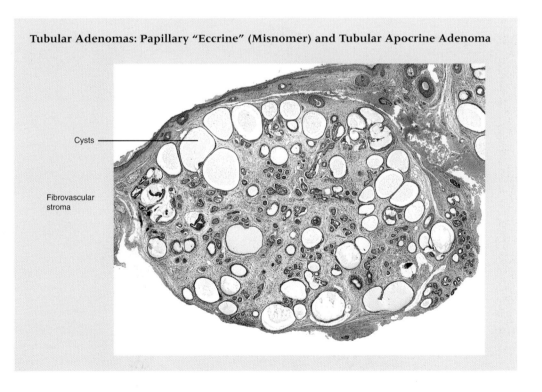

Tubular Adenomas: Papillary "Eccrine" (Misnomer) and Tubular Apocrine Adenoma

Cysts

Fibrovascular stroma

NEVI, HYPERPLASIAS, AND BENIGN ADNEXAL NEOPLASMS

Tubular Adenomas: Papillary "Eccrine" (Misnomer) and Tubular Apocrine Adenoma

Two layers of
cuboidal cells

Papillary
projections

Eosinophilic
debris

Apocrine
secretion

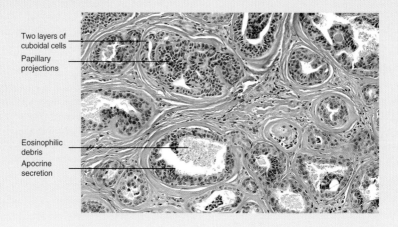

Tubular Adenomas: Papillary "Eccrine" (Misnomer) and Tubular Apocrine Adenoma

Dermal tumor
with tubular
and cystic
components

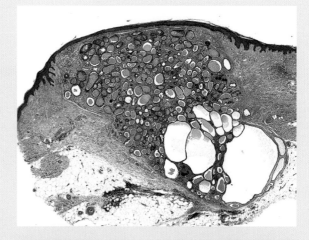

Ductal
structures with
double-layered
cyst wall.
Apocrine
secretion and
eosinophilic
debris

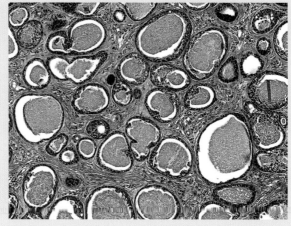

NEVI, HYPERPLASIAS, AND BENIGN ADNEXAL NEOPLASMS

Apocrine tubular adenoma and eccrine papillary adenoma are closely related and differ mainly by localisation and predominant type of secretion. The presence of ducts is a clue to apocrine origin.

Cl: Well-circumscribed intradermal papule with preferential localisation on the extremities or scalp.

Hi:

- Intradermal tumor, consisting of small tubular strands and cysts, embedded in fibrous stroma
- The ductal epithelium has two layers of cuboidal cells
- Small intraluminal papillary projections (pseudopapillae)
- Signs of apocrine secretion ("epithelial snouts") may be present
- Minimal necrosis
- No mitotic activity

References

Ansai, S.I., Anan, T., Fukumoto, T., and Saeki, H. (2016) Tubulopapillary cystic adenoma with apocrine differentiation: a unifying concept for syringocystad- enoma papilliferum, apocrine gland cyst, and tubular papillary adenoma. *Am J Dermatopathol* **39**(11): 829–37.

Ito, T., Nomura, T., Fujita, Y., Abe, R., and Shimizu, H. (2014) Tubular apocrine adenoma clinically and der- moscopically mimicking basal cell carcinoma. *J Am Acad Dermatol* **71**(2): e45–6.

Kazakov, D.V., Bisceglia, M., Calonje, E., et al. (2007) Tubular adenoma and syringocystadenoma papilliferum: a reappraisal of their relationship. An interobserver study of a series, by a panel of dermatopathologists. *Am J Dermatopathol* **29**(3): 256–63.

Kazakov, D.V., Mukensnabl, P., and Michal, M. (2006) Tubular adenoma of the skin with follicular and seba- ceous differentiation: a report of two cases. *Am J Dermatopathol* **28**(2): 142–6.

Montalli, V.A., Martinez, E., Tincani, A., et al. (2014) Tubular variant of basal cell adenoma shares immunophenotypical features with normal inter- calated ducts and is closely related to intercalated duct lesions of salivary gland. *Histopathology* **64**(6): 880–9.

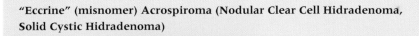

"Eccrine" (misnomer) Acrospiroma (Nodular Clear Cell Hidradenoma, Solid Cystic Hidradenoma)

Dermal nodule on the scalp (left)

Well circumscribed dermal nodule (right)

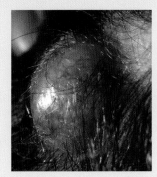
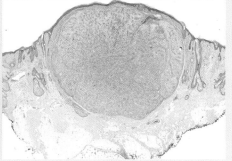

NEVI, HYPERPLASIAS, AND BENIGN ADNEXAL NEOPLASMS

"Eccrine" (misnomer) Acrospiroma (Nodular Clear Cell Hidradenoma, Solid Cystic Hidradenoma)

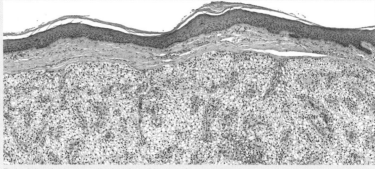

Pale (clear) tumor cells (mid and bottom)

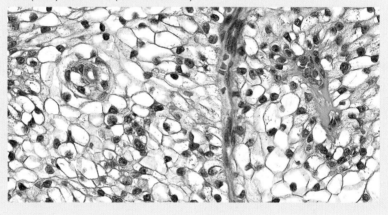

Cl: Nodular tumor with smooth surface that may occur at any localisation and at any age,

Hi:

- Well-circumscribed dermal tumor
- Aggregates of confluent epithelial lobules
- Characteristic feature: sclerotic tumor stroma between tumor nests
- Tumor cells with alternating morphology: pale clear cells and smaller cells with eosinophilic cytoplasm
- Minimal amounts of squamous differentiation
- Cystic and tubular structures may be focally present
- Low mitotic activity
- Transition to incipient malignancy may occur only focally (step sections!) with crowded nuclei (hyperchromasia), pleomorphism, increased mitotic activity

References

Ahmed, A., Kim, W., and Speiser, J. (2017) Mucinous hidradenoma in a child: a case report and review of the literature. *J Cutan Pathol* Apr 21. doi: 10.1111/cup.12957 [epub ahead of print].

Nandeesh, B.N. and Rajalakshmi, T. (2012) A study of histopathologic spectrum of nodular hidradenoma. *Am J Dermatopathol* **34**(5): 461–70.

Tingaud, C., Costes, V., Frouin, E., et al. (2016) Lymph node location of a clear cell hidradenoma: report of a patient and review of literature. *J Cutan Pathol* **43**(8): 702–6.

Yu, G., Goodloe, S. Jr, D'Angelis, C.A., McGrath, B.E., and Chen, F. (2010) Giant clear cell hidradenoma of the knee. *J Cutan Pathol* **37**(9): e37–41.

NEVI, HYPERPLASIAS, AND BENIGN ADNEXAL NEOPLASMS

Spiradenoma

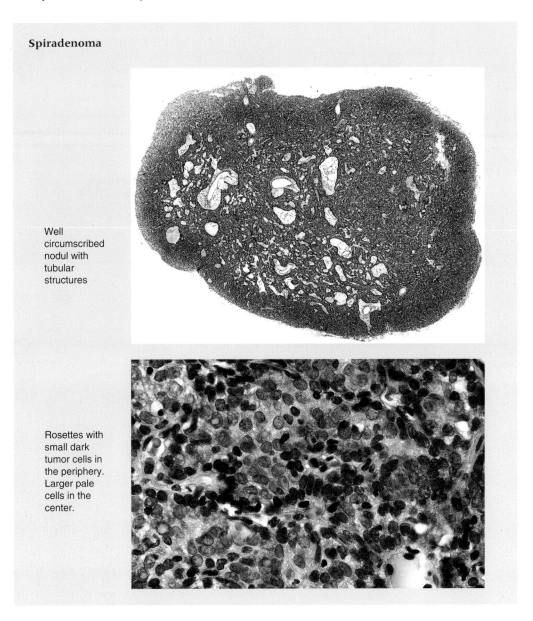

Well circumscribed nodul with tubular structures

Rosettes with small dark tumor cells in the periphery. Larger pale cells in the center.

Cl: Solitary or sometimes multiple grouped intradermal nodules in young adults with non-specific clinical appearance; mostly painful upon palpation. Frequent association with trichoepitheliomas and cylindromas suggests a genetic background. Apocrine and malignant variants (spiradenocarcinoma) exist.

Hi:
- Well-circumscribed nodule, may resemble lymph node in scanning magnification
- Two distinct cell populations of intermingled epithelial tumor cells ("pepper and salt" pattern):
  - Small lymphocyte-like dark epithelial cells amidst
  - Larger pale epithelial cells with vesicular nuclei
- Thick basement membrane (PAS) surrounding the tumor
- Ductal structures with PAS positivity
- There may be morphological overlap with cylindroma (thick basement membrane)

References

Ben Brahim, E., Sfia, M., Tangour, M., Makhlouf, R., Cribier, B., and Chatti, S. (2010) Malignant eccrine spiradenoma: a new case report. *J Cutan Pathol* **37**(4): 478–81.

NEVI, HYPERPLASIAS, AND BENIGN ADNEXAL NEOPLASMS

Kaku, Y., Fukumoto, T., and Kimura, T. (2015) Spiradenocarcinoma in preexisting spiradenoma with a large in situ adenocarcinoma component. *Am J Dermatopathol* **37**(10): e122–5.

Sellheyer, K. (2015) Spiradenoma and cylindroma originate from the hair follicle bulge and not from the eccrine sweat gland: an immunohistochemical study with CD200 and other stem cell markers. *J Cutan Pathol* **42**(2): 90–101.

Cylindroma (Turban Tumor)

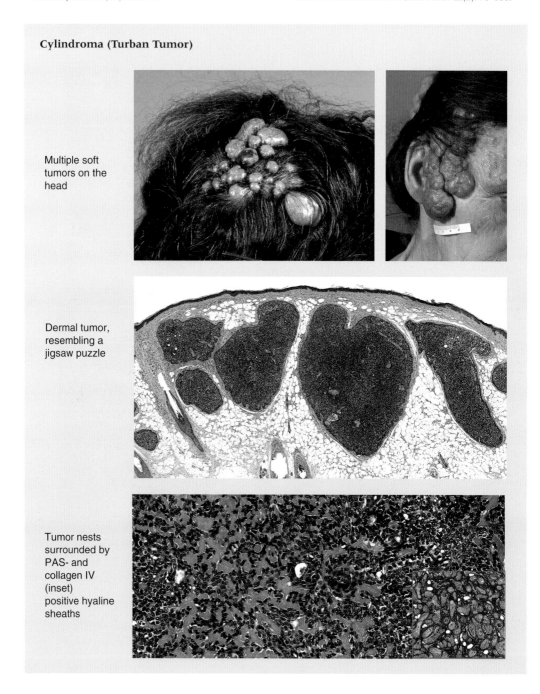

Multiple soft tumors on the head

Dermal tumor, resembling a jigsaw puzzle

Tumor nests surrounded by PAS- and collagen IV (inset) positive hyaline sheaths

Cl: This autosomal inherited tumor occurs in childhood and usually presents as multiple, slowly growing, hairless soft nodules preferentially on the scalp. Morphological relationship to eccrine spiradenoma and trichoepithelioma. There is some evidence that cylindroma and spiradenoma may originate from the follicular bulge rather than from eccrine sweat glands.

NEVI, HYPERPLASIAS, AND BENIGN ADNEXAL NEOPLASMS

Hi:

- Multiple islands of tumor cells arranged in a dense, jigsaw puzzle-like pattern
- Tumor nests are surrounded by PAS-positive hyaline sheaths
- The predominant tumor cell shows a roundish basaloid morphology with a small vesicular nucleus
- Tiny tubular structures may be present
- Malignant variants exist

References

Donner, L.R. (2012) Well-differentiated malignant cylindroma. *Am J Dermatopathol* **34**(6): 677.

Sellheyer, K. (2015) Spiradenoma and cylindroma originate from the hair follicle bulge and not from the eccrine sweat gland: an immunohistochemical study with CD200 and other stem cell markers. *J Cutan Pathol* **42**(2): 90 101.

Anogenital Mammary-Like Gland

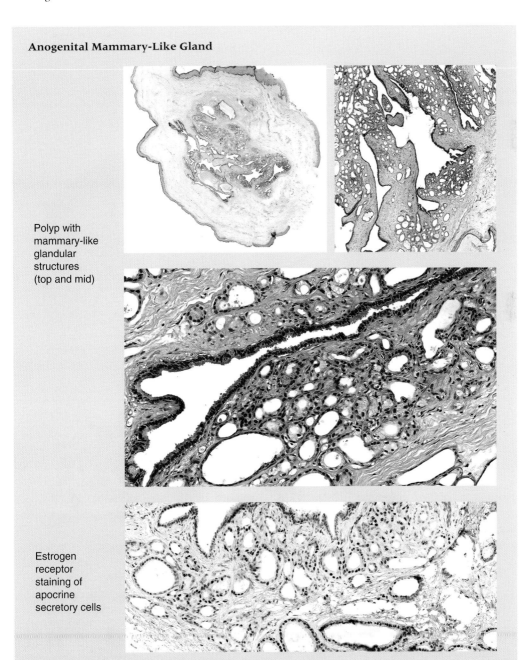

Polyp with mammary-like glandular structures (top and mid)

Estrogen receptor staining of apocrine secretory cells

NEVI, HYPERPLASIAS, AND BENIGN ADNEXAL NEOPLASMS

Cl: Polypous lesion in the anogenital area, originating from apocrine glands. Tumor evolution into extramammary Paget's disease may occur.

Hi: Aggregates of ectopic mammary gland structures in the dermis, surrounded by a fibrous stromal reaction.

References

Charfi, S., Sevestre, H., Dumont, F., Regimbeau, J.M., and Chatelain, D. (2009) Atypical apocrine proliferation involving anogenital mammary-like glands of the perianal region. *J Cutan Pathol* **36**(Suppl 1): 52–5.

Kazakov, D.V., Bisceglia, M., Sima, R., and Michal, M. (2006) Adenosis tumor of anogenital mammary-like glands: a case report and demonstration of clonality by HUMARA assay. *J Cutan Pathol* **33**(1): 43–6.

Kazakov, D.V., Hugel, H., Vanecek, T., and Michal, M. (2006) Unusual hyperplasia of anogenital mammary-like glands. *Am J Dermatopathol* **28**(2): 134–7.

Konstantinova, A.M., Kyrpychova, L., Belousova, I.E., et al. (2017) Anogenital mammary-like glands: a study of their normal histology with emphasis on glandular depth, presence of columnar epithelial cells, and distribution of elastic fibers. *Am J Dermatopathol* **39**(9): 663–667.

Konstantinova, A.M., Stewart, C.J., Kyrpychova, L., Belousova, I.E., Michal, M., and Kazakov, D.V. (2017) An immunohistochemical study of anogenital mammary-like glands. *Am J Dermatopathol* **39**(8): 599–605.

Hidradenoma Papilliferum (Apocrine Papillary Cystadenoma)

Cystic lesion with intraluminar papillary projections (papillae and pseudo-papillae)

Decapitation secretion

Fibrovascular stroma

NEVI, HYPERPLASIAS, AND BENIGN ADNEXAL NEOPLASMS

Cl: Typically located in the genital region (labia) of young women; rarely in other locations (chest).

Hi:
- Cystic lesion with sharp circumscription and anastomosing lacunae and cystic spaces
- No connection with the overlying epidermis
- Focal epithelial intraluminal papillae
- Double layer of cuboidal epithelial cells with apocrine secretion (inner layer) and myoepithelial immunophenotype (outer layer)
- Decapitation secretion throughout the entire tumor

DD: Syringocystadenoma papilliferum; anogenital mammary-like glands.

References

Elbendary, A., Cochran, E., Xie, Q., et al. (2016) Hidradenoma papilliferum with oncocytic metaplasia: a histopathological and immunohistochemical study. *Am J Dermatopathol* **38**(6): 444–7.

El-Khoury, J., Renald, M.H., Plantier, F., Avril, M.F., and Moyal-Barracco, M. (2016) Vulvar hidradenoma papilliferum (HP) is located on the sites of mammary-like anogenital glands (MLAGs): analysis of the photographs of 52 tumors. *J Am Acad Dermatol* **75**(2): 380–4.

Fernandez-Acenero, M.J., Sanchez, T.A., Sanchez, M.C., and Requena, L. (2003) Ectopic hidradenoma papilliferum: a case report and literature review. *Am J Dermatopathol* **25**(2): 176–8.

Kazakov, D.V., Mikyskova, I., Kutzner, H., et al. (2005) Hidradenoma papilliferum with oxyphilic metaplasia: a clinicopathological study of 18 cases, including detection of human papillomavirus. *Am J Dermatopathol* **27**(2): 102–10.

Konstantinova, A.M., Michal, M., Kacerovska, D., et al. (2016) Hidradenoma papilliferum: a clinicopathologic study of 264 tumors from 261 patients, with emphasis on mammary-type alterations. *Am J Dermatopathol* **38**(8): 598–607.

Nishie, W., Sawamura, D., Mayuzumi, M., Takahashi, S., and Shimizu, H. (2004) Hidradenoma papilliferum with mixed histopathologic features of syringocystadenoma papilliferum and anogenital mammary-like glands. *J Cutan Pathol* **31**(8): 561–4.

Parks, A., Branch, K.D., Metcalf, J., Underwood, P., and Young, J. (2012) Hidradenoma papilliferum with mixed histopathologic features of syringocystadenoma papilliferum and anogenital mammary-like glands: report of a case and review of the literature. *Am J Dermatopathol* **34**(1): 104–9.

Tanaka, M., and Shimizu, S. (2003) Hidradenoma papilliferum occurring on the chest of a man. *J Am Acad Dermatol* **48**(2 Suppl): S20–1.

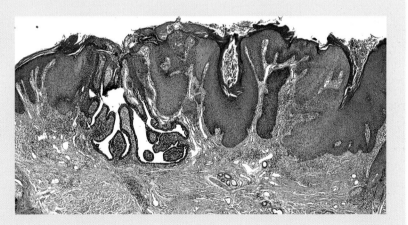

Syringocystadenoma Papilliferum

Acanthosis, papillomatosis and hyperkeratosis

NEVI, HYPERPLASIAS, AND BENIGN ADNEXAL NEOPLASMS

Syringocystadenoma Papilliferum

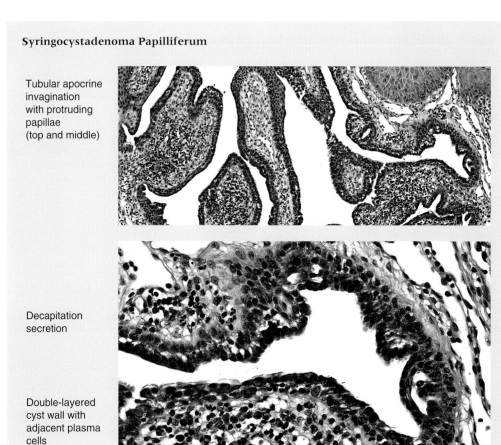

Tubular apocrine invagination with protruding papillae (top and middle)

Decapitation secretion

Double-layered cyst wall with adjacent plasma cells

Cl: Verrucous papules on the face or head, often developing in sebaceous nevus of the scalp but also as sporadic lesions in a linear or plaque-like configuration. Crust formation due to secretion through draining fistulae.

Hi:

- Verrucous hyperkeratotic surface
- Finger-like double-layered tubules and ducts evolving from the surface epidermis and protruding into the deep dermis
- Small papillary projections protruding into the ductal lumina
- Connection with surface epithelium sometimes through dilated ostiofollicular spaces (seen in serial sections)
- Ducts and cystic spaces lined by double layer of apocrine epithelia with outer layer of myoepithelia
- Stromal reaction with inflammatory infiltrate containing many plasma cells

DD: Hidradenoma papilliferum; syringocystadenocarcinoma papilliferum, which shows an identical pattern to the benign variant but with additional marked pleomorphism and high mitotic activity of epithelial tumor cells.

References

Ansai, S.I., Anan, T., Fukumoto, T., and Saeki, H. (2017) Tubulopapillary cystic adenoma with apocrine differentiation: a unifying concept for syringocystadenoma papilliferum, apocrine gland cyst, and tubular papillary adenoma. *Am J Dermatopathol* **39**(11): 829–37.

Boni, R., Xin, H., Hohl, D., Panizzon, R., and Burg, G. (2001).Syringocystadenoma papilliferum: a study of potential tumor suppressor genes. *Am J Dermatopathol* **23**(2): 87–9.

Ghazeeri, G., and Abbas, O. (2014) Syringocystadenoma papilliferum developing over hyperkeratosis of the nipple in a pregnant woman. *J Am Acad Dermatol* **70**(4): e84–5.

MALIGNANT NEOPLASMS

Hsu, P.J., Liu, C.H., and Huang, C.J. (2003) Mixed tubu-lopapillary hidradenoma and syringocystadenoma papilliferum occurring as a verrucous tumor. *J Cutan Pathol* **30**(3): 206–10.

Kasashima, S., Kawashima, A., and Fujii, T. (2016) Syringocystadenoma papilliferum of the male nipple. *J Cutan Pathol* **43**(8): 679–83.

Kazakov, D. V., Bisceglia, M., Calonje, E., et al. (2007) Tubular adenoma and syringocystadenoma papilliferum: a reappraisal of their relationship. An interobserver study of a series, by a panel of dermatopathologists. *Am J Dermatopathol* **29**(3): 256–63.

Nishie, W., Sawamura, D., Mayuzumi, M., Takahashi, S., and Shimizu, H. (2004) Hidradenoma papilliferum with mixed histopathologic features of syringocystadenoma papilliferum and anogenital mammary-like glands. *J Cutan Pathol* **31**(8): 561–4.

Patterson, J.W., Straka, B.F., and Wick, M.R. (2001) Linear syringocystadenoma papilliferum of the thigh. *J Am Acad Dermatol* **45**(1): 139–41.

Singh, U.R. (2000) Syringocystadenoma papilliferum mimicking breast carcinoma. *Am J Dermatopathol* **22**(1): 91.

Xu, X.L., Zhang, G.Y., Zeng, X.S., Wang, Q., and Sun, J.F. (2010) A case of zonal syringocystadenoma papilliferum of the axilla mimicking verruca vulgaris. *Am J Dermatopathol* **32**(1): 49–51.

Malignant Adnexal Neoplasms
Eccrine Differentiation

Microcystic Adnexal Carcinoma (Syringomatous Carcinoma, Sclerosing Sweat Ductal Carcinoma)

Scarring lesion on the lower lip (left)

Deep reaching dermal infiltrate (right)

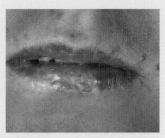
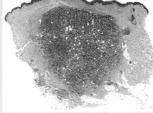

Epithelial strands, cysts and follicular structures amidst desmoplastic stroma

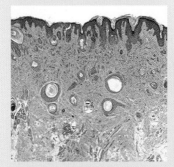
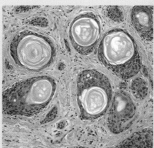

Tumor strands embedded in sclerosing stroma (left)

AE1/AE3 positive tumor cells (right)

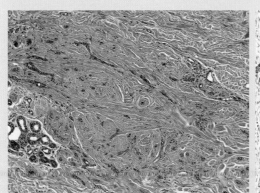
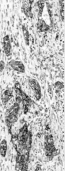

MALIGNANT NEOPLASMS

Cl: Small nodule or plaque, presenting usually on the face (chin, lip, cheek). Locally slowly growing but aggressive with deep invasion.

Hi: Predominant hallmarks: sclerotic collagenous stroma, microcysts, and pale elongated tumor strands. Biphasic differentiation (eccrine and follicular), allowing them in many cases to be distinguished from desmoplastic trichoepithelioma and from syringoma.

- Invasive, poorly circumscribed tumor with nests and strands of epithelial cells in the dermis
- Often with characteristic subepidermal tumor-free grenz zone
- Prominent subepidermal follicular microcysts
- Deeper parts with elongated slender strands of pale basaloid tumor cells
- Little cytological atypia, no mitoses, little proliferative activity (Ki67)
- Perineural involvement is common
- Immunophenotype: BerEP4 may be focally positive
- Pale cell variants may occur

DD: Morpheaform basal cell carcinoma; desmoplastic trichoepithelioma.

References

Cooper, P.H., Mills, S.E., Leonard, D.D., et al. (1985) Sclerosing sweat duct (syringomatous) carcinoma. *Am J Surg Pathol* **9**(6): 422–33.

Jedrych, J. and McNiff, J.M. (2013) Expression of p75 neurotrophin receptor in desmoplastic trichoepithelioma, infiltrative basal cell carcinoma, and microcystic adnexal carcinoma. *Am J Dermatopathol* **35**(3): 308–15.

Lai, J.H., Limacher, J.J., and Richards, R.N. (2014) Solid carcinoma revisited: a possible variant of microcystic adnexal carcinoma. *Am J Dermatopathol* **36**(11): 925–7.

McCalmont, T.H. and Ye, J. (2011) Eosinophils as a clue to the diagnosis of microcystic adnexal carcinoma. *J Cutan Pathol* **38**(11): 849, 850–2.

Sellheyer, K., Nelson, P., Kutzner, H., and Patel, R.M. (2013) The immunohistochemical differential diagnosis of microcystic adnexal carcinoma, desmoplastic trichoepithelioma and morpheaform basal cell carcinoma using BerEP4 and stem cell markers. *J Cutan Pathol* **40**(4): 363–70.

Tse, J.Y., Nguyen, A.T., Le, L.P., and Hoang, M.P. (2013) Microcystic adnexal carcinoma versus desmoplastic trichoepithelioma: a comparative study. *Am J Dermatopathol* **35**(1): 50–5.

Verdier-Sevrain, S., Thomine, E., Lauret, P., and Hemet, J. (1995) [Syringomatous carcinoma a propos of three cases with a review of the literature]. *Ann Pathol* **15**(4): 280–4.

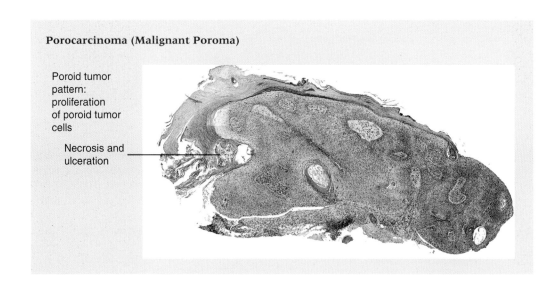

Porocarcinoma (Malignant Poroma)

Poroid tumor pattern: proliferation of poroid tumor cells

Necrosis and ulceration

MALIGNANT NEOPLASMS

Porocarcinoma (Malignant Poroma)

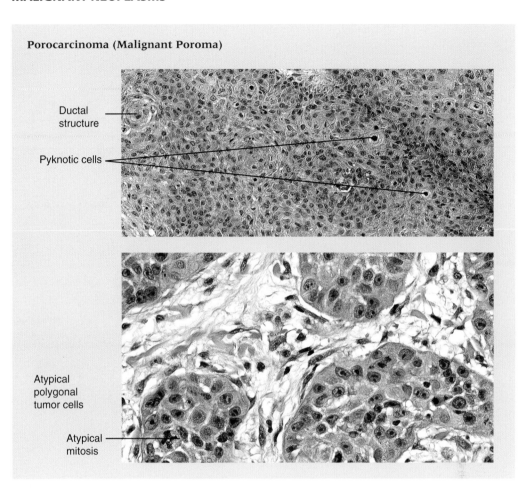

Ductal structure

Pyknotic cells

Atypical polygonal tumor cells

Atypical mitosis

Cl: Ulcerated tumor, preferentially localized on the legs of elderly individuals. Tendency to local epidermotropic and lymph node metastases. Poor prognosis. May evolve from a pre-existing poroma.

Hi:

- Invasive poroid tumor with marked pleomorphism and sharp lateral dermarcation towards regular epidermis

- Often multicentric with closely grouped tumor strands evolving from epidermis
- Poroid proliferation of pleomorphic tumor cells
- Marked cellular atypia with hyperchromatic nuclei similar to Bowen carcinoma
- Multiple mitoses
- Ductal differentiation and features of eccrine poroma may be lacking

Eccrine (Mucinous) Carcinoma

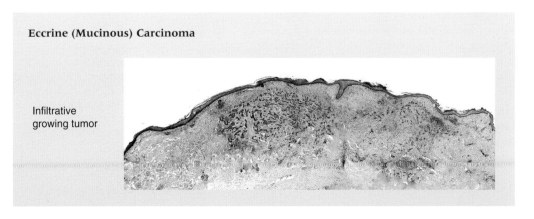

Infiltrative growing tumor

MALIGNANT NEOPLASMS

Eccrine (Mucinous) Carcinoma

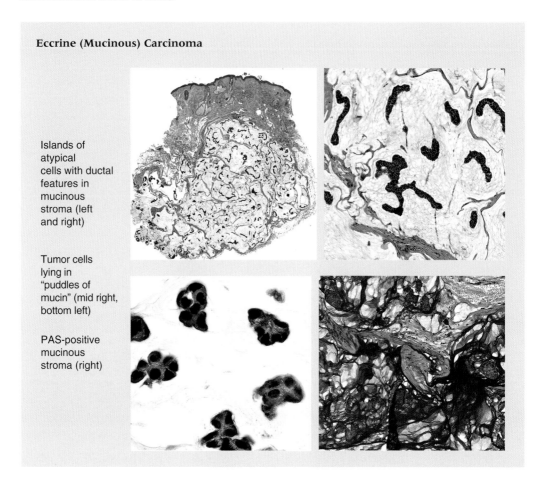

Islands of atypical cells with ductal features in mucinous stroma (left and right)

Tumor cells lying in "puddles of mucin" (mid right, bottom left)

PAS-positive mucinous stroma (right)

Cl: Skin-colored or red nodule, preferentially in the head and neck region. Some of the cases may represent cutaneous metastases of internal carcinoma (breast, gastrointestinal).

Hi:
- Both infiltrative and nodular tumor with ill-defined margins
- Irregular nests and anastomosing slender strands of atypical basaloid tumor cells with hyperchromatic nuclei
- Large amounts of mucin representing most of the tumor stroma
- Basaloid epithelial tumor strands and nests lying in "puddles of mucin"
- Moderate mitotic activity

DD: Metastasis from mucinous carcinoma of the breast or gastrointestinal tract; mucin-rich cystic basal cell carcinoma; endocrine mucin-producing tumor.

References

Abdulkader, M., Kuhar, M., Hattab, E., and Linos, K. (2016) GATA3 positivity in endocrine mucin-producing sweat gland carcinoma and invasive mucinous carcinoma of the eyelid: report of 2 cases. *Am J Dermatopathol* **38**(10): 789–91.

Caputo, V., Colombi, R., Ribotta, M., and Rongioletti, F. (2011) Cutaneous squamous cell carcinoma with mucinous metaplasia on the sole associated with high-risk human papillomavirus type 18. *Am J Dermatopathol* **33**(3): 317–22.

Levy, G., Finkelstein, A., and McNiff, J.M. (2010) Immunohistochemical techniques to compare primary vs. metastatic mucinous carcinoma of the skin. *J Cutan Pathol* **37**(4): 411–15.

Matin, R.N., Gibbon, K., Rizvi, H., Harwood, C.A., and Cerio, R. (2011) Cutaneous mucinous carcinoma arising in extramammary Paget disease of the perineum. *Am J Dermatopathol* **33**(7): 705–9.

MALIGNANT NEOPLASMS

Apocrine Differentiation

Apocrine (Hidr-)Adenocarcinoma (Mucinous)

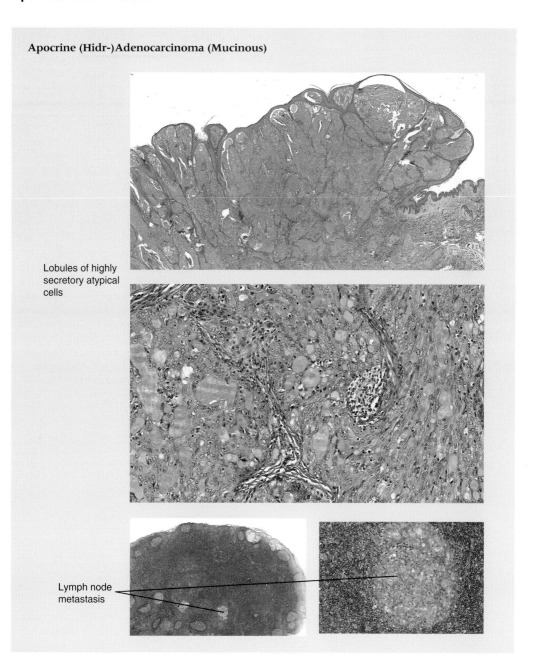

Lobules of highly secretory atypical cells

Lymph node metastasis

Cl: Nodule, sometimes ulcerated, preferentially in the head and neck area or the extremities. Frequent metastases in the regional lymph nodes.

Hi: Malignant counterpart of solid hidradenoma.

- Multilobulated acrospiroma-like tumor with clonal pleomorphism and high mitotic activity, which may be restricted to clonal parts of the tumor
- Focal hyperchromasia in conjunction with pleomorphism and many mitoses are leading features
- Infiltrative growth pattern in advanced lesions
- Focal necroses in advanced lesions

HYPERPLASIAS AND HAMARTOMAS

References

Honda, Y., Tanigawa, H., Harada, M., et al. (2013) Hidradenocarcinoma showing prominent mucinous and squamous differentiation and associated pagetoid cells. *J Cutan Pathol* **40**(5): 503–8.

Kazakov, D.V., Ivan, D., Kutzner, H., et al. (2009) Cutaneous hidradenocarcinoma: a clinicopathological, immunohistochemical, and molecular biologic study of 14 cases, including Her2/neu gene expression/ amplification, TP53 gene mutation analysis, and t(11;19) translocation. *Am J Dermatopathol* **31**(3): 236–47.

Ko, C.J., Cochran, A.J., Eng, W., and Binder, S.W. (2006) Hidradenocarcinoma: a histological and immunohistochemical study. *J Cutan Pathol* **33**(11): 726–30.

Nash, J.W., Barrett, T.L., Kies, M., et al. (2007).Metastatic hidradenocarcinoma with demonstration of Her-2/ neu gene amplification by fluorescence in situ hybridization: potential treatment implications. *J Cutan Pathol* **34**(1): 49–54.

Sebaceous Differentiation

Epithelial tumors with sebaceous differentiation usually present with lobules of mature sebocytes, in particular in the sebaceomas which comprise the entities formerly known as sebaceous epithelioma and sebaceous adenoma. However, there is a vast array of other epithelial tumors, such as basal cell carcinoma, that may show discrete signs of sebaceous differentiation that may easily be overlooked. As a rule of thumb, a single epithelial cell with intracytoplasmic adipophilin-positive vacuoles may be taken as an indicator of sebaceous differentiation in a benign or malignant epithelial tumor. Usually, there are small clusters of adipophilin-positive tumor cells which allow straightforward differentiation from necrotic carcinoma cells that may also show sebaceous and fatty deposits within the cytoplasm. Immunohistochemical staining for adipophilin in the context of an epithelial tumor has evolved as the method of choice for defining sebaceous differentiation.

References

Boussahmain, C., Mochel, M.C., and Hoang, M.P. (2013) Perilipin and adipophilin expression in sebaceous carcinoma and mimics. *Hum Pathol* **44**(9): 1811–16.

Ostler, D.A., Prieto, V.G., Reed, J.A., Deavers, M.T., Lazar, A.J., and Ivan, D. (2010).Adipophilin expression in sebaceous tumors and other cutaneous lesions with clear cell histology: an immunohistochemical study of 117 cases. *Mod Pathol* **23**(4): 567–73.

Tetzlaff, M.T. (2018) Immunohistochemical markers informing the diagnosis of sebaceous carcinoma and its distinction from its mimics: adipophilin and Factor XIIIa to the rescue? *J Cutan Pathol* **45**(1): 29–32.

HYPERPLASIAS AND HAMARTOMAS

Hyperplasias and Hamartomas

Ectopic (Heterotopic) Sebaceous Glands (Fordyce Glands)

Fordyce glands on the lip (left) and on the penile sulcus coronarius (right)

Fordyce glands (lip)

Montgomery glands of the areola mammae

Hyperplastic penile ectopic sebaceous glands

HYPERPLASIAS AND HAMARTOMAS

Various localisations: lip (Fordyce's spot); Montgomery glands of the areola mammae; ectopic glands on the penile sulcus coronarius.

Cl: Small, 2–3 mm yellow papules on the buccal mucosa of the lips and on the external mucosa of the genitalia. They are present in most individuals and do not have any nosological impact.

Hi: Transitional or mucosal epithelium showing normal sebaceous glands or hyperplasia of sebaceous glands. There are no associated hair follicles ("isolated sebaceous glands").

References

Moosbrugger, E.A. and Adams, B.B. (2011) Disseminated eruption of ectopic sebaceous glands following Stevens-Johnson syndrome. *J Am Acad Dermatol* **65**(2): 446–8.

Tschen, J.A., Schulze, K.E., and Chiao, N. (2006) Ectopic sebaceous gland: a developmental anomaly. *J Cutan Pathol* **33**(7): 519–21.

(Senile) Sebaceous Gland Hyperplasia

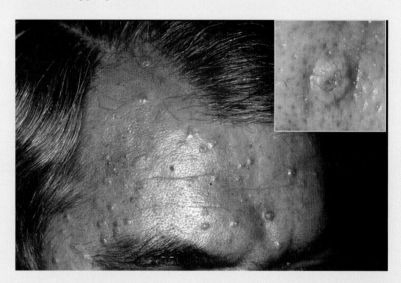

Yellow papules with central dell (inset)

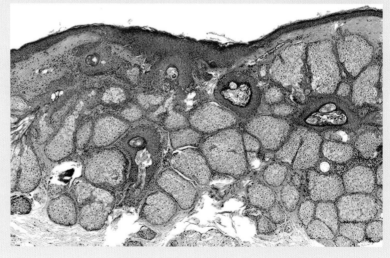

Hyperplastic sebaceous glands connected with the epidermis through a single follicular duct

HYPERPLASIAS AND HAMARTOMAS

Cl: Multiple disseminated yellow or skin-colored papules with central dent, preferentially on the forehead or cheeks of elderly men. No malignant potential.

Hi:

- Aggregates of hyperplastic sebaceous glands
- Single follicular sebaceous duct leading to the surface
- Mature sebaceous epithelia
- Holocrine secretion

DD: Verrucae planae; molluscum contagiosum.

References

De Villez, R.L. and Roberts, L.C. (1982) Premature sebaceous gland hyperplasia. *J Am Acad Dermatol* **6**(5): 933–5.

Kudoh, K., Hosokawa, M., Miyazawa, T., and Tagami, H. (1988) Giant solitary sebaceous gland hyperplasia clinically simulating epidermoid cyst. *J Cutan Pathol* **15**(6): 396 8.

Vergara, G., Belinchon, I., Silvestre, J.F., Albares, M.P., and Pascual, J.C. (2003) Linear sebaceous gland hyperplasia of the penis: a case report. *J Am Acad Dermatol* **48**(1): 149–50.

Nevus Sebaceous (Jadassohn)

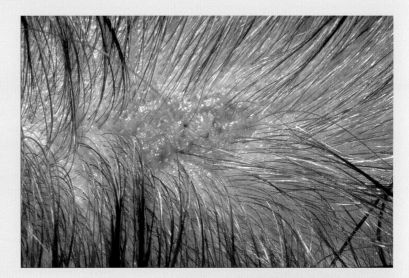

Yellow plaque with papillomatous surface

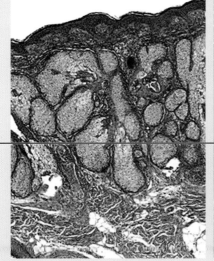
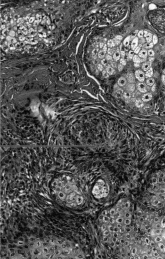

Multiple hyperplastic sebaceous glands. Lack of hair follicles (left)

Rudimentary papilla; trichoepithelial structure

BENIGN NEOPLASMS

Cl: Hairless yellowish plaque with papillomatous surface, preferentially on the scalp, present since birth. Ductal, sebaceous, and hair follicle tumors may arise in sebaceous nevi.

Hi: Clusters of sebaceous glands but no mature hair follicles. Basaloid and follicular induction may occur. The surface can be papillomatous and acanthotic and resemble a seborrheic keratosis. There may be strong similarity with superficial basal cell carcinoma and morphological overlap with trichoblastoma. Genuine trichoblastoma – usually larger and hyperpigmented – and trichoblastoma-like hamartomatous tumors may be inherent parts of nevus sebaceous. Trichilemmoma and tubular apocrine adenomas of smaller size are other autochthonous tissue components of large nevus sebaceous.

DD: Verrucous epidermal nevus.

References

Cribier, B., Scrivener, Y., and Grosshans, E. (2000) Tumors arising in nevus sebaceus: a study of 596 cases. *J Am Acad Dermatol* **42**(2 Pt 1): 263–8.

Dore, E., Noe, M.H., and Swick, B.L. (2015) Trichoblastoma, syringocystadenoma papilliferum, desmoplastic trichilemmoma and tumor of the follicular infundibulum with signet-ring cells, all arising in nevus sebaceus. *J Cutan Pathol* **42**(9): 645–51.

Idriss, M.H. and Elston, D.M. (2014) Secondary neoplasms associated with nevus sebaceus of Jadassohn: a study of 707 cases. *J Am Acad Dermatol* **70**(2): 332–7.

Kaddu, S., Schaeppi, H., Kerl, H., and Soyer, H.P. (2000) Basaloid neoplasms in nevus sebaceus. *J Cutan Pathol* **27**(7): 327–37.

Sellheyer, K., Cribier, B., Nelson, P., Kutzner, H., and Rutten, A. (2013) Basaloid tumors in nevus sebaceus revisited: the follicular stem cell marker PHLDA1 (TDAG51) indicates that most are basal cell carcinomas and not trichoblastomas. *J Cutan Pathol* **40**(5): 455–62.

Variant: Pilo-Sebaceous Hamartoma

Cl: Variant of nevus sebaceous showing a conglomerate of sebaceous and pilar components. Hair follicles are present.

Hi:
- Intradermally located tumor
- Centrally located mesenchymal part: fat, blood vessels, fibrous tissue
- Malformed follicles with prominent sebaceous glands in the periphery

Reference

Raghu, P., Tran, T.A., Rady, P., Tyring, S., and Carlson, J.A. (2012) Ileostomy-associated chronic papillomatous dermatitis showing nevus sebaceous-like hyperplasia, HPV 16 infection, and lymphedema: a case report and literature review of ostomy-associated reactive epidermal hyperplasias. *Am J Dermatopathol* **34**(7): e97–102.

Benign Neoplasms
Sebaceous Adenoma

This term should not be confused with adenoma sebaceum, which is angiofibroma in tuberous sclerosis. Recently, benign sebaceous tumors have been subsumed under the umbrella term *sebaceoma* that comprises sebaceous adenoma (pale sebaceous tumor with predominance of mature sebocytes) and sebaceous epithelioma (dark sebaceous tumor with predominance of basophilic germinative sebocytes).

Cl: Yellowish, occasionally eroded and crusted papule or nodule preferentially on the periorbital area of the face or on the scalp of adult patients, but also in other localisations. Association with Muir–Torre syndrome possible.

Hi:
- Nodule composed of enlarged sebaceous glands
- Sebaceous-ductal connection with the epidermis
- Arrangement around a central follicle
- Sebaceous maturation with foamy holocrine sebocytes in the center
- Basaloid germinative sebocytes in the periphery

DD: Basal cell carcinoma; sebaceous hyperplasia; mixed sebaceous tumor (tubular adenoma of the skin with follicular and sebaceous differentiation) has been reported.

References

Azevedo, R.S., Almeida, O.P., Netto, J.N., et al. (2009) Comparative clinicopathological study of intraoral sebaceous hyperplasia and sebaceous adenoma. *Oral Surg Oral Med Oral Pathol Oral Radiol Endod* **107**(1): 100–4.

Kazakov, D.V., Mukensnabl, P., and Michal, M. (2006) Tubular adenoma of the skin with follicular and sebaceous differentiation: a report of two cases. *Am J Dermatopathol* **28**(2): 142–6.

Marques-da-Costa, J., Campos-do-Carmo, G., Ormiga, P., Ishida, C., Cuzzi, T., and Ramos-e-Silva, M. (2015)

BENIGN NEOPLASMS

Sebaceous adenoma: clinics, dermatoscopy, and histopathology. *Int J Dermatol* **54**(6): e200–202.

Somashekara, K.G., Lakshmi, S., and Priya, N.S. (2011) A rare case of sebaceous adenoma of the palate, with literature review. *J Laryngol Otol* **125**(7): 750–2.

Takayama, K., Usui, Y., Ito, M., Goto, H., and Takeuchi, M. (2013) A case of sebaceous adenoma of the eyelid showing excessively rapid growth. *Clin Ophthalmol* **7**: 667–70.

Terrell, S., Wetter, R., Fraga, G., Kestenbaum, T., and Aires, D.J. (2007) Penile sebaceous adenoma. *J Am Acad Dermatol* **57**(2 Suppl): S42–3.

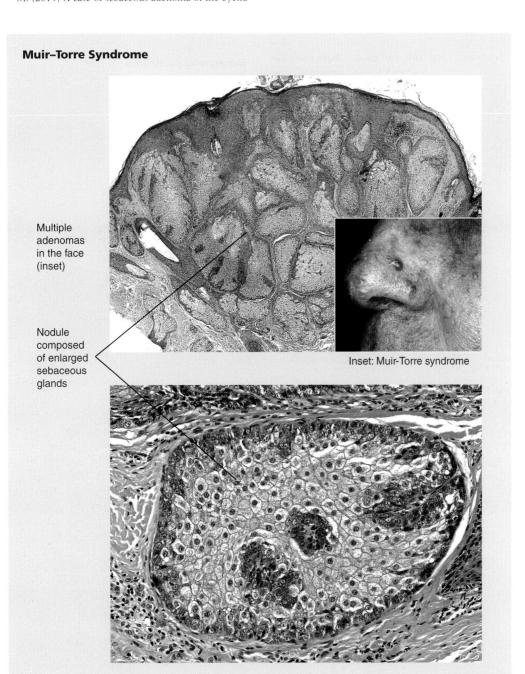

Muir–Torre Syndrome

Multiple adenomas in the face (inset)

Nodule composed of enlarged sebaceous glands

Inset: Muir-Torre syndrome

BENIGN NEOPLASMS

Cl: Germline mutation, leading to association of multiple sebaceous tumors (sebaceous hyperplasias, sebaceous adenomas, and carcinomas) and/or extrafacial (mostly trunk) keratoacanthomas with visceral carcinomas (mostly colon).

Hi: In most cases, histopathological changes correspond to banal sebaceous hyperplasias, sebaceous adenomas or straightforward sebaceous carcinomas. A specific Muir–Torre-associated "landmark tumor" is cystic sebaceous tumor (former classification: cystic sebaceous adenoma or adenocarcinoma). Cystic sebaceous tumor is large, nodular, proliferates like an epidermal cyst, and shows large

masses of mature adipocytes within its cyst wall and in the cyst cavity, which may be totally obstructed. There is a sharp and smooth outer border with germinative sebocytes.

Comment: Immunohistochemical testing for expression of DNA mismatch repair proteins in sebaceous tumors of Muir–Torre patients and suspected patients is paramount: in Muir–Torre-associated sebaceous lesions, at least one set of the DNA mismatch repair proteins MSH2/MSH6 and MLH1/PMS2 is not expressed. These findings should be corroborated by additional molecular test for microsatellite instability.

Sebaceous Epithelioma (Sebaceoma)

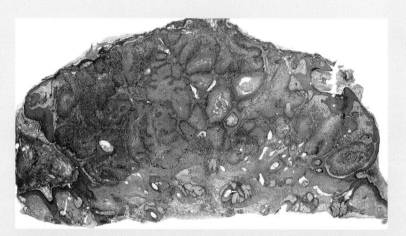

Nodule composed of enlarged sebaceous glands

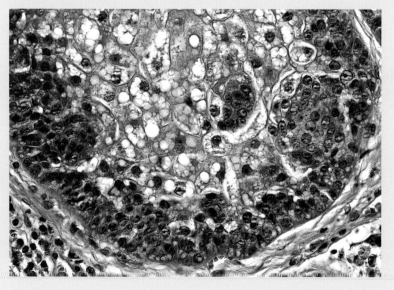

Foamy sebaceous cells in the center, surrounded by basaloid germinative cells in the periphery

BENIGN NEOPLASMS

Sebaceous Epithelioma (Sebaceoma)

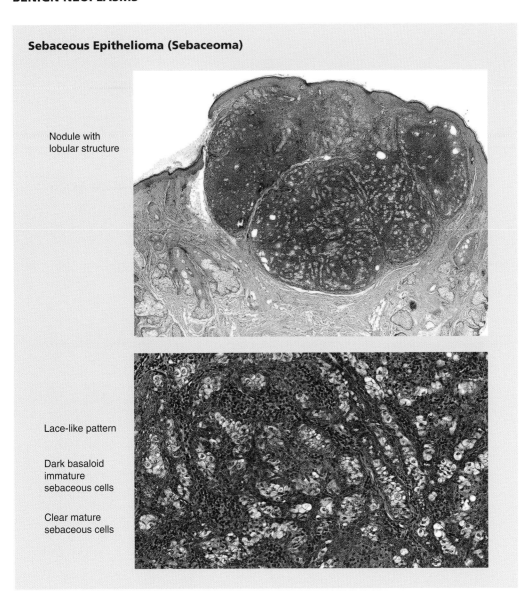

Nodule with lobular structure

Lace-like pattern

Dark basaloid immature sebaceous cells

Clear mature sebaceous cells

Cl: Slowly growing papule or nodule with preferential localisation in the head and neck area, clinically simulating basal cell epithelioma or other epithelial tumors.

Hi:
- Basal cell carcinoma-like basaloid epithelial tumor with focal sebaceous differentiation (germinative sebocytes)
- Rippled pattern of basaloid germinative sebocytes showing EMA-positivity and little or no intracytoplasmic adipophilin-positive fatty deposits.
- Focal, mostly peripheral, sebaceous differentiation (germinative sebocytes)

- BerEP4 negative in contrast to basal cell carcinoma
- Adipophilin expression within germinative sebocytes

Immunohistochemistry: Adipophilin serves as a useful marker of sebaceous differentiation in various epithelial tumors.

References

Chuang, H.C., Kao, P.H., Huang, Y.L., Lee, L.Y., and Kuo, T.T. (2014) Desmoplastic sebaceoma arising from nevus sebaceus: a new variant. *J Cutan Pathol* **41**(6): 509–12.

MALIGNANT NEOPLASMS

Fan, Y.S., Carr, R.A., Sanders, D.S., Smith, A.P., Lazar, A.J., and Calonje, E. (2007) Characteristic Ber-EP4 and EMA expression in sebaceoma is immunohistochemically distinct from basal cell carcinoma. *Histopathology* **51**(1): 80–6.

Misago, N. and Narisawa, Y. (2001) Rippled-pattern sebaceoma. *Am J Dermatopathol* **23**(5): 437–43.

Malignant Neoplasms

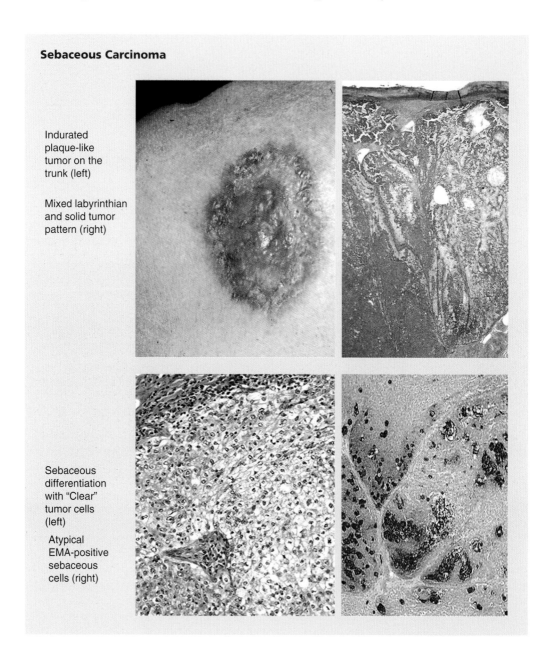

Sebaceous Carcinoma

Indurated plaque-like tumor on the trunk (left)

Mixed labyrinthian and solid tumor pattern (right)

Sebaceous differentiation with "Clear" tumor cells (left)

Atypical EMA-positive sebaceous cells (right)

NEVI, HYPERPLASIA, AND HAMARTOMAS

Cl: Aggressive tumor occurring on the eyelid and in extraocular localisations. Risk for metastases is high; mortality rate 10–20%. Predilection for Asian individuals. Ocular sebaceous carcinoma usually is considered to be more aggressive than extraocular sebaceous carcinoma.

Hi:
- Tumors showing basaloid, sebaceous, and/or squamous differentiation
- Morphological blending with classic squamous cell carcinoma pattern may occur
- Presence of atypical foamy or vacuolated atypical sebocytes in all variants of sebaceous carcinoma
- Intraepidermal pagetoid spread of clear cell-like atypical sebocytes is restricted to the ocular variant of sebaceous carcinoma; it can be mistaken for pagetoid solar keratosis or carcinoma *in situ*
- Extraocular sebaceous carcinoma shows solid, highly pleomorphic tumor pattern with high proliferative activity

Immunohistochemistry: Common denominator of all sebaceous carcinoma variants is expression of adipophilin by neoplastic sebocytes.

DD: Cutaneous PEComa*; metastatic clear cell carcinomas of visceral origin (renal cell carcinoma); clear cell variants of other tumors (melanoma, carcinoma); genuine squamous cell carcinoma with necrotic keratinocytes that may imitate immature sebocytes (adipophilin-positive necrosis).

* PEComa family comprises a group of related mesenchymal neoplasms, including angiomyolipoma, lymphangiomyomatosis, and clear cell tumor of the lung.

References

Ansai, S., Takeichi, H., Arase, S., Kawana, S., and Kimura, T. (2011) Sebaceous carcinoma: an immunohistochemical reappraisal. *Am J Dermatopathol* **33**(6): 579–87.

Candelario, N.M., Sanchez, J.E., Sanchez, J.L., Martin-Garcia, R.F., and Rochet, N.M. (2016) Extraocular sebaceous carcinoma – a clinicopathologic reassessment. *Am J Dermatopathol* **38**(11): 809–12.

Crandall, M., Satter, E.K., and Hurt, M. (2012) Extraocular sebaceous carcinoma arising in a nevus sebaceous during pregnancy. *J Am Acad Dermatol* **67**(3): e111–13.

Kazakov, D.V., Kutzner, H., Spagnolo, D.V., Rutten, A., Mukensnabl, P., and Michal, M. (2010).What is extraocular cutaneous sebaceous carcinoma in situ? *Am J Dermatopathol* **32**(8): 857–8.

Kramer, J.M. and Chen, S. (2010) Sebaceous carcinoma in situ. *Am J Dermatopathol* **32**(8): 854–5.

Kyllo, R.L., Brady, K.L., and Hurst, E.A. (2015) Sebaceous carcinoma: review of the literature. *Dermatol Surg* **41**(1): 1–15.

Plaza, J.A., Mackinnon, A., Carrillo, L., Prieto, V.G., Sangueza, M., and Suster, S. (2015) Role of immunohistochemistry in the diagnosis of sebaceous carcinoma: a clinicopathologic and immunohistochemical study. *Am J Dermatopathol* **37**(11): 809–21.

Prieto-Granada, C. and Rodriguez-Waitkus, P. (2016) Sebaceous carcinoma of the eyelid. *Cancer Control* **23**(2): 126–32.

Hair Follicle Differentiation

Nevi, Hyperplasia, and Hamartomas
Hair Follicle Nevus

Cl: Localisation: head, neck; area of hypertrichosis.
Hi: Group of normal vellus hairs.

Conical Infundibular Acanthoma (Giant Dilated Pore of Winer)

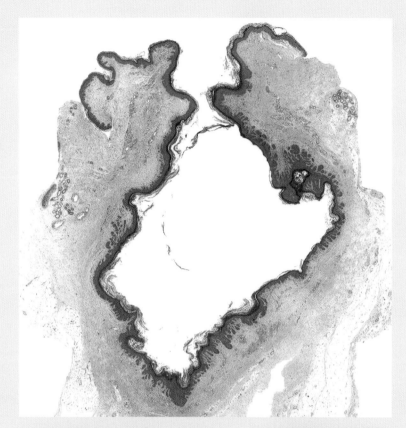

Cavity, widely
open to the skin
surface

Slight irregular
acanthosis and
papillomatosis

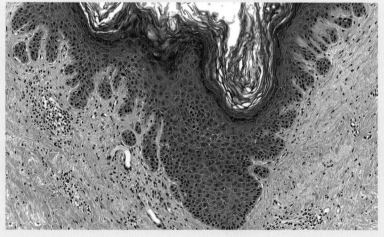

BENIGN NEOPLASMS

Cl: Conical triangular, comedo-like dilation of a follicle on the face, neck or upper part of the chest of older individuals.

Hi:

- Dilated ostiofollicular cyst
- Wide open to the skin surface
- Dilated ostium may be filled with cornified material
- Cavity wall is normal or shows irregularly acanthotic infundibular rete ridges
- Slightly papillomatous
- Small sebaceous glands or vellus hair may be included in the wall

- Melanin pigmentation

DD: Pilar sheath acanthoma; superficial follicular epithelial cyst.

References

Misago, N., Sada, A., and Narisawa, Y. (2006) Trichoblastoma with a dilated pore. *J Am Acad Dermatol* **54**(2): 357–8.

Steffen, C. (2001) Winer's dilated pore: the infundibuloma. *Am J Dermatopathol* **23**(3): 246–53.

Benign Neoplasms

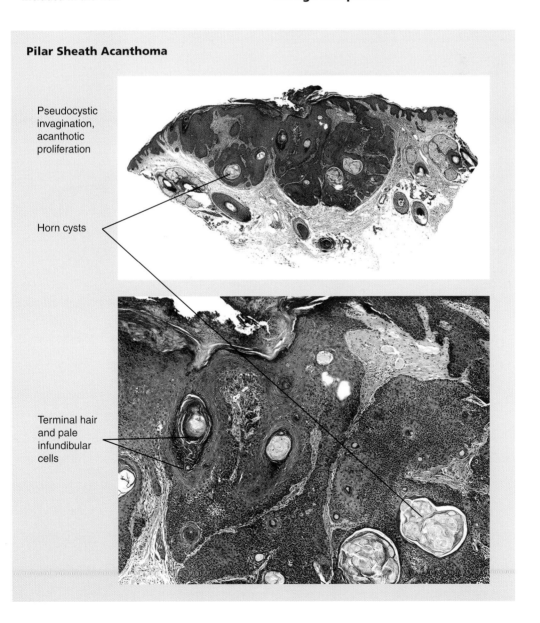

Pilar Sheath Acanthoma

Pseudocystic invagination, acanthotic proliferation

Horn cysts

Terminal hair and pale infundibular cells

BENIGN NEOPLASMS

Cl: Solitary broad-based papule or nodule, preferentially on the upper lip of older individuals. There may be a central porus-like cyst filled with keratotic material.

Hi:

- Cystic invagination of the epidermis, filled with keratotic material
- Acanthotic epithelial cyst wall with markedly enlarged rete ridges
- Epithelia showing root sheath differentiation
- No mature hair follicle present

Immunohistochemistry: Homogeneous positivity for CK17.

DD: Trichofolliculoma; conical infundibular acanthoma; dilated pore of Winer; giant comedo.

References

Bhawan, J. (1979) Pilar sheath acanthoma. A new benign follicular tumor. *J Cutan Pathol* **6**(5): 438–40.

Bruscino, N., Tripo, L., Corradini, D., Urso, C., and Palleschi, G.M. (2014) Pilar sheath acanthoma simulating basal cell carcinoma. *G Ital Dermatol Venereol* **149**(1): 155–6.

Lee, J.Y. and Hirsch, E. (1987) Pilar sheath acanthoma. *Arch Dermatol* **123**(5): 569–70.

Mehregan, A.H. and Brownstein, M.H. (1978) Pilar sheath acanthoma. *Arch Dermatol* **114**(10): 1495–7.

Smolle, J. and Kerl, H. (1983) [Pilar sheath acanthoma – a benign follicular hamartoma]. *Dermatologica* **167**(6): 335–8.

Vakilzadeh, F. (1987) [Pilar sheath acanthoma]. *Hautarzt* **38**(1): 40–2.

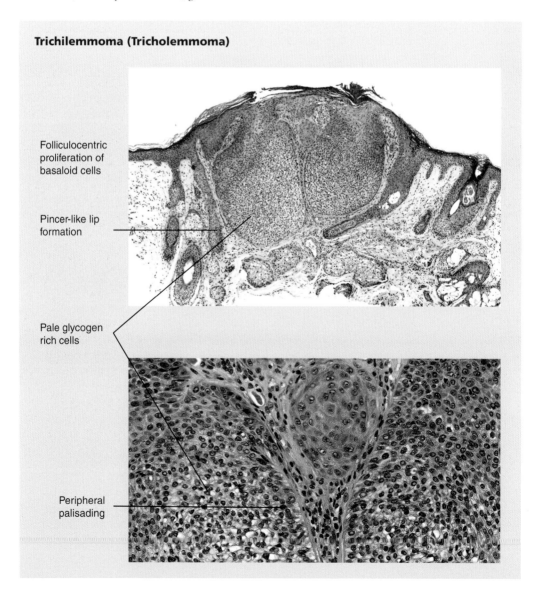

Trichilemmoma (Tricholemmoma)

Folliculocentric proliferation of basaloid cells

Pincer-like lip formation

Pale glycogen rich cells

Peripheral palisading

BENIGN NEOPLASMS

Cl: Solitary trichilemmoma presents mostly in adults as a small exophytic verrucous papule, several mm in size and located preferentially in the head and neck region. Multiple trichilemmomas are found in Cowden's disease (multifocal hamartomatous polyposis of the intestine; autosomal PTEN mutation).

Hi:

- Circumscribed folliculocentric proliferation of pale basaloid isomorphic cells with no proliferative activity
- Bilateral epidermal collarette
- Thickened basement membrane beneath the proliferation may be a good diagnostic criterion
- Tumor silhouette may simulate a superficial pale cell basal cell carcinoma
- Normal basal layer with peripheral palisading ("BCC-like")
- Negative for (BCC-marker) BerEP4
- Desmoplastic stroma in desmoplastic trichilemmoma

DD: Verruca vulgaris; inverted follicular keratosis; acrospiroma; basal cell carcinoma.

References

Cabral, E.S. and Cassarino, D.S. (2007) Desmoplastic tricholemmoma of the eyelid misdiagnosed as sebaceous carcinoma: a potential diagnostic pitfall. *J Cutan Pathol* **34**(Suppl 1): 22–5.

Dore, E., Noe, M.H., and Swick, B.L. (2015) Trichoblastoma, syringocystadenoma papilliferum, desmoplastic trichilemmoma and tumor of the follicular infundibulum with signet-ring cells, all arising in nevus sebaceus. *J Cutan Pathol* **42**(9): 645–51.

Martinez-Ciarpaglini, C. and Monteagudo, C. (2016) Pigmented desmoplastic trichilemmoma. *J Cutan Pathol* **43**(6): 535–7.

Misago, N., Toda, S., and Narisawa, Y. (2011) CD34 expression in human hair follicles and tricholemmoma: a comprehensive study. *J Cutan Pathol* **38**(8): 609–15.

Misago, N., Toda, S., and Narisawa, Y. (2012) Tricholemmoma and clear cell squamous cell carcinoma (associated with Bowen's disease): immunohistochemical profile in comparison to normal hair follicles. *Am J Dermatopathol* **34**(4): 394–9.

Navarrete-Dechent, C., Uribe, P., and Gonzalez, S. (2017) Desmoplastic trichilemmoma dermoscopically mimicking molluscum contagiosum. *J Am Acad Dermatol* **76**(2S1): S22–S24.

BENIGN NEOPLASMS

Tumor of the Follicular Infundibulum (Infundibuloma)

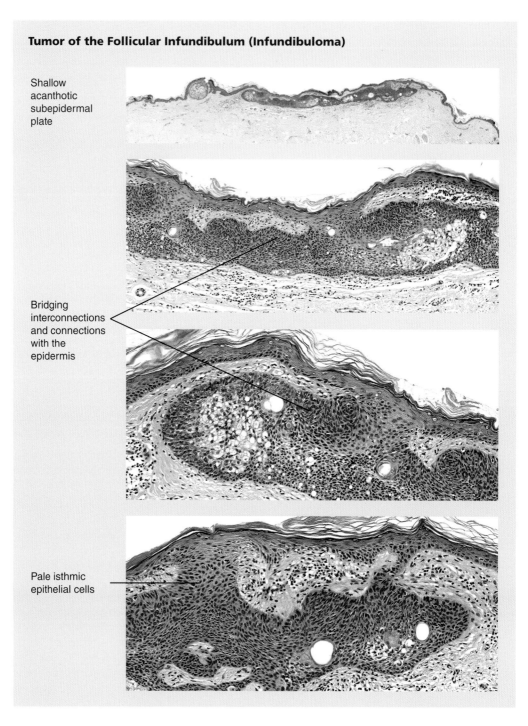

Shallow acanthotic subepidermal plate

Bridging interconnections and connections with the epidermis

Pale isthmic epithelial cells

Cl: Papule or plaque on the head or face of elderly individuals. Multiple eruptive lesions can occur in other localisations. It is considered by some to be a variant of basal cell carcinoma.

Hi:
- Interconnecting "streamer-like" pale basaloid epithelial strands in a horizontal array, restricted to the subepidermal cutis

BENIGN NEOPLASMS

- Multifocal connections to the overlaying epidermis
- Predominant pale basaloid epithelia corresponding to outer root sheath epithelia
- Various types of appendageal differentiation may be present
- Positivity for calretinin

DD: Basal cell carcinoma; trichilemmoma; flat seborrheic keratosis.

References

Abbas, O. and Mahalingam, M. (2009) Tumor of the follicular infundibulum: an epidermal reaction pattern? *Am J Dermatopathol* **31**(7): 626–33.

Baquerizo Nole, K.L., Lopez-Garcia, D.R., Teague, D.J., et al. (2015) Is tumor of follicular infundibulum a reaction to dermal scarring? *Am J Dermatopathol* **37**(7): 535–8.

Dore, E., Noe, M.H., and Swick, B.L. (2015) Trichoblastoma, syringocystadenoma papilliferum, desmoplastic trichilemmoma and tumor of the follicular infundibulum with signet-ring cells, all arising in nevus sebaceus. *J Cutan Pathol* **42**(9): 645–51.

Grosshans, E. and Hanau, D. (1981) [The infundibular adenoma: a follicular poroma with sebaceous and apocrine differentiation (author's transl)]. *Ann Dermatol Venereol* **108**(1): 59–66.

Koch, B. and Rufli, T. (1991) Tumor of follicular infundibulum. *Dermatologica* **183**(1): 68–9.

Kossard, S., Finley, A.G., Poyzer, K., and Kocsard, E. (1989) Eruptive infundibulomas. A distinctive presentation of the tumor of follicular infundibulum. *J Am Acad Dermatol* **21**(2 Pt 2): 361–6.

Mahalingam, M., Bhawan, J., Finn, R., and Stefanato, C.M. (2001) Tumor of the follicular infundibulum with sebaceous differentiation. *J Cutan Pathol* **28**(6): 314–17.

Manonukul, J., Omeapinyan, P., and Vongjirad, A. (2009) Mucoepidermoid (adenosquamous) carcinoma, trichoblastoma, trichilemmoma, sebaceous adenoma, tumor of follicular infundibulum and syringocystadenoma papilliferum arising within 2 persistent lesions of nevus sebaceous: report of a case. *Am J Dermatopathol* **31**(7): 658–63.

Mehregan, A.H. (1971) Tumor of follicular infundibulum. *Dermatologica* **142**(3): 177–83.

Steffen, C. (2001) Winer's dilated pore: the infundibuloma. *Am J Dermatopathol* **23**(3): 246–53.

Weyers, W., Horster, S., and Diaz-Cascajo, C. (2009) Tumor of follicular infundibulum is basal cell carcinoma. *Am J Dermatopathol* **31**(7): 634–41.

Trichoepithelioma (Superficial Trichoblastoma)

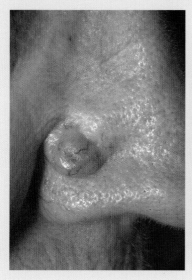
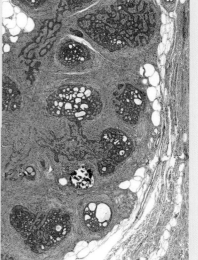

Tumor with telangiectases on the nose (left)

Strands and nests of basaloid cells (right)

Trichoepithelioma (Superficial Trichoblastoma)

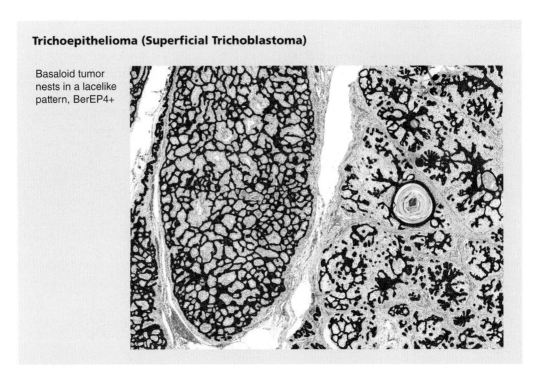

Basaloid tumor nests in a lacelike pattern, BerEP4+

Cl: Skin-colored or yellowish-red, slowly growing papule, preferentially on the face of children or young adults. Presence of multiple lesions is typically seen in Spiegler Brooke syndrome (angiofibromas of epithelioma adenoides cysticum).

Hi:

- Lobules of strands and nests of basaloid cells in lace-like or cribriform pattern
- Peripheral palisading
- Keratinous microcysts
- Focal differentiation into hair bulbs
- Stromal reaction showing eosinophilic dense collagenous tissue
- Focal differentiation of papillary mesenchymal bodies, i.e. nestin-positive conglomerates of hair papilla-like fibroblasts with adjacent basaloid epithelia, simulating an abortive hair bulb

DD: Basal cell carcinoma; trichofolliculoma; basaloid follicular hamartoma.

References

Kazakov, D.V. and Michal, M. (2006) Trichoepithelioma with giant and multinucleated neoplastic epithelial cells. *Am J Dermatopathol* **28**(1): 63–4.

Kyrpychova, L., Kacerovska, D., Michal, M., and Kazakov, D.V. (2017) Sporadic trichoblastomas and those occurring in the setting of multiple familial trichoepithelioma/Brooke-Spiegler syndrome show no BAP1 loss. *Am J Dermatopathol* **39**(10): 793–4.

Lum, C.A. and Binder, S.W. (2004) Proliferative characterization of basal-cell carcinoma and trichoepithelioma in small biopsy specimens. *J Cutan Pathol* **31**(8): 550–4.

Melly, L., Lawton, G., and Rajan, N. (2012) Basal cell carcinoma arising in association with trichoepithelioma in a case of Brooke-Spiegler syndrome with a novel genetic mutation in CYLD. *J Cutan Pathol* **39**(10): 977–8.

Pham, T.T., Selim, M.A., Burchette, J.L. Jr, Madden, J., Turner, J., and Herman, C. (2006) CD10 expression in trichoepithelioma and basal cell carcinoma. *J Cutan Pathol* **33**(2): 123–8.

Rivet, J., Rogez, C., and Wechsler, J. (2001) Trichoepithelioma with "monster" stromal cells. *J Cutan Pathol* **28**(7): 379–82.

Sellheyer, K. and Nelson, P. (2011) Follicular stem cell marker PHLDA1 (TDAG51) is superior to cytokeratin-20 in differentiating between trichoepithelioma and basal cell carcinoma in small biopsy specimens. *J Cutan Pathol* **38**(7): 542–50.

BENIGN NEOPLASMS

Trichoblastoma (Trichoblastic Fibroma; Immature Trichoepithelioma)

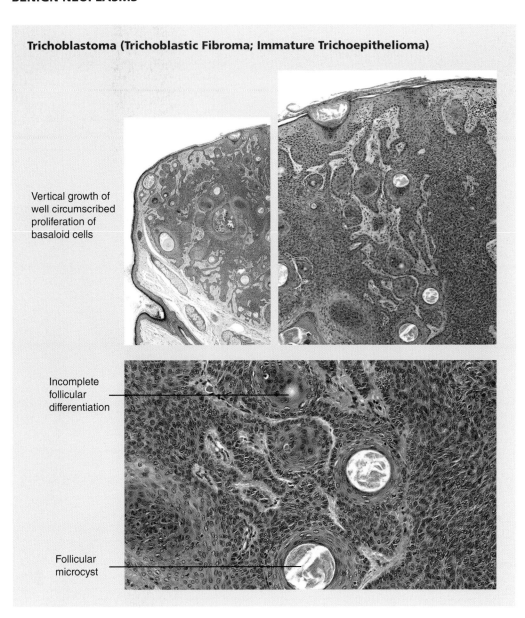

Vertical growth of well circumscribed proliferation of basaloid cells

Incomplete follicular differentiation

Follicular microcyst

Cl: Trichoblastoma frequently originates in a sebaceous nevus; it can occur at any site and may reach large size. Ulceration is exceedingly rare. Many trichoblastomas occur independent of the nevus on the scalp of middle-aged to elderly men.

Hi:
- Well-circumscribed vertically growing tumor, with basaloid tumor cells arranged in cords, sheets or clusters, branching and anastomosing
- Connected to the epidermis
- Characteristic zonation of individual tumor nests and lobules ("pizza sign") with an outer

rim of deep basophilic epithelia and a pale center, often containing melanophages
- Nestin-positive papillary mesenchymal bodies
- CK20-positive Merkel cells distributed throughout the tumor in a starry sky-like pattern
- Amorphous eosinophilic debris and mucomyxoid stromal alterations may be present
- Different histological patterns exist:
  ○ Small nodular
  ○ Large nodular
  ○ Adamantinoid trichoblastoma, with lymphocytic infiltrate within tumor nests (outdated

BENIGN NEOPLASMS

synonyms are lymphoepithelial tumor or cutaneous lymphadenoma)
- ◦ Cystic
- ◦ Papillary trichoblastoma
- ◦ Racemiform (like an elk's antlers)
- ◦ Cribriform (like a sieve)
- ◦ Retiform (like a net)
- ◦ Rippled pattern
- ◦ Clear cell trichoblastoma
- ◦ Pigmented trichoblastoma
- ◦ Desmoplastic trichoblastoma (see below)

DD: Basal cell carcinoma.

Trichoblastoma, Small and Large Nodular

Well circumscribed tumor with small (left) or large (right) nodules of basaloid cells and compact stroma

"Pizza sign": palisading dark cells around pale center; hair germs and primitive hair papillae

BENIGN NEOPLASMS

Adamantinoid Trichoblastoma (Cutaneous Cystadenoma)

Well circumscribed tumor with small nodules of basaloid cells and dense stroma

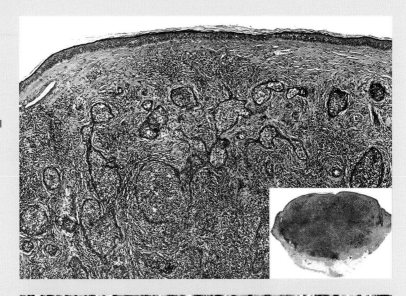

"Pizza sign": Palisading border, pale center

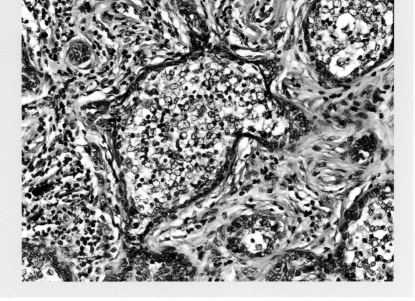

BENIGN NEOPLASMS

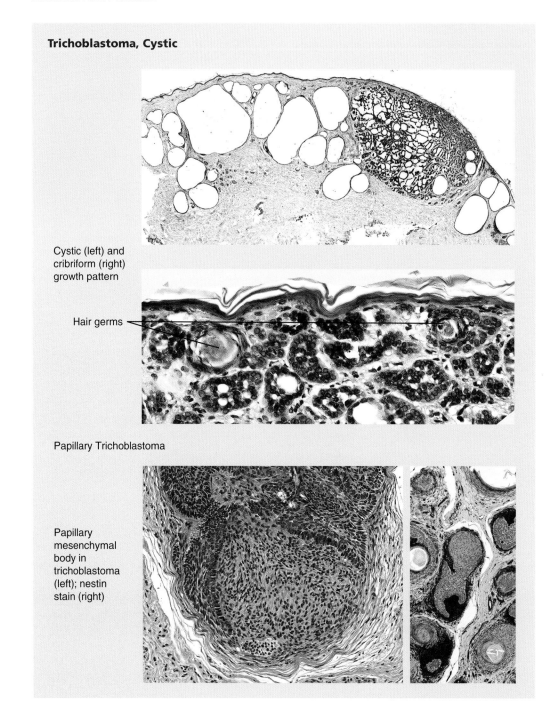

Trichoblastoma, Cystic

Cystic (left) and cribriform (right) growth pattern

Hair germs

Papillary Trichoblastoma

Papillary mesenchymal body in trichoblastoma (left); nestin stain (right)

BENIGN NEOPLASMS

References

Battistella, M., Peltre, B., and Cribier, B. (2014) PHLDA1, a follicular stem cell marker, differentiates clear-cell/granular-cell trichoblastoma and clear-cell/granular cell basal cell carcinoma: a case-control study, with first description of granular-cell trichoblastoma. *Am J Dermatopathol* **36**(8): 643–50.

Goyal, A., Solus, J.F., Chan, M.P., et al. (2016) Cytokeratin 17 is highly sensitive in discriminating cutaneous lymphadenoma (a distinct trichoblastoma variant) from basal cell carcinoma. *J Cutan Pathol* **43**(5): 422–9.

Hamasaki, H., Koga, K., Hamasaki, M., et al. (2011) Immunohistochemical analysis of laminin 5-gamma2 chain expression for differentiation of basal cell carcinoma from trichoblastoma. *Histopathology* **59**(1): 159–61.

Jaqueti, G., Requena, L., and Sanchez Yus, E. (2000) Trichoblastoma is the most common neoplasm developed in nevus sebaceus of Jadassohn: a clinicopathologic study of a series of 155 cases. *Am J Dermatopathol* **22**(2): 108–18.

Juarez, A., Rutten, A., Kutzner, H., and Requena, L. (2012) Cystic trichoblastoma (so-called trichoblastic infundibular cyst): a report of three new cases. *J Cutan Pathol* **39**(6): 631–6.

Kanitakis, J., Brutzkus, A., Butnaru, A.C., and Claudy, A. (2002) Melanotrichoblastoma: immunohistochemical study of a variant of pigmented trichoblastoma. *Am J Dermatopathol* **24**(6): 498–501.

Kazakov, D.V., Banik, M., Kacerovska, D., and Michal, M. (2011) A cutaneous adnexal neoplasm with features of adamantinoid trichoblastoma (lymphadenoma) in the benign component and lymphoepithelial-like carcinoma in the malignant component: a possible case of malignant transformation of a rare trichoblastoma variant. *Am J Dermatopathol* **33**(7): 729–32.

Kazakov, D.V., Mentzel, T., Erlandson, R.A., Mukensnabl, P., and Michal, M. (2006) Clear cell trichoblastoma: a clinicopathological and ultrastructural study of two cases. *Am J Dermatopathol* **28**(3): 197–201.

Kurzen, H., Esposito, L., Langbein, L., and Hartschuh, W. (2001) Cytokeratins as markers of follicular differentiation: an immunohistochemical study of trichoblastoma and basal cell carcinoma. *Am J Dermatopathol* **23**(6): 501–9.

Swick, B.L., Baum, C.L., and Walling, H.W. (2009) Rippled-pattern trichoblastoma with apocrine differentiation arising in a nevus sebaceus: report of a case and review of the literature. *J Cutan Pathol* **36**(11): 1200–5.

Tronnier, M. (2001) Clear cell trichoblastoma in association with a nevus sebaceus. *Am J Dermatopathol* **23**(2): 143–5.

Wang, L., Wang, G., Yang, L., and Gao, T. (2009) Multiple clear cell trichoblastoma. *J Cutan Pathol* **36**(3): 370–3.

Trichoepithelioma (Sclerosing Epithelial Hamartoma)

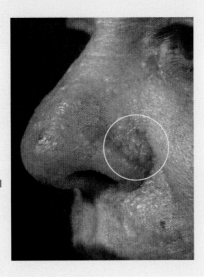
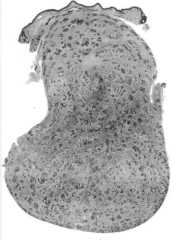

Flat tumor with telangiectases on the nose (left)

Sclerosing dermal tumor with small strands of basaloid cells (right)

Trichoepithelioma (Sclerosing Epithelial Hamartoma)

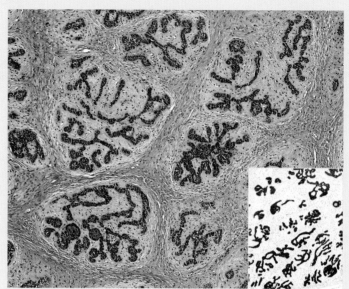

Arborising strands
of basaloid tumor
cells in a densely
collagenized
stroma

Tumor cells are
AE1/AE3 positive
(inset)

Desmoplastic Trichoepithelioma (Sclerosing Epithelial Hamartoma)

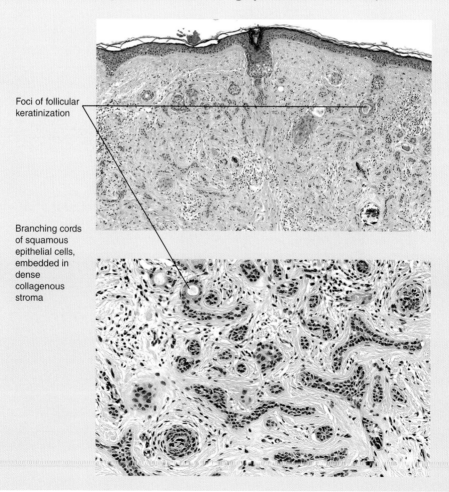

Foci of follicular
keratinization

Branching cords
of squamous
epithelial cells,
embedded in
dense
collagenous
stroma

BENIGN NEOPLASMS

Cl: Scar-like, discoid, centrally indented solitary skin-colored tumor with raised borders, preferentially localized in the face of young women.

Hi:

- Symmetrical, poorly circumscribed tumor
- Small cords of squamous epithelium
- Superficial adnexal microcysts
- Dense collagenous paucicellular eosinophilic stroma (desmoplastic variant)

DD: Syringoma; morphea-like basal cell carcinoma; microcystic adnexal carcinoma.

References

Costache, M., Bresch, M., and Boer, A. (2008) Desmoplastic trichoepithelioma versus morphoeic basal cell carcinoma: a critical reappraisal of histomorphological and immunohistochemical criteria for differentiation. *Histopathology* **52**(7): 865–76.

Jedrych, J. and McNiff, J.M. (2013) Expression of p75 neurotrophin receptor in desmoplastic trichoepithelioma, infiltrative basal cell carcinoma, and microcystic adnexal carcinoma. *Am J Dermatopathol* **35**(3), 308–315.

Jedrych, J., Leffell, D., and McNiff, J. M. (2012). Desmoplastic trichoepithelioma with perineural involvement: a series of seven cases. *J Cutan Pathol* **39**(3): 317–23.

McCalmont, T.H. and Humberson, C. (2012) Neurotropism in association with desmoplastic trichoepithelioma. *J Cutan Pathol* **39**(3): 312–14.

McFaddin, C., Sirohi, D., Castro-Echeverry, E., and Fernandez, M.P. (2015) Desmoplastic trichoepithelioma with pseudocarcinomatous hyperplasia: a report of three cases. *J Cutan Pathol* **42**(2): 102–7.

Sellheyer, K., Nelson, P., Kutzner, H., and Patel, R.M. (2013) The immunohistochemical differential diagnosis of microcystic adnexal carcinoma, desmoplastic trichoepithelioma and morpheaform basal cell carcinoma using BerEP4 and stem cell markers. *J Cutan Pathol* **40**(4): 363–70.

Tse, J.Y., Nguyen, A.T., Le, L.P., and Hoang, M.P. (2013) Microcystic adnexal carcinoma versus desmoplastic trichoepithelioma: a comparative study. *Am J Dermatopathol* **35**(1): 50–5.

Vollmer, R.T. (2009) Panel vs. single marker for discriminating desmoplastic trichoepithelioma from morpheaform/infiltrative basal cell carcinoma. *J Cutan Pathol* **36**(2): 283; author reply 284.

Trichofolliculoma (Folliculosebaceous Cystic Hamartoma)

Central pore with keratotic material and miniature hair shafts

Radial branching of tiny hair follicles

BENIGN NEOPLASMS

Trichofolliculoma (Folliculosebaceous Cystic Hamartoma)

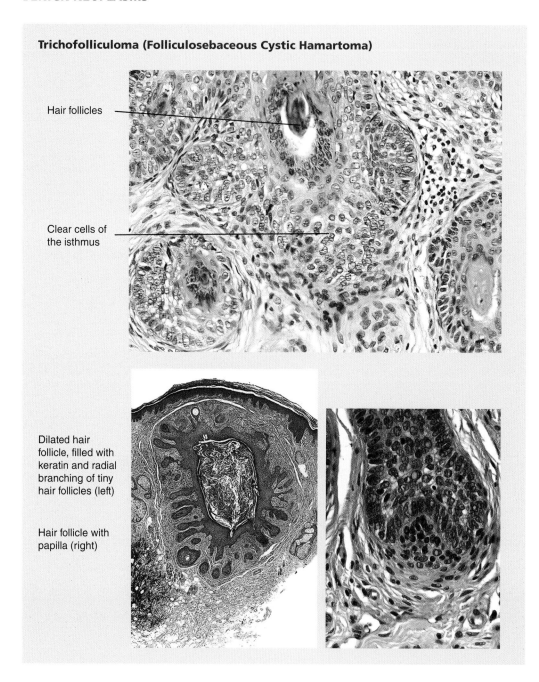

Hair follicles

Clear cells of the isthmus

Dilated hair follicle, filled with keratin and radial branching of tiny hair follicles (left)

Hair follicle with papilla (right)

BENIGN NEOPLASMS

Trichofolliculoma (Folliculosebaceous Cystic Hamartoma)

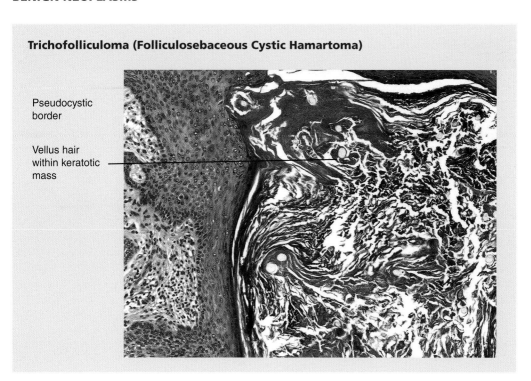

Pseudocystic border

Vellus hair within keratotic mass

Cl: Solitary papule preferentially on the nose of adults or in other localisations of the head and neck. Multiple small abortive hair follicles emerge centrifugally from a central horn-filled follicular cystic dilation. Folliculosebaceous cystic hamartoma is considered to be a variant of trichofolliculoma or sebaceous trichofolliculoma with many sebaceous glands.

Hi:

- Dilated and branching follicular structure, opening to the surface
- Abortive small hair follicles branching out from the outer follicular layer
- Branches contain immature and well-differentiated follicles with hair papillae
- Sebaceous differentiation (small lobules) rare

DD: Basal cell carcinoma; trichoepithelioma; fibrofolliculoma.

References

Ansai, S., Kimura, T., and Kawana, S. (2010) A clinico-pathologic study of folliculosebaceous cystic hamartoma. *Am J Dermatopathol* **32**(8): 815–20.

Cole, P., Kaufman, Y., Dishop, M., Hatef, D.A., and Hollier, L. (2008) Giant, congenital folliculosebaceous cystic hamartoma: a case against a pathogenetic relationship with trichofolliculoma. *Am J Dermatopathol* **30**(5): 500–3.

Lee, S.Y., Lee, D.R., You, C.E., Park, M.Y., and Son, S.J. (2006) Folliculosebaceous cystic hamartoma on the nipple. *Am J Dermatopathol* **28**(3): 205–7.

Lim, P. and Kossard, S. (2009) Trichofolliculoma with mucinosis. *Am J Dermatopathol* **31**(4): 405–6.

Misago, N., Kimura, T., Toda, S., Mori, T., and Narisawa, Y. (2010) A revaluation of trichofolliculoma: the histopathological and immunohistochemical features. *Am J Dermatopathol* **32**(1): 35–43.

Misago, N., Kimura, T., Toda, S., Mori, T., and Narisawa, Y. (2010) A revaluation of folliculosebaceous cystic hamartoma: the histopathological and immunohistochemical features. *Am J Dermatopathol* **32**(2): 154–61.

Nguyen, C.M., Skupsky, H., and Cassarino, D. (2015) Folliculosebaceous cystic hamartoma with spindle cell lipoma-like stromal features. *Am J Dermatopathol* **37**(12): e140–2.

Wu, Y.H. (2008) Folliculosebaceous cystic hamartoma or trichofolliculoma? A spectrum of hamartomatous changes inducted by perifollicular stroma in the follicular epithelium. *J Cutan Pathol* **35**(9): 843–8.

BENIGN NEOPLASMS

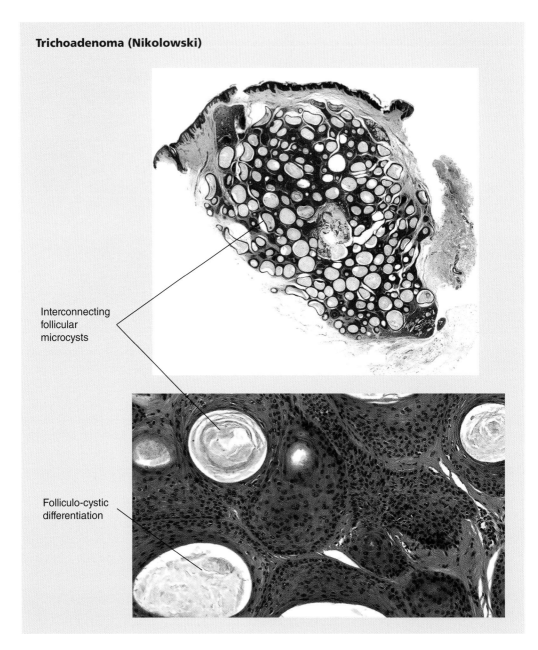

Trichoadenoma (Nikolowski)

Interconnecting follicular microcysts

Folliculo-cystic differentiation

Cl: Solitary firm nodule; rare.

Hi:

- Eosinophilic tumor composed of multiple small round follicular horn-filled cysts, interconnected by small epithelial bridges
- No connection with the epidermis
- Granular layer usually absent
- Dense collagenous stroma

DD: Trichoepithelioma; microcystic adnexal carcinoma; basal cell carcinoma.

References

Gonzalez-Vela, M.C., Val-Bernal, J.F., Garcia-Alberdi, E., Gonzalez-Lopez, M.A., and Fernandez-Llaca, J.H. (2007).Trichoadenoma associated with an intradermal melanocytic nevus: a combined malformation. *Am J Dermatopathol* **29**(1): 92–5.

BENIGN NEOPLASMS

Reibold, R., Undeutsch, W., and Fleiner, J. (1998) [Trichoadenoma of Nikolowski – review of four decades and seven new cases]. *Hautarzt* **49**(12): 925–8.

Shimanovich, I., Krahl, D., and Rose, C. (2010) Trichoadenoma of Nikolowski is a distinct neoplasm within the spectrum of follicular tumors. *J Am Acad Dermatol* **62**(2): 277–83.

Pilomatricoma (Calcifying Epithelioma Malherbe)

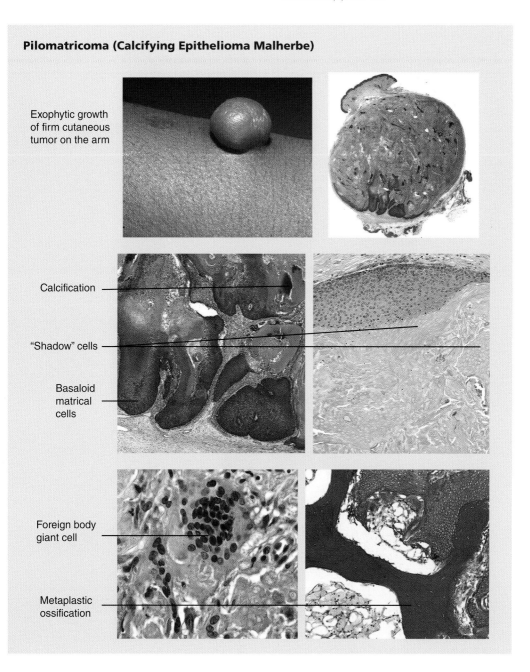

Exophytic growth of firm cutaneous tumor on the arm

Calcification

"Shadow" cells

Basaloid matrical cells

Foreign body giant cell

Metaplastic ossification

BENIGN NEOPLASMS

Cl: Solitary firm cutaneous or subcutaneous nodule, preferentially on face, upper extremities and shoulder of children, simulating an epidermoid cyst.

Hi:

- Nodular tumor mostly consisting of irregularly shaped lobules of basaloid germinative cells
- Deep basophilic basaloid germinative cells showing differentiation towards hair matrix cells
- Gradual transition from germinative cells to "shadow cells" to necrotic debris
- Metaplastic calcification and ossification may occur
- High proliferative activity with many mitoses
- Inflammatory granulomatous foreign body reaction with multinucleated giant cells

Immunocytochemistry: Characteristic co-expression of high molecular weight cytokeratin and beta-catenin.

DD: Epidermoid cyst; trichilemmal cyst; trichilemmal carcinoma; squamous cell carcinoma; basal cell carcinoma; pilomatrical carcinoma.

References

Byun, J.W., Bang, C.Y., Yang, B.H., et al. (2011) Proliferating pilomatricoma. *Am J Dermatopathol* **33**(7): 754–5.

Cribier, B., Worret, W.I., Braun-Falco, M., Peltre, B., Langbein, L., and Schweizer, J. (2006) Expression patterns of hair and epithelial keratins and transcription factors HOXC13, LEF1, and beta-catenin in a malignant pilomatricoma: a histological and immunohistochemical study. *J Cutan Pathol* **33**(1): 1–9.

de Souza, E.M., Ayres Vallarelli, A.F., Cintra, M.L., Vetter-Kauczok, C.S., and Brocker, E.B. (2009) Anetodermic pilomatricoma. *J Cutan Pathol* **36**(1): 67–70.

Li, L., Zeng, Y., Fang, K., et al. (2012) Anetodermic pilomatricoma: molecular characteristics and trauma in the development of its bullous appearance. *Am J Dermatopathol* **34**(4): e41–5.

Lozzi, G.P., Soyer, H.P., Fruehauf, J., Massone, C., Kerl, H., and Peris, K. (2007) Giant pilomatricoma. *Am J Dermatopathol* **29**(3): 286–9.

Yiqun, J. and Jianfang, S. (2004) Pilomatricoma with a bullous appearance. *J Cutan Pathol* **31**(8): 558–60.

Zamecnik, M., Michal, M., and Mukensnabl, P. (2000) Cell death in pilomatricoma. *J Cutan Pathol* **27**(2): 100.

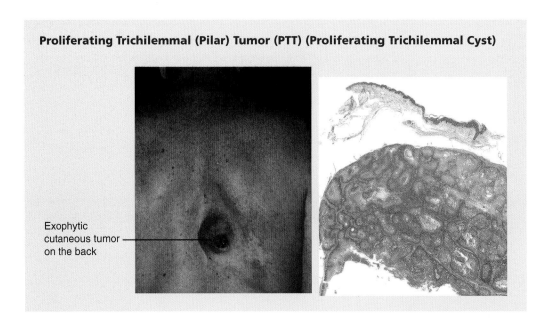

Proliferating Trichilemmal (Pilar) Tumor (PTT) (Proliferating Trichilemmal Cyst)

Exophytic cutaneous tumor on the back

BENIGN NEOPLASMS

Proliferating Trichilemmal (Pilar) Tumor (PTT) (Proliferating Trichilemmal Cyst)

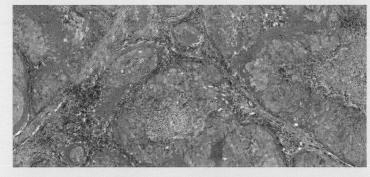

Sharply circumscribed tumor with smooth outer margin (right top)

Confluent sheets with trichilemmal keratinization (middle)

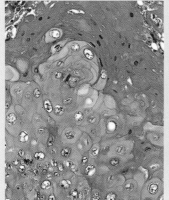

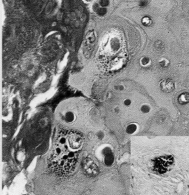

Squamous epithelium, showing trichilemmal keratinization (left)

Atypical squamous cells, eosinophilic keratotic mass (right). Focal calcification (inset)

Kossa

Cl: Large, dermal or subcutaneous, slowly growing, exophytic tumor on the scalp, sometimes on the back of elderly individuals, arising from pre-existing trichilemmal cyst. Untreated, it may become inflamed and ulcerated. Prognosis usually excellent. Malignant transformation with metastases may occur in exceptionally large lesions.

Hi:

- Sharply circumscribed, partially cystic and lobulated tumor, extending into the subcutis
- Inward-bound lobular growth pattern of cells with trichilemmal keratinization (isthmus-catagen type of epithelia), correlating to trichilemmal cyst
- Irregular lobular architecture suggesting carcinomatous growth, albeit without dysplasia, mitotic activity, and marked necroses
- Proliferative activity (Ki67) limited to the basal zones of individual lobules
- Cystic spaces may be filled with inflammatory infiltrate and amorphous horn masses
- Foci of dystrophic calcification

DD: Trichilemmal cyst; squamous cell carcinoma; trichilemmal carcinoma; pilomatricomas; basal cell carcinomas; epithelioma cuniculatum. Malignant proliferating trichilemmal cyst is the most important differential diagnosis, showing very large size (>5 cm), poor outer circumscription with focal invasive growth, increased mitotic activity – in particular within suprabasal layers and massive central necrosis.

References

Burg, G. and Landthaler, M. (1988) [Proliferating tricholemmal tumor]. *Hautarzt* **39**(2): 117–19.

Haas, N., Audring, H., and Sterry, W. (2002) Carcinoma arising in a proliferating trichilemmal cyst expresses fetal and trichilemmal hair phenotype. *Am J Dermatopathol* **24**(4): 340–4.

Lindsey, S F., Aickara, D., Price, A., et al. (2017) Giant proliferating trichilemmal cyst arising from a nevus sebaceus growing for 30 years. *J Cutan Pathol* Apr 17. doi: 10.1111/cup.12951 [epub ahead of print].

MALIGNANT NEOPLASMS

Lopez-Rios, F., Rodriguez-Peralto, J.L., Aguilar, A., Hernandez, L., and Gallego, M. (2000) Proliferating trichilemmal cyst with focal invasion: report of a case and a review of the literature. *Am J Dermatopathol* **22**(2): 183–7.

Mori, O., Hachisuka, H., and Sasai, Y. (1990).Proliferating trichilemmal cyst with spindle cell carcinoma. *Am J Dermatopathol* **12**(5): 479–84.

Noto, G., Pravata, G., and Arico, M. (1997) Malignant proliferating trichilemmal tumor. *Am J Dermatopathol* **19**(2): 202–4.

Park, B.S., Yang, S.G., and Cho, K.H. (1997) Malignant proliferating trichilemmal tumor showing distant metastases. *Am J Dermatopathol* **19**(5): 536–9.

Plumb, S.J. and Stone, M.S. (2002) Proliferating trichilemmal tumor with a malignant spindle cell component. *J Cutan Pathol* **29**(8): 506–9.

Sakamoto, F., Ito, M., Nakamura, A., and Sato, Y. (1991). Proliferating trichilemmal cyst with apocrine-acrosyringeal and sebaceous differentiation. *J Cutan Pathol* **18**(2): 137–41.

Val-Bernal, J.F., Garijo, M.F., and Fernandez, F. (1998) Malignant proliferating trichilemmal tumor. *Am J Dermatopathol* **20**(4): 433–4.

Malignant Neoplasms

Malignant Pilomatricoma (Pilomatrical Carcinoma)

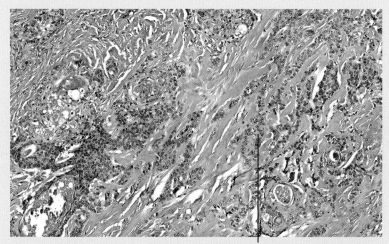

Infiltrating growth of atypical pilomatrical cells

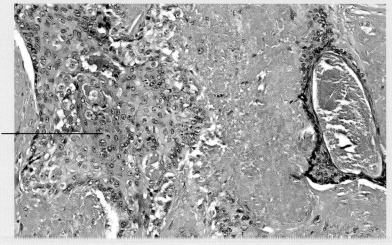

Focal necrosis. Prominent lack of shadow cells

MALIGNANT NEOPLASMS

Cl: Rare malignant variant of pilomatricoma.

Hi:

- Large size (>5 cm)
- Infiltrating growth pattern
- Marked loss of shadow cells – with abrupt transition from germinative cells to necrotic debris

- Hyperchromasia and pleomorphism involving all parts of the tumor
- Many mitoses

DD: Squamous cell carcinoma, pilomatricoma.

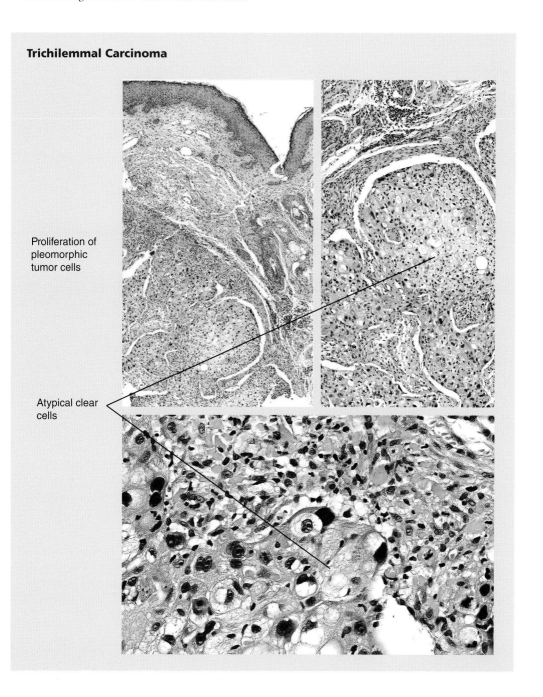

Trichilemmal Carcinoma

Proliferation of pleomorphic tumor cells

Atypical clear cells

MALIGNANT NEOPLASMS

Trichilemmal carcinoma is considered to be a pleomorphic clear cell variant of squamous cell carcinoma showing features of trichilemmal differentiation.

References

Arsenovic, N., Sen, S., Naik, V., Reed, M., and Moreira, R. (2009) Trichilemmal cyst with carcinoma in situ within an atypical fibroxanthoma. *Am J Dermatopathol* **31**(6): 587–90.

Cassarino, D.S., Derienzo, D.P., and Barr, R.J. (2006) Cutaneous squamous cell carcinoma: a comprehensive clinicopathologic classification. Part one. *J Cutan Pathol* **33**(3): 191–206.

Cassarino, D.S., Derienzo, D.P., and Barr, R.J. (2006) Cutaneous squamous cell carcinoma: a comprehensive clinicopathologic classification. Part two. *J Cutan Pathol* **33**(4): 261–79.

Fernandez-Figueras, M.T., Casalots, A., Puig, L., Llatjos, R., Ferrandiz, C., and Ariza, A. (2001) Proliferating trichilemmal tumour: p53 immunoreactivity in association with p27Kip1 over-expression indicates a low-grade carcinoma profile. *Histopathology* **38**(5): 454–7.

Haas, N., Audring, H., and Sterry, W. (2002) Carcinoma arising in a proliferating trichilemmal cyst expresses fetal and trichilemmal hair phenotype. *Am J Dermatopathol* **24**(4): 340–4.

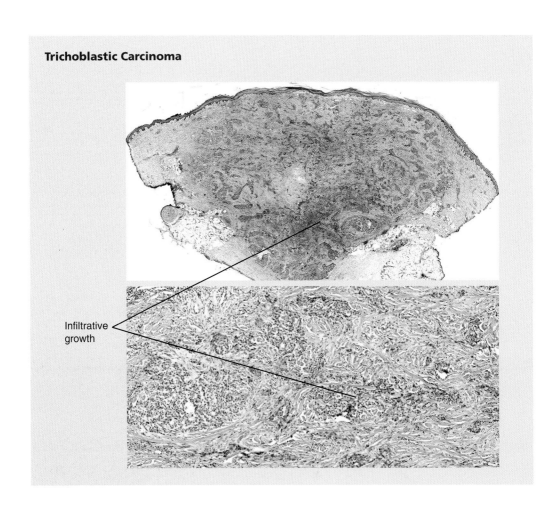

Trichoblastic Carcinoma

Infiltrative growth

BENIGN NEOPLASM

Trichoblastic Carcinoma

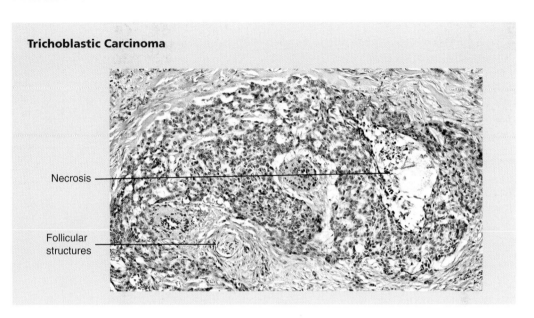

Necrosis

Follicular
structures

Trichoblastic carcinoma is the malignant variant of trichoblastoma, which most commonly develops in sebaceous nevus of Jadassohn. Infiltrative growth pattern, cellular atypia and focal necrosis are found.

Pilosebaceous Mesenchyme

Benign Neoplasm

Trichodiscoma (Follicular Fibroma, Fibrofolliculoma, Perifollicular Fibroma)

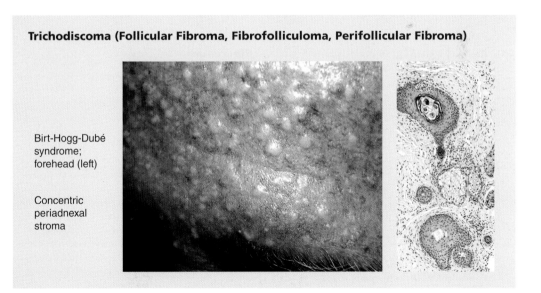

Birt-Hogg-Dubé
syndrome;
forehead (left)

Concentric
periadnexal
stroma

BENIGN NEOPLASM

Spindle Cell Predominant Trichodiscoma (Follicular Fibroma, Fibrofolliculoma, Perifollicular Fibroma)

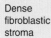

Dense fibroblastic stroma

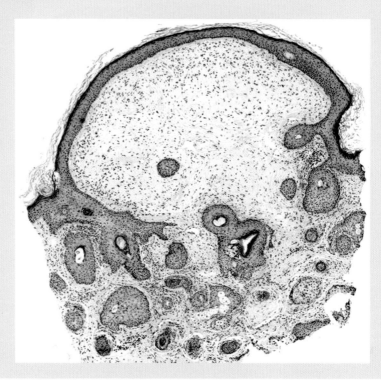

Cl: Fibrofolliculoma, perifollicular fibroma, and trichodiscoma are proliferations of the dermal perifollicular mesenchyme, and are considered to be different stages of evolution of a single tumor entity that clinically mostly presents with small papules, preferentially in the head and neck area. Trichodiscoma may appear as a sporadic variant with solitary protuberant lesions in the nasolabial area, or as multiple small whitish agminated lesions in the setting of Birt–Hogg–Dubé syndrome (associated with tumors of the kidney and pulmonary cysts).

Hi:

- Exophytic tumor with adnexal (sebaceous) and stromal (fibroblasts) components
- Aggregated and fascicularly oriented CD34-positive fibroblasts with interspersed adipocytes in the center
- Mucin-rich stroma (imitating spindle cell lipoma)
- Hyperplastic sebaceous glands on either side of the tumor
- Mature hair follicle missing; rarely small vellus hair at the outer periphery

References

Chartier, M., Reed, M.L., Mandavilli, S., Fung, M., Grant-Kels, J., and Murphy, M. (2007) CD34-reactive trichodiscoma. *J Cutan Pathol* **34**(10): 808.

Kacerovska, D., Kazakov, D.V., and Michal, M. (2010) Spindle-cell predominant trichodiscoma with a palisaded arrangement of stromal cells. *Am J Dermatopathol* **32**(7): 743–4.

Kacerovska, D., Michal, M., and Kazakov, D. V. (2010) Trichodiscoma with lipomatous metaplasia and pleomorphic stromal cells. *J Cutan Pathol* **37**(10): 1110–11.

Kutzner, H., Requena, L., Rutten, A., and Mentzel, T. (2006) Spindle cell predominant trichodiscoma: a fibrofolliculoma/trichodiscoma variant considered formerly to be a neurofollicular hamartoma: a clinicopathological and immunohistochemical analysis of 17 cases. *Am J Dermatopathol* **28**(1): 1–8.

Misago, N., Kimura, T., and Narisawa, Y. (2009) Fibrofolliculoma/trichodiscoma and fibrous papule (perifollicular fibroma/angiofibroma): a revaluation of the histopathological and immunohistochemical features. *J Cutan Pathol* **36**(9): 943–51.

Tran, T.A. and Carlson, J.A. (2016) Composite fibrofolliculoma/trichodiscoma with vascular mesenchymal stromal overgrowth. *Am J Dermatopathol* **38**(7): 562–5.

CHAPTER 3

Paget's Disease

Atlas of Dermatopathology: Tumors, Nevi, and Cysts, First Edition. Günter Burg, Heinz Kutzner,
Werner Kempf, Josef Feit, and Bruce R. Smoller.
© 2019 John Wiley & Sons Ltd. Published 2019 by John Wiley & Sons Ltd.

Mammary Paget's Disease

Cl: Eczema-like or psoriasiform or bowenoid lesions unilaterally in or around one nipple of the breast, mostly in females. They reflect intraepidermal metastasis of ductal adenocarcinoma of the breast.

Hi:

- Intraepidermal pagetoid spread of large clear cells with pale cytoplasm and prominent nucleus
- All epidermal layers favored, in contrast to superficial spreading melanoma, in which the basal layer is favored

- Cells are positive for PAS and CK7, EMA, and CAM5.2
- Small amounts of mucin
- Lack of dyskeratosis
- Superficial erosion, covered with crust
- Increased number of melanocytes may occur

DD: Pagetoid melanoma (S100; melanoma-specific markers); Bowen's disease; pagetoid reticulosis. Toker cells (CK7+) are regular non-neoplastic autochthonous intraepidermal clear cells, which are found in 10% of normal nipple epidermis.

Extramammary Paget's Disease

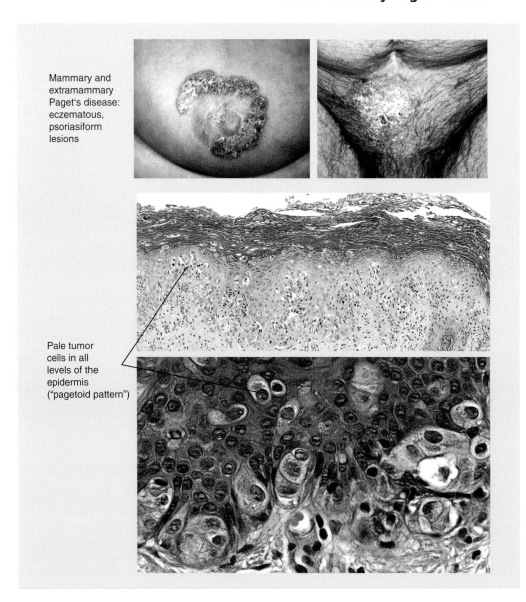

Mammary and extramammary Paget's disease: eczematous, psoriasiform lesions

Pale tumor cells in all levels of the epidermis ("pagetoid pattern")

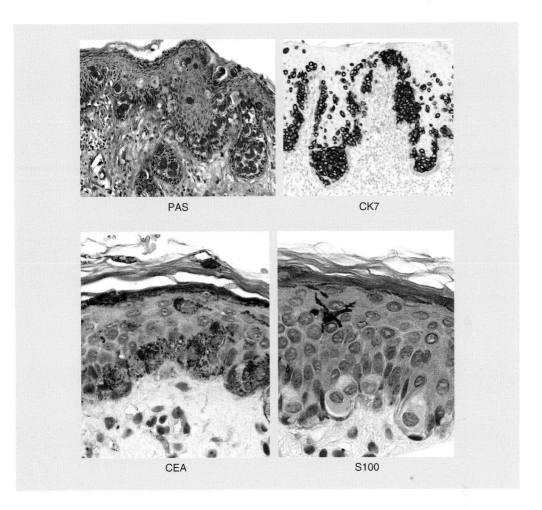

PAS

CK7

CEA

S100

More than 20% of these are associated with visceral malignancies of the GU or GI tract.

Cl: Scaling eczematous or psoriasiform lesions in the anogenital region, axilla or other areas with apocrine glands. Oozing and crust formation.

Hi: Similar to mammary Paget. PAS-positive tumor cells within all layers of the epidermis and within follicular epithelium.

DD: Superficial spreading melanoma; Bowen's disease; pagetoid reticulosis; apocrine carcinoma of the groin with intraepidermal pagetoid dissemination; metastasizing urothelial and vesicular carcinoma (uroplakin-positive); rectal and colon carcinoma (CDX2-positive); prostate carcinoma (PSA-positive).

References

Belousova, I.E., Kazakov, D.V., Michal, M., and Suster, S. (2006) Vulvar toker cells: the long-awaited missing link: a proposal for an origin-based histogenetic classification of extramammary paget disease. *Am J Dermatopathol* **28**(1): 84–6.

Castelli, E., Wollina, U., Anzarone, A., Morello, V., and Tomasino, R.M. (2002) Extramammary Paget disease of the axilla associated with comedo-like apocrine carcinoma in situ. *Am J Dermatopathol* **24**(4): 351–7.

Chang, J., Prieto, V.G., Sangueza, M., and Plaza, J.A. (2014) Diagnostic utility of p63 expression in the differential diagnosis of pagetoid squamous cell carcinoma in situ and extramammary Paget disease: a histopathologic study of 70 cases. *Am J Dermatopathol* **36**(1): 49–53.

De la Garza Bravo, M.M., Curry, J.L., Torres-Cabala, C.A., et al. (2014) Pigmented extramammary Paget disease of the thigh mimicking a melanocytic tumor: report of a case and review of the literature. *J Cutan Pathol* **41**(6): 529–35.

Elbendary, A., Xue, R., Valdebran, M., et al. (2017) Diagnostic criteria in intraepithelial pagetoid neoplasms: a histopathologic study and evaluation of select features in Paget disease, Bowen disease, and melanoma in situ. *Am J Dermatopathol* **39**(6): 419–27.

Fujimura, T., Kambayashi, Y., Kakizaki, A., Furudate, S., and Aiba, S. (2016) RANKL expression is a useful marker for differentiation of pagetoid squamous cell carcinoma in situ from extramammary Paget disease. *J Cutan Pathol* **43**(9): 772–5.

Konstantinova, A.M., Hayes, M.M., Stewart, C.J., et al. (2016a) Syringomatous structures in extramammary Paget disease: a potential diagnostic pitfall. *Am J Dermatopathol* **38**(9): 653–7.

Konstantinova, A.M., Shelekhova, K.V., Stewart, C.J., et al. (2016b) Depth and patterns of adnexal involvement in primary extramammary (anogenital) Paget disease: a study of 178 lesions from 146 patients. *Am J Dermatopathol* **38**(11): 802–8.

Matsumoto, M., Ishiguro, M., Ikeno, F., et al. (2007) Combined Bowen disease and extramammary Paget disease. *J Cutan Pathol* **34**(Suppl 1): 47–51.

Ohashi, T., Takenoshita, H., and Yamamoto, T. (2014) Acantholysis in mammary Paget disease. *Am J Dermatopathol* **36**(10): 856–7.

Perrotto, J., Abbott, J.J., Ceilley, R.I., and Ahmed, I. (2010) The role of immunohistochemistry in discriminating primary from secondary extramammary Paget disease. *Am J Dermatopathol* **32**(2): 137–43.

Petersson, F., Ivan, D., Kazakov, D.V., Michal, M., and Prieto, V.G. (2009) Pigmented Paget disease – a diagnostic pitfall mimicking melanoma. *Am J Dermatopathol* **31**(3): 223–6.

Plaza, J.A., Torres-Cabala, C., Ivan, D., and Prieto, V.G. (2009) HER-2/neu expression in extramammary Paget disease: a clinicopathologic and immunohistochemistry study of 47 cases with and without underlying malignancy. *J Cutan Pathol* **36**(7): 729–33.

Terada, T. (2016) Extramammary Paget disease of signet ring cell carcinoma type: a case report. *Am J Dermatopathol* **38**(3): 249–51.

Villada, G., Farooq, U., Yu, W., Diaz, J.P., and Milikowski, C. (2015) Extramammary Paget disease of the vulva with underlying mammary-like lobular carcinoma: a case report and review of the literature. *Am J Dermatopathol* **37**(4): 295–8.

CHAPTER 4

Melanocytes

Atlas of Dermatopathology: Tumors, Nevi, and Cysts, First Edition. Günter Burg, Heinz Kutzner,
Werner Kempf, Josef Feit, and Bruce R. Smoller.
© 2019 John Wiley & Sons Ltd. Published 2019 by John Wiley & Sons Ltd.

Non-Neoplastic Hyperpigmentations

Ephelides (Genuine Freckles)

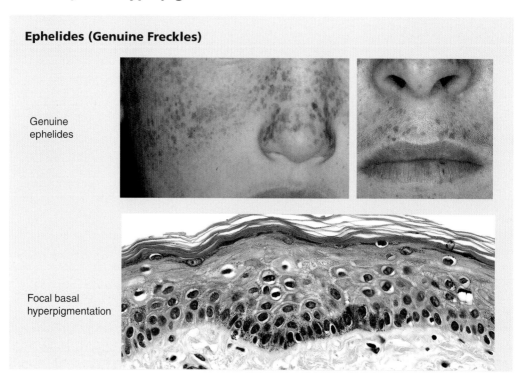

Genuine
ephelides

Focal basal
hyperpigmentation

Cl: Small brown roundish macules, preferentially in sun-exposed areas of the face and shoulders in fair-skinned individuals (Fitzpatrick type I or II). Genetic predisposition.

Hi: Focal hyperpigmentation of the epidermal basal layer. The number of melanocytes is normal.

DD: Café-au-lait spots; syndromatic melanotic macules; ink spot; actinic lentigo.

References

Bastiaens, M., ter Huurne, J., Gruis, N., et al. (2001) The melanocortin-1-receptor gene is the major freckle gene. *Hum Mol Genet* **10**(16): 1701–8.

Rhodes, A.R., Albert, L.S., Barnhill, R.L., and Weinstock, M.A. (1991) Sun-induced freckles in children and young adults. A correlation of clinical and histopathologic features. *Cancer* **67**(7): 1990–2001.

PUVA (Psoralen UVA) Lentigo

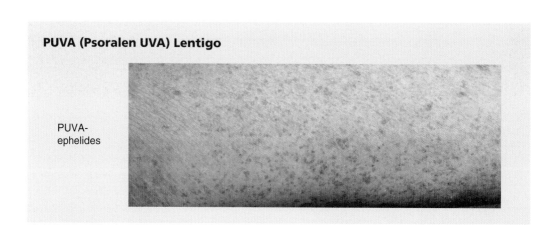

PUVA-
ephelides

PUVA (Psoralen UVA) Lentigo

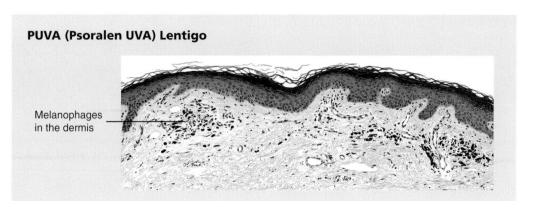

Melanophages in the dermis

Cl: Small light-brown splash-like macules resulting from long-lasting therapy with psoralen and UVA (PUVA).

Hi: Hyperpigmented melanophages in the upper dermis.

References

Kanerva, L., Niemi, K.M., and Lauharanta, J. (1984). A semiquantitative light and electron microscopic analysis of histopathologic changes in photochemotherapy-induced freckles. *Arch Dermatol Res* **276**(1): 2–11.

Kanerva, L., Lauharanta, J., Niemi, K.M., Juvakoski, T., and Lassus, A. (1983) Persistent ashen-gray maculae and freckles induced by long-term PUVA treatment. *Dermatologica* **166**(6): 281–6.

"Nevus" Spilus (Speckled Lentiginous Nevus; Café-Au-Lait Spot)

"Ink-Spot" Lentigo (Reticulated Melanocytic Macule)

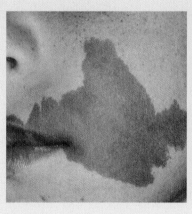

Nevus spilus (left)

Ink spot (right)

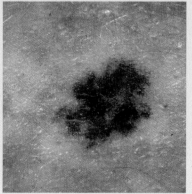

"Nevus" Spilus

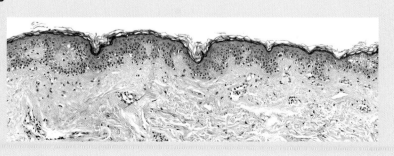

Slight acanthosis, melanocytes and pigment loaded keratinocytes

Cl: Widespread or segmental macules of variable size and uniform light-brown color, usually persisting from birth throughout life without change. There may be multiple disseminated hyperpigmented spots (melanocytic nevi of various sizes) within the macule. Melanoma arising in a nevus spilus has been reported.

Hi:

- Slight acanthosis with elongated rete ridges
- Melanin in keratinocytes
- Slight increase of the number of melanocytes
- Within the lentiginous zone, multiple interspersed nevi (junctional, compound, large congenital) of various sizes may be present

References

Haenssle, H.A., Kaune, K.M., Buhl, T., et al. (2009) Melanoma arising in segmental nevus spilus: detection by sequential digital dermatoscopy. *J Am Acad Dermatol* **61**(2): 337–41.

Kurban, R.S., Preffer, F.I., Sober, A.J., Mihm, M.C. Jr, and Barnhill, R.L. (1992) Occurrence of melanoma in "dysplastic" nevus spilus: report of case and analysis by flow cytometry. *J Cutan Pathol* **19**(5): 423–8.

Tavoloni Braga, J.C., Gomes, E., Macedo, M.P., et al. (2014) Early detection of melanoma arising within nevus spilus. *J Am Acad Dermatol* **70**(2): e31–2.

Torres, K.G., Carle, L., and Royer, M. (2017) Nevus spilus (speckled lentiginous nevus) in the oral cavity: report of a case and review of the literature. *Am J Dermatopathol* **39**(1): e8–12.

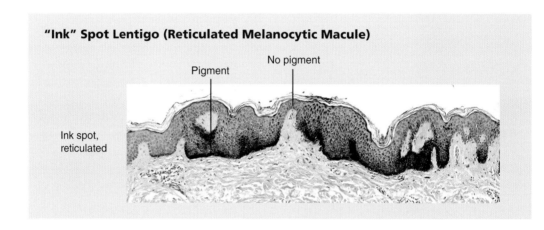

"Ink" Spot Lentigo (Reticulated Melanocytic Macule)

Cl: Small black bizarre spot with jagged borders ("black splash"), mostly in sun-exposed areas of adults.

Hi:

- Heavy hyperpigmentation of the epidermis, particularly at the tips of rete ridges
- Minimal increase of number of melanocytes
- Prominent hypopigmented skip zones between hyperpigmented rete ridges

Reference

Bolognia, J.L. (1992) Reticulated black solar lentigo ('ink spot' lentigo). *Arch Dermatol* **128**(7): 934–40.

Senile Freckles (Solar [Actinic] Lentigo)

Lentiginous spots on the back of the hand

Bud-like elongated rete ridges with basal hyperpigmentation ("dirty feet")

Solar elastosis

Pseudopod-like epidermal proliferations with hyperpigmentation

Cl: These common flat, pigmented lesions, preferentially located in sun-exposed areas of elderly individuals, are considered to be flat seborrheic keratosis.

Hi:
- Elongated pseudopod-like projections and lentiginous proliferation of rete ridges
- Increased pigment in keratinocytes at base of rete ridges ("dirty feet" sign)
- Number of melanocytes normal or slightly increased
- Solar elastosis in the upper dermis

DD: Lentigo maligna, other pigmented lentiginous lesions.

References

Black, W.H., Thareja, S.K., Blake, B.P., Chen, R., Cherpelis, B.S., and Glass, L.F. (2011) Distinction of melanoma in situ from solar lentigo on sundamaged skin using morphometrics and MITF immunohistochemistry. *Am J Dermatopathol* **33**(6): 573–8.

Feinmesser, M., Tsabari, C., Fichman, S., Hodak, E., Sulkes, J., and Okon, E. (2003) Differential expression of proliferation- and apoptosis-related markers in lentigo maligna and solar keratosis keratinocytes. *Am J Dermatopathol* **25**(4): 300–7.

Fraga, G.R. and Amin, S.M. (2014) Large cell acanthoma: a variant of solar lentigo with cellular hypertrophy. *J Cutan Pathol* **41**(9): 733–9.

Hillesheim, P.B., Slone, S., Kelley, D., Malone, J., and Bahrami, S. (2011) An immunohistochemical comparison between MiTF and MART-1 with Azure blue counterstaining in the setting of solar lentigo and melanoma in situ. *J Cutan Pathol* **38**(7): 565–9.

Sethi, M., Craythorne, E., Al-Arashi, M.Y., Bhawan, J., and Stefanato, C.M. (2014) Macromelanosomes: their significantly greater presence in the margins of a lentigo maligna versus solar lentigo. *Am J Dermatopathol* **36**(6): 490–2.

Mucosal Lentiginous Spots (Lip, Buccal, and Genital Mucosa)

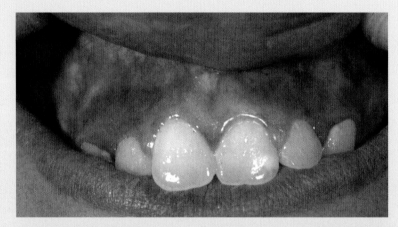

Gingiva

Labial lentigo

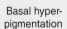

Basal hyper-pigmentation

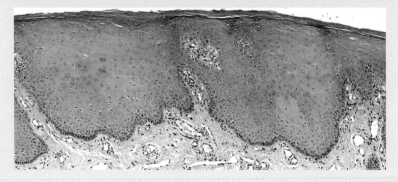

COMMON ACQUIRED MELANOCYTIC NEVI

Cl: These lesions may be solitary or syndromic (Peutz–Jeghers syndrome; Laugier–Hunziger syndrome).

Hi:
- Regular mucosa
- Basal hyperpigmentation
- No significant increase of number of melanocytes

DD: Incipient mucosal melanoma: increased number of irregularly spaced single melanocytes in the basal zone ("mycosis fungoides" pattern).

Nevi

Common Acquired Melanocytic Nevi

Melanosis Neviformis (Pigmented Hairy Epidermal Nevus; Becker Nevus)

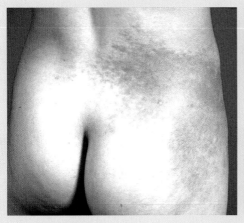 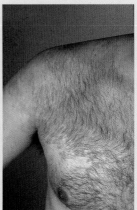

Hairless (left) and hairy (right) pigmented nevi

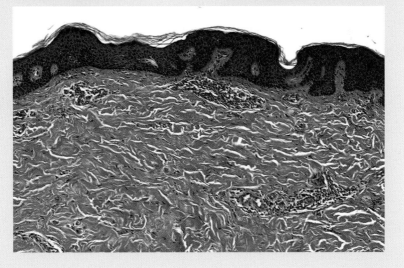

Acanthosis with basal hyper-pigmentation

"Flat bottom" rete tips

Cl: Even though the lesions exist from birth, they become apparent mostly in puberty as slightly hyperpigmented, irregular but sharply demarcated macules with growth of terminal hairs. Back and shoulder are favored sites.

Hi:
- Elongation of rete ridges with characteristic "flat bottom" rete tips throughout the lesion
- Normal number of melanocytes
- Melanin in basal keratinocytes
- Increased number of hair follicles and bundles of smooth muscle in the dermis

COMMON ACQUIRED MELANOCYTIC NEVI

Junctional Nevus

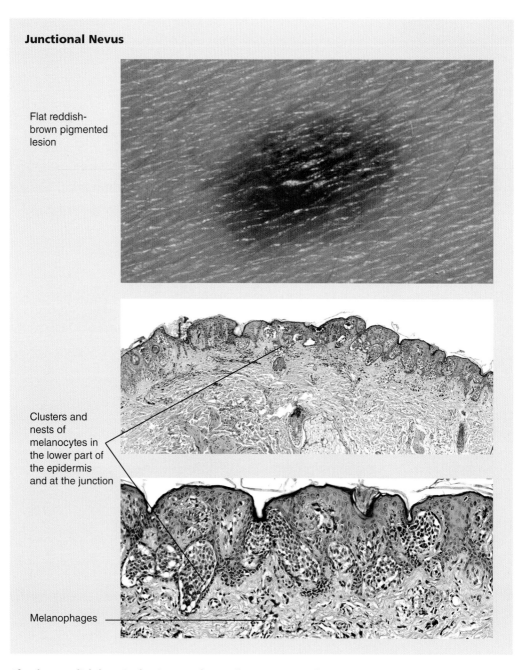

Flat reddish-brown pigmented lesion

Clusters and nests of melanocytes in the lower part of the epidermis and at the junction

Melanophages

Cl: Flat or slightly raised, pigmented macule; blurred border. Initial forms are referred to as lentigo simplex or even "jentigo" (junctional nevus/lentigo).

Hi:

- Melanocytes in single clusters and in nests
- Restricted to the lower part of the epidermis and the dermoepidermal junction
- Lateral borders ("shoulder") taper out with small peripheral nests

- No melanocytic atypia
- No melanocytes within the dermis
- Melanophages are often present
- Slight lymphocytic infiltrate may be present in the upper dermis

DD: Activated or proliferating junctional nevus, showing compact horny layer, replete with melanin granules, melanocytic activity at the base, broad band of melanophages and inflammatory infiltrate in the upper dermis.

COMMON ACQUIRED MELANOCYTIC NEVI

Compound Nevus

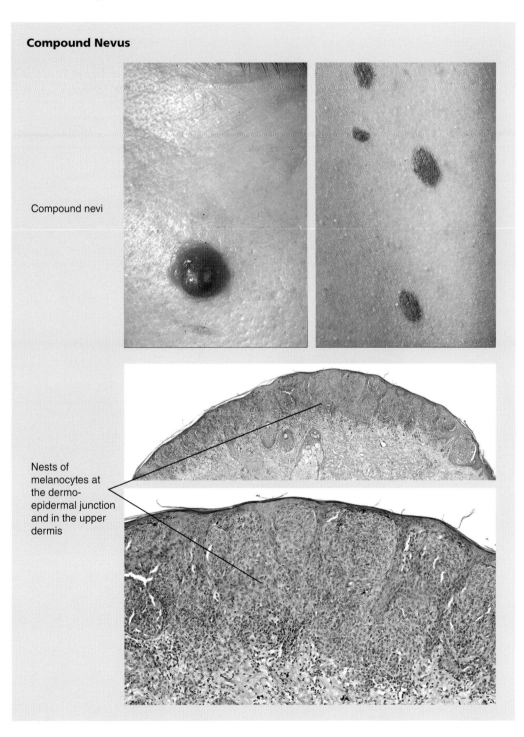

Compound nevi

Nests of melanocytes at the dermo-epidermal junction and in the upper dermis

Cl: Mostly pigmented papules of variable size, sometimes hairy.

Hi:
- Symmetrical melanocytic lesion with sharp borders

- Junctional part: intraepidermal nests of melanocytes
- Dermal part: dermal nests of melanocytes
- Broad papillae, filled with melanocytes
- Elongated rete ridges
- No single melanocytes above the basal layer

COMMON ACQUIRED MELANOCYTIC NEVI

Comment: Nevi on palms or soles (acral nevi) can have some melanocytes and pigment scattered intraepidermally. There may be transepidermal elimination of pigment and cells in these special localisations. MANIAC (melanocytic acral nevus with intraepidermal ascent of cells) is considered to be a melanoma impostor due to small melanocytic nests with transepidermal elimination. Overall features of MANIAC, however, are those of a dysplastic compound nevus in acral skin.

Dermal Nevus

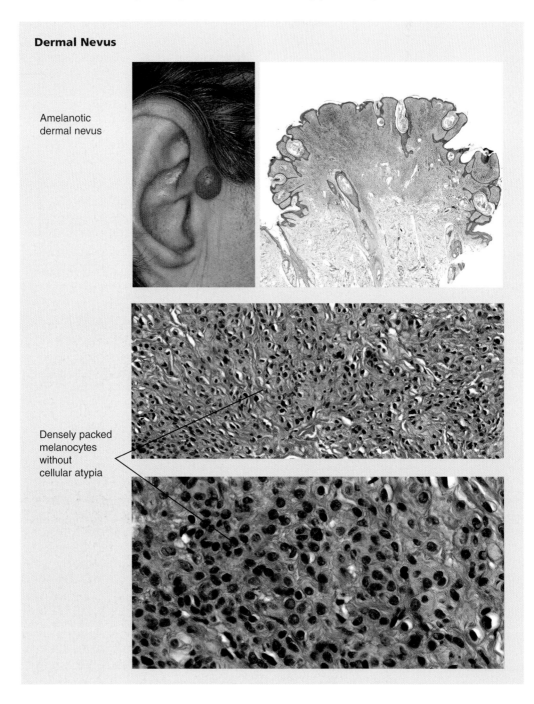

Amelanotic dermal nevus

Densely packed melanocytes without cellular atypia

COMMON ACQUIRED MELANOCYTIC NEVI

Dermal Nevus, with Maturation

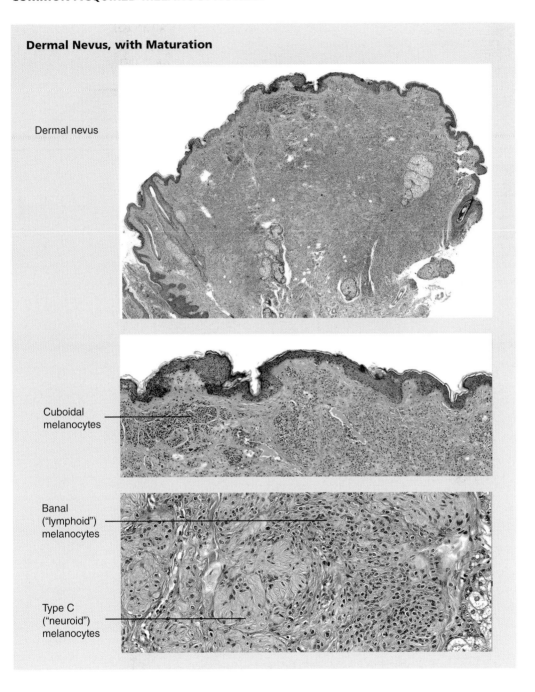

Dermal nevus

Cuboidal melanocytes

Banal ("lymphoid") melanocytes

Type C ("neuroid") melanocytes

COMMON ACQUIRED MELANOCYTIC NEVI

Dermal Nevus, with Maturation

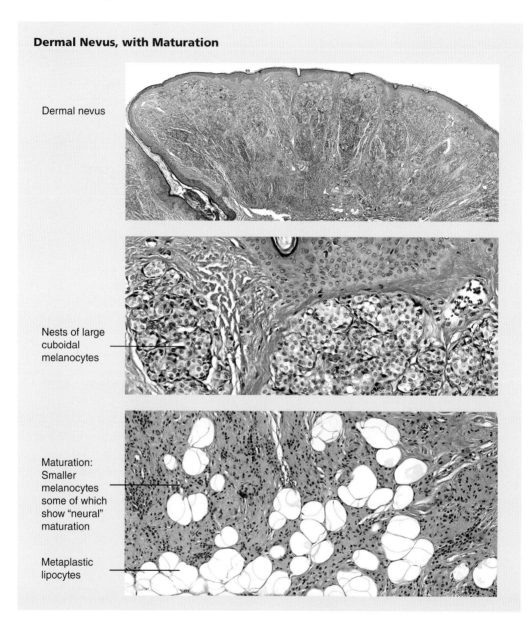

Dermal nevus

Nests of large
cuboidal
melanocytes

Maturation:
Smaller
melanocytes
some of which
show "neural"
maturation

Metaplastic
lipocytes

Cl: Papule, variably pigmented or amelanotic and skin-colored.

Hi:

• Nests and sheets of densely packed melanocytes within the dermis

• Melanocytes show well-defined cytoplasm; nuclei are roundish or oval with fine chromatin

• Multinuclear melanocytes are sometimes found

• The amount of melanin is variable

Comment: Dermal melanocytes "mature" (i.e. get smaller) when descending from upper dermal levels to deeper layers; large melanocytes eventually may evolve into smaller cells with roundish or epithelioid, sometimes even neuroid cell-like morphology (type C melanocytes).

Variant: Miescher's Nevus (Dermal Nevus)

Cl: Clinical variant, showing a broad-based skin-colored nodular lesion, usually on the face, head, and neck.

COMMON ACQUIRED MELANOCYTIC NEVI

Variant: Balloon Cell Nevus

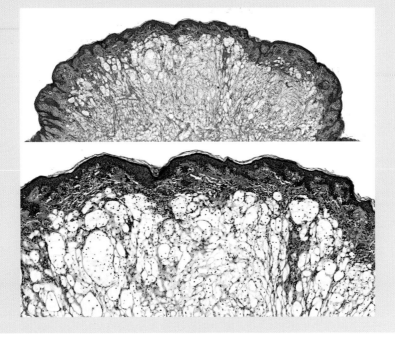

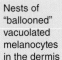
Nests of "ballooned" vacuolated melanocytes in the dermis

Cl: Histological variant of a melanocytic nevus.

Hi:

- Symmetry and sharp borders as in common melanocytic nevus
- The hallmarks are well-circumscribed nests and clusters of large melanocytes with pale cytoplasm
- Small, peripherally localized multinuclear balloon giant cells are frequently seen

References

Chiang, Y.Y., Tsai, H.H., Lee, W.R., and Wang, K.H. (2009) Clear cell fibrous papule: report of a case mimicking a balloon cell nevus. *J Cutan Pathol* **36**(3): 381–4.

Huang, Y.Y. and Vandergriff, T. (2017) Balloon cell change in common blue nevus. *J Cutan Pathol* **44**(4): 407–9.

McGowan, J.W., Smith, M.K., Ryan, M., and Hood, A.F. (2006) Proliferative nodules with balloon-cell change in a large congenital melanocytic nevus. *J Cutan Pathol* **33**(3): 253–5.

Urso, C. (2008) Nodal melanocytic nevus with balloon-cell change (nodal balloon-cell nevus). *J Cutan Pathol* **35**(7): 672–6.

Variant: "Activated" Acral (Lentiginous) Melanocytic Nevus

Columns of pigment in the compact cornified layer

Marked proliferation of large isomorphic melanocytes in the basal layer. Only minimal transepidermal elimination of single cells

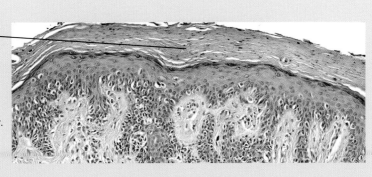

COMMON ACQUIRED MELANOCYTIC NEVI

Cl: The hairless skin of palms and soles with thick horny layers are favored sites.

Hi:

- Histological features of junctional nevus
- Sharp borders
- Narrow columns of pigment in the cornified layer
- In early lesions, only a few single melanocytes may be encountered above the basal layer. However, pagetoid spread of melanocytes is not a feature of acral nevus

DD: Acral lentiginous melanoma: increased numbers of irregularly spaced, single melanocytes in the basal layer without accompanying nest formation usually heralds early acrolentiginous melanoma *in situ* (mycosis fungoides-like pattern of early acrolentiginous melanoma). Intracorneal thrombotic deposits ("black heel") are a common clinical impostor of atypical melanocytic proliferation at palms and soles.

Reference

Saida, T., Koga, H., Goto, Y., and Uhara, H. (2011) Characteristic distribution of melanin columns in the cornified layer of acquired acral nevus: an important clue for histopathologic differentiation from early acral melanoma. *Am J Dermatopathol* **33**(5): 468–73.

Variant: (Atypical) Genital Melanocytic Nevus

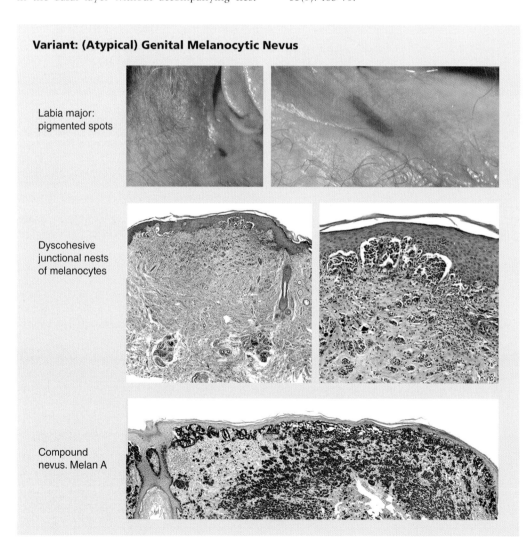

Labia major: pigmented spots

Dyscohesive junctional nests of melanocytes

Compound nevus. Melan A

COMMON ACQUIRED MELANOCYTIC NEVI

Cl: Mostly flat, clinically "atypical" lesions of the vulva, present in up to 5% of women.

Hi:
- Well-circumscribed symmetrical lesions
- Junctional or compound features
- Enlarged junctional nests of melanocytes
- Intraepidermal (pagetoid) melanocytes
- Slight cytological atypia

DD: Melanoma; epithelioid cell nevus (Spitz).

References

Brenn, T. (2011) Atypical genital nevus. *Arch Pathol Lab Med* **135**(3): 317–20.

Hunt, R.D., Orlow, S J., and Schaffer, J.V. (2014) Genital melanocytic nevi in children: experience in a pediatric dermatology practice. *J Am Acad Dermatol* **70**(3): 429–34.

Pinto, A., McLaren, S.H., Poppas, D.P., and Magro, C.M. (2012) Genital melanocytic nevus arising in a background of lichen sclerosus in a 7-year-old female: the diagnostic pitfall with malignant melanoma. A literature review. *Am J Dermatopathol* **34**(8): 838–43.

Polat, M., Topcuoglu, M.A., Tahtaci, Y., Hapa, A., and Yilmaz, F. (2009) Spitz nevus of the genital mucosa. *Indian J Dermatol Venereol Leprol* **75**(2): 167–9.

Quddus, M.R., Rashid, L.B., Sung, C.J., Robinson-Bostom, L., and Lawrence, W.D. (2010) Atypical melanocytic nevi of genital type: a distinctive pigmented lesion of the genital tract often confused with malignant melanoma. *Dermatol Online J* **16**(2): 9.

Ribe, A. (2008) Melanocytic lesions of the genital area with attention given to atypical genital nevi. *J Cutan Pathol* **35**(Suppl 2): 24–7.

Tseng, D., Kim, J., Warrick, A., et al. (2014) Oncogenic mutations in melanomas and benign melanocytic nevi of the female genital tract. *J Am Acad Dermatol* **71**(2): 229–36.

Variant: Halo Nevus (Leukoderma Centrifugum Acquisitum; Sutton Nevus)

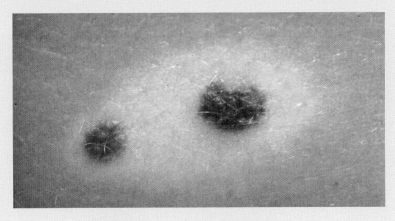

Depigmentation around compound nevi

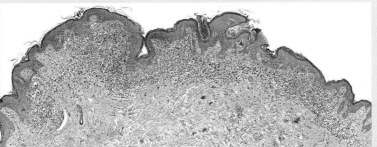

Dome-shaped lesion with dense lymphocytic infiltrate with melanophages

COMMON ACQUIRED MELANOCYTIC NEVI

Variant: Halo Nevus (Leukoderma Centrifugum Acquisitum; Sutton Nevus)

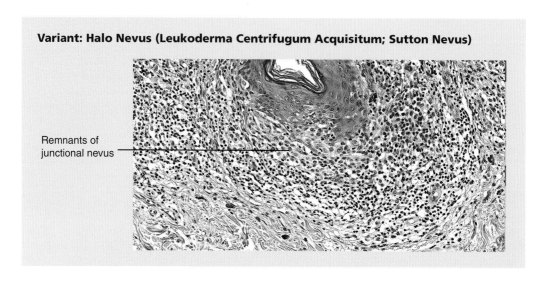

Remnants of
junctional nevus

Cl: Solitary or multiple, mostly in children and young adults. Depigmented outer ring around a nevus or remnants of an involuted nevus in the center. Late lesions of Sutton nevus quite often are repigmented and the diagnosis can only be established histologically.

Hi:

- Remnants of irregularly shaped junctional, compound or dermal nevus cell nests
- Diminished/absent melanocytes at the periphery of the lesion
- Dense infiltrate composed of lymphocytes, camouflaging the pre-existing melanocytic nests
- Inflammatory cells throughout the nevus, sometimes with signs of incipient regression at the shoulders
- Focal epithelial atrophy with adjacent bands of confluent melanocytes (incomplete consumption of the epidermis)
- Moderate melanocytic polymorphism without mitoses
- Melanophages are not a leading feature
- Rete ridges preserved. Lesion always slightly dome-shaped, never flat

Immunophenotype: SOX-10, MART-1 or other stains for melanocytes.

DD: Malignant melanoma; Spitz nevus; lichen planus.

References

Harvey, N.T., Millward, M., Macgregor, K., Bucat, R.P., and Wood, B.A. (2016) Cutaneous metastatic melanoma resembling a halo nevus, in the setting of PD-1 inhibition. *Am J Dermatopathol* **38**(12): e159–62.

Lee, N.R., Chung, H.C., Hong, H., Lee, J.W., and Ahn, S.K. (2015) Spontaneous involution of congenital melanocytic nevus with halo phenomenon. *Am J Dermatopathol* **37**(12): e137–9.

Moretti, S., Spallanzani, A., Pinzi, C., Prignano, F., and Fabbri, P. (2007) Fibrosis in regressing melanoma versus nonfibrosis in halo nevus upon melanocyte disappearance: could it be related to a different cytokine microenvironment? *J Cutan Pathol* **34**(4): 301–8.

Steffen, C. and Thomas, D. (2003) The man behind the eponyms: Richard L Sutton: periadenitis mucosa necrotica recurrens (Sutton's ulcer) and leukoderma acquisitum centrifugum-Sutton's (halo) nevus. *Am J Dermatopathol* **25**(4): 349–54.

COMMON ACQUIRED MELANOCYTIC NEVI

Variant: Eczematoid Melanocytic (Meyerson's) Nevus

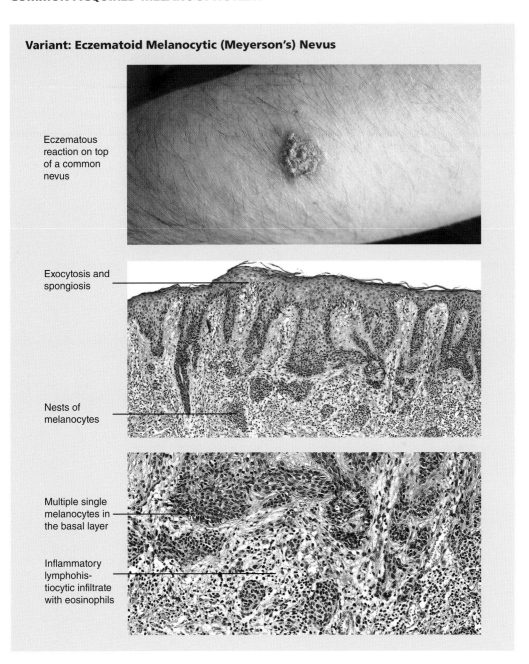

Eczematous reaction on top of a common nevus

Exocytosis and spongiosis

Nests of melanocytes

Multiple single melanocytes in the basal layer

Inflammatory lymphohis-tiocytic infiltrate with eosinophils

Cl: Common nevus with eczematous oozing and crusty surface. No history of injury.

Hi:

- Acanthosis and spongiosis of the epidermis reflecting eczematous changes that are restricted to the site of the melanocytic proliferation, stopping at the shoulders
- Common junctional, compound or congenital nevus in the upper dermis
- Junctional and early lesions with a multitude of isomorphic single melanocytes, some of them above the basal layer
- Homogeneous proliferation pattern
- Lymphohistiocytic infiltrate with eosinophils in the upper dermis between nests of melanocytes

COMMON ACQUIRED MELANOCYTIC NEVI

References

Conde-Taboada, A., de la Torre, C., Feal, C., Mayo, E., Gonzalez-Sixto, B., and Cruces, M. J. (2005) Meyerson's naevi induced by interferon alfa plus ribavirin combination therapy in hepatitis C infection. *Br J Dermatol* **153**(5): 1070–2.

Cook-Norris, R.H., Zic, J.A., and Boyd, A.S. (2008) Meyerson's naevus: a clinical and histopathological study of 11 cases. *Australas J Dermatol* **49**(4): 191–5.

Dawn, G. and Burden, A.D. (2002) Meyerson's phenomenon around a seborrhoeic keratosis. *Clin Exp Dermatol* **27**(1): 73.

Girard, C., Bessis, D., Blatire, V., Guilhou, J.J., and Guillot, B. (2005) Meyerson's phenomenon induced by interferon-alfa plus ribavirin in hepatitis C infection. *Br J Dermatol* **152**(1): 182–3.

Meyerson, L.B. (1971) A peculiar papulosquamous eruption involving pigmented nevi. *Arch Dermatol* **103**(5): 510–12.

Pizem, J., Stojanovic, L., and Luzar, B. (2012) Melanocytic lesions with eczematous reaction (Meyerson's phenomenon) – a histopathologic analysis of 64 cases. *J Cutan Pathol* **39**(10): 901–10.

Ramon, R., Silvestre, J.F., Betlloch, I., Banuls, J., Botella, R., and Navas, J. (2000) Progression of Meyerson's naevus to Sutton's naevus. *Dermatology* **200**(4): 337–8.

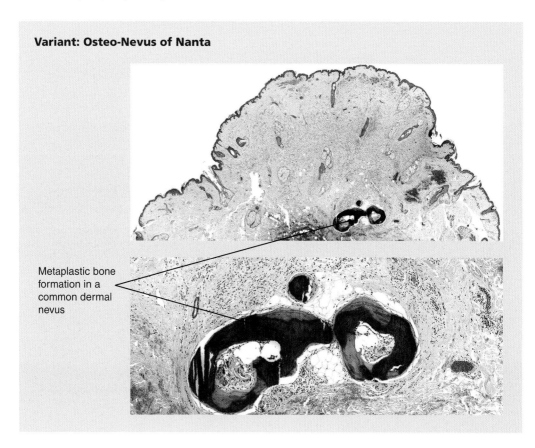

Variant: Osteo-Nevus of Nanta

Metaplastic bone formation in a common dermal nevus

Cl: Common nevus.

Hi: Osteoma cutis in association with a common dermal nevus; metaplastic ossification within or at the base of the lesion.

References

Abessi, B., Meyer, D.R., and Carlson, J.A. (2012) Osteoma cutis (nevus of nanta) of the eyebrow. *Ophthal Plast Reconstr Surg* **28**(1): 74–5.

Al-Daraji, W. (2007) Osteo-nevus of Nanta (osseous metaplasia in a benign intradermal melanocytic nevus): an uncommon phenomenon. *Dermatol Online J* **13**(4): 16.

Bezic, J., Karaman, I., Zekic Tomas, S., Zivkovic, P.M., and Bozic, J. (2016) Osteonevus of Nanta revisited: clinicopathological features of 33 cases. *Am J Dermatopathol* **38**(11): 859–61.

Keida, T., Hayashi, N., Kawakami, M., and Kawashima, M. (2005) Transforming growth factor beta and connective tissue growth factor are involved in the evolution of nevus of Nanta. *J Dermatol* **32**(6): 442–5.

COMMON ACQUIRED MELANOCYTIC NEVI

Variant: Combined Epithelioid Spitzoid Nevus, "Wiesner Nevus" (BAP-1 Deficient Epithelioid Melanocytic Tumor)

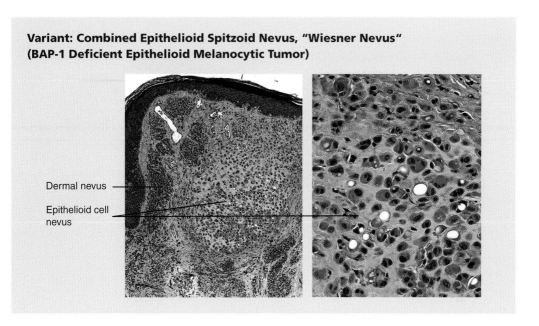

Dermal nevus

Epithelioid cell nevus

Hi: Features of a common junctional or dermal nevus combined with a banal or cellular blue nevus. Both nevus variants may lie side by side, or gradually blend into each other.

Variant: Recurrent (Persistent) Melanocytic Nevus (Pseudomelanoma)

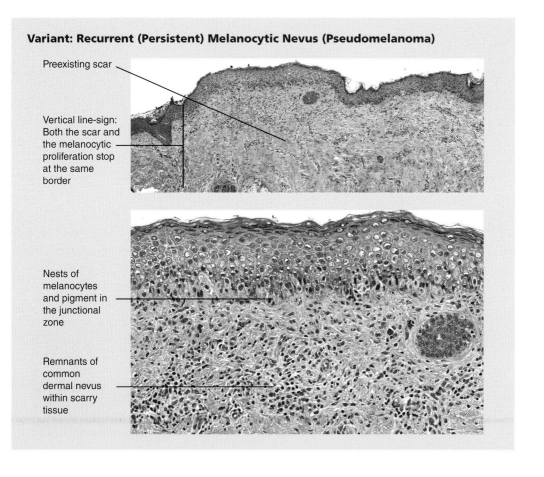

Preexisting scar

Vertical line-sign: Both the scar and the melanocytic proliferation stop at the same border

Nests of melanocytes and pigment in the junctional zone

Remnants of common dermal nevus within scarry tissue

COMMON ACQUIRED MELANOCYTIC NEVI

Variant: Recurrent (Persistent) Melanocytic Nevus (Pseudomelanoma)

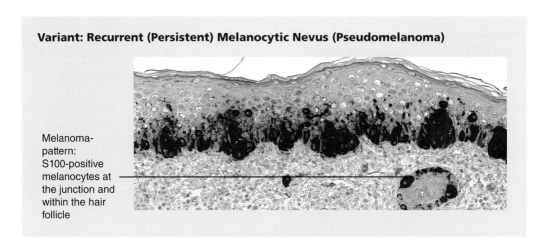

Melanoma-pattern: S100-positive melanocytes at the junction and within the hair follicle

Cl: Scar, usually showing irregular pigmentation, following incomplete surgical removal (shave) or injury with accidental partial removal of a former common melanocytic nevus.

Hi:

- Well-circumscribed melanocytic proliferation, strictly overlying a pre-existing scar
- No lateral spread: junctional melanocytic nests stop at either end of the scar ("screeching halt" sign)
- Effacement of the epidermal rete ridges
- Irregular nests of melanocytes in the junctional zone simulating evolving melanoma
- Moderate cytological atypia but no mitoses
- No transepidermal elimination of single melanocytes
- A few scattered melanocytes may be seen above the dermal epidermal junction directly over the scar
- Residual banal dermal nevus nests may be present beneath the overlying dermal scar

DD: Malignant melanoma.

References

Boer, A., Wolter, M., and Kaufmann, R. (2003) [Pseudomelanoma following laser treatment or laser-treated melanoma?] *J Dtsch Dermatol Ges* **1**(1): 47–50.

Grunwald, M.H., Gat, A., and Amichai, B. (2006) Pseudomelanoma after Solcoderm treatment. *Melanoma Res* **16**(5): 459–60.

Hwang, K., Lee, W.J., and Lee, S.I. (2002) Pseudomelanoma after laser therapy. *Ann Plast Surg* **48**(5): 562–4.

Lee, H.W., Ahn, S.J., Lee, M.W., Choi, J.H., Moon, K.C., and Koh, J.K. (2006) Pseudomelanoma following laser therapy. *J Eur Acad Dermatol Venereol* **20**(3): 342–4.

Variant: Nevus in Pregnancy

"Atypical" nevi in pregnancy

COMMON ACQUIRED MELANOCYTIC NEVI

Variant: Nevus in Pregnancy

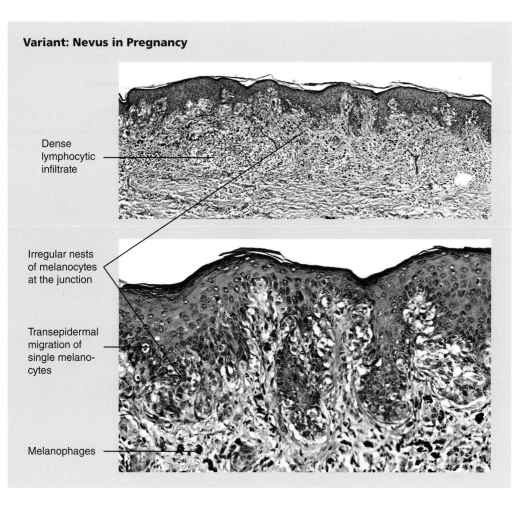

Dense lymphocytic infiltrate

Irregular nests of melanocytes at the junction

Transepidermal migration of single melanocytes

Melanophages

Cl: Atypical changes can be seen in some melanocytic nevi during pregnancy.

Hi:

- The lesion is symmetrical and sharply demarcated, showing features of an activated nevus
- Junctional "activity" with irregular melanocytic nests
- Few single melanocytes above the basal layer, but no pagetoid melanocytic pattern
- Low mitotic activity may be present
- Melanophages and inflammatory infiltrate in the dermis

DD: Malignant melanoma; melanoma arising in a pre-existing nevus.

References

Katz, V.L., Farmer, R.M., and Dotters, D. (2002) Focus on primary care: from nevus to neoplasm: myths of melanoma in pregnancy. *Obstet Gynecol Surv* **57**(2): 112–19.

Lee, H.J., Ha, S.J., Lee, S.J., and Kim, J.W. (2000) Melanocytic nevus with pregnancy-related changes in size accompanied by apoptosis of nevus cells: a case report. *J Am Acad Dermatol* **42**(5 Pt 2): 936–8.

Nading, M.A., Nanney, L.B., and Ellis, D.L. (2009) Pregnancy and estrogen receptor beta expression in a large congenital nevus. *Arch Dermatol* **145**(6): 691–4.

Trayanov, I., Trayanova, E., Chokoeva, A., and Tchernev, G. (2015) [Congenital melanocytic nevus of the shoulder with rapid growth progression during pregnancy. Successful surgical approach]. *Akush Ginekol (Sofiia)* **54**(8): 51–6.

Wilford, C.E., Brantley, J.S., and Diwan, A.H. (2014) Atypical histopathologic features in a melanocytic nevus after cryotherapy and pregnancy. *J Cutan Pathol* **41**(10): 802–5.

COMMON ACQUIRED MELANOCYTIC NEVI

Variant: Ancient Nevus

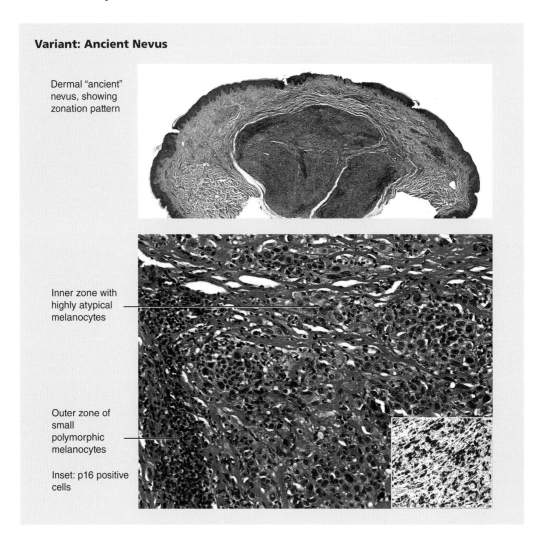

Dermal "ancient" nevus, showing zonation pattern

Inner zone with highly atypical melanocytes

Outer zone of small polymorphic melanocytes

Inset: p16 positive cells

Cl: Simulator of malignant melanoma. Head and neck area of adults. Papular or nodular lesion resembling common dermal (Miescher) nevus. Named in analogy to ancient schwannoma.

Hi:

- Pleomorphic dermal nevus with prominent zonation pattern
- Outer zone composed of small- to medium-sized, slightly polymorphic melanocytes with moderate accompanying inflammatory infiltrate
- Inner zone composed of confluent nests and sheets with highly atypical and pleomorphic melanocytes, some of them with spitzoid and rhabdoid features
- Very few mitoses (<2 per section)

Immunohistochemistry: Loss of nuclear BAP-1 expression in conjunction with cytoplasmic VE1 positivity (*BRAF* V600E mutation).

DD: Malignant melanoma; melanoma metastasis; atypical spitzoid tumor.

Comment: Recently, ancient nevus has been subsumed under the heading of BAP1-deficient melanocytic proliferations ("BAP-oma") which may occur sporadically as well as in the context of a germline mutation with accompanying familial cancer syndrome. Gradual transition from ancient nevus to malignant melanoma in a multistep process is possible.

References

Kerl, H., Wolf, I.H., Kerl, K., Cerroni, L., Kutzner, H., and Argenyi, Z.B. (2011) Ancient melanocytic nevus: a simulator of malignant melanoma. *Am J Dermatopathol* **33**(2): 127–30.

BLUE NEVI

Kerl, H., Soyer, H.P., Cerroni, L., Wolf, I.H., and Ackerman, A.B. (1998) Ancient melanocytic nevus. *Semin Diagn Pathol* **15**(3): 210–15.

Wiesner, T., Obenauf, A.C., Murali, R., et al. (2011) Germline mutations in BAP1 predispose to melanocytic tumors. *Nat Genet* **43**(10): 1018–21.

Blue Nevi

Several morphological variants exist, depending on the degree of stroma fibrosclerosis and melanocytic cellularity.

Common Blue Nevus

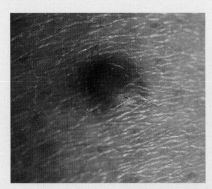
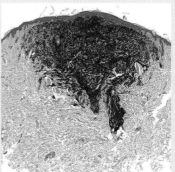

Sharply demarcated hyperpigmented melanocytic lesion in the dermis

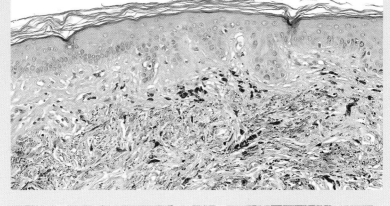

Pigmented, dendritic and stellate melanocytes together with melanophages

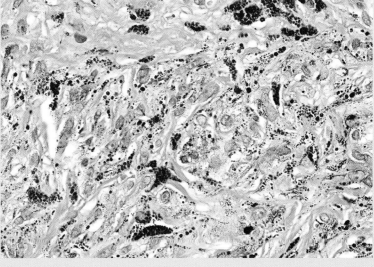

Accumulation of melanin dispersed within melanocytes and within melanophages

VARIANTS OF COMMON BLUE NEVUS

Cl: The typical lesion is a well-circumscribed dome-shaped bluish-black papule. The color is due to the localisation of dispersed pigment in mid and deep dermis.

Hi:

- Normal epidermis
- No junctional melanocytic nests
- Single or fascicularly arranged elongated, bipolar or stellate dendritic melanocytes between densely packed dermal collagen

- Dense accumulation of fine melanin dispersed within the melanocytes and within melanophages
- Melanocytes sometimes aggregating around appendages and neurovascular tissue
- Variable degree of fibrosis; sclerotic stroma in most cases

Common Blue Nevus

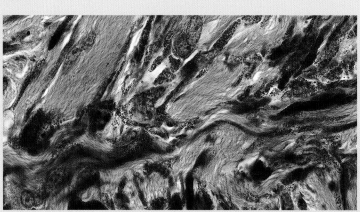

Pigmented bipolar, dendritic and stellate melanocytes

- Superficial variant is limited to the upper half of the dermis
- Remarkably, junctional activity is always completely missing, with the exception of deep penetrating nevus
- Deep penetrating nevus affects the whole thickness of the dermis, including the dermal-epidermal junction, and may reach into the subcutaneous fat
- Combined nevus (see above): collision of two types of nevus, mostly banal congenital nevus and common blue cellular nevus
- Pigmented epithelioid melanocytoma and Carney's syndrome-associated blue nevus: large atypical spitzoid melanocytes may be present, albeit without mitoses
- Presence of any necrosis may suggest malignant transformation
- Cellular blue nevus (neuro-nevus) showing deep-reaching, dumb bell-shaped pale cellular fascicles of melanocytes with overlying common blue nevus in the upper dermis (see below)

DD: Malignant blue nevus is a morphological variant of heavily pigmented malignant melanoma; blue nevus-like metastasis of malignant melanoma: patches of atypical hyperpigmented melanocytes in a blue nevus-like pattern, often accompanied by inflammatory infiltrate and mitoses; dermal melanocytosis, indistiguishable from nevus Ota or nevus Ito; nodular melanoma; hydrocystome noire; hemosiderotic dermatofibroma.

References

Bhawan, J. and Cao, S.L. (1999) Amelanotic blue nevus: a variant of blue nevus. *Am J Dermatopathol* **21**(3): 225–8.

Bui, J., Ardakani, N.M., Tan, I., Crocker, A., Khattak, M.A., and Wood, B.A. (2017) Metastatic cellular blue nevus: a rare case with metastasis beyond regional nodes. *Am J Dermatopathol* **39**(8): 618–21.

Busam, K.J. and Lohmann, C.M. (2004) Congenital pauci-melanotic cellular blue nevus. *J Cutan Pathol* **31**(4): 312–17.

VARIANTS OF COMMON BLUE NEVUS

Campa, M., Patel, M., Aubert, P., Hosler, G., and Witheiler, D. (2016) Blue nevus-like metastasis of a cutaneous melanoma identified by fluorescence in situ hybridization. *Am J Dermatopathol* **38**(9): 695–7.

Carr, S., See, J., Wilkinson, B., and Kossard, S. (1997) Hypopigmented common blue nevus. *J Cutan Pathol* **24**(8): 494–8.

Dohse, L. and Ferringer, T. (2010) Nodal blue nevus: a pitfall in lymph node biopsies. *J Cutan Pathol* **37**(1): 102–4.

Ferrara, G., Soyer, H.P., Malvehy, J., et al. (2007) The many faces of blue nevus: a clinicopathologic study. *J Cutan Pathol* **34**(7): 543–51.

Huang, Y.Y. and Vandergriff, T. (2017) Balloon cell change in common blue nevus. *J Cutan Pathol* **44**(4): 407–9.

Kacerovska, D., Michal, M., and Kazakov, D.V. (2008) Sebocyte-like melanocytes in desmoplastic blue nevus. *Am J Dermatopathol* **30**(5): 509–10.

Kuhn, A., Groth, W., Gartmann, H., and Steigleder, G.K. (1988) Malignant blue nevus with metastases to the lung. *Am J Dermatopathol* **10**(5): 436–41.

Mones, J.M. and Ackerman, A.B. (2004) "Atypical" blue nevus, "malignant" blue nevus, and "metastasizing" blue nevus: a critique in historical perspective of three concepts flawed fatally. *Am J Dermatopathol* **26**(5): 407–30.

Moreno, C., Requena, L., Kutzner, H., de la Cruz, A., Jaqueti, G., and Yus, E.S. (2000) Epithelioid blue nevus: a rare variant of blue nevus not always associated with the Carney complex. *J Cutan Pathol* **27**(5): 218–23.

North, J.P., Yeh, I., McCalmont, T.H., and LeBoit, P.E. (2012).Melanoma ex blue nevus: two cases resembling large plaque-type blue nevus with subcutaneous cellular nodules. *J Cutan Pathol* **39**(12): 1094–9.

Perez, M.T. and Suster, S. (1999) Balloon cell change in cellular blue nevus. *Am J Dermatopathol* **21**(2): 181–4.

Piana, S., Grenzi, L., and Albertini, G. (2009) Cellular blue nevus with satellitosis: a possible diagnostic pitfall. *Am J Dermatopathol* **31**(4): 401–2.

Schopper, H.K., Stone, M.S., and Wanat, K.A. (2015) Blue nevus with tubule and pseudoacini formation. *J Cutan Pathol* **42**(11): 914–15.

Temple-Camp, C.R., Saxe, N., and King, H. (1988) Benign and malignant cellular blue nevus. A clinicopathological study of 30 cases. *Am J Dermatopathol* **10**(4): 289–96.

Tran, T.A., Carlson, J.A., Basaca, P.C., and Mihm, M.C. (1998) Cellular blue nevus with atypia (atypical cellular blue nevus): a clinicopathologic study of nine cases. *J Cutan Pathol* **25**(5): 252–8.

Zyrek-Betts, J., Micale, M., Lineen, A., et al. (2008) Malignant blue nevus with lymph node metastases. *J Cutan Pathol* **35**(7): 651–7.

Variant: Deep Penetrating Blue Nevus

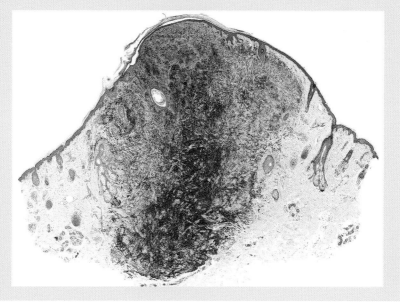

Melanocytes and pigment throughout the dermis reaching into the subcutis

VARIANTS OF COMMON BLUE NEVUS

Variant: Deep Penetrating Blue Nevus

Enlarged melanocytes with vesicular nuclei. Some epithelioid hyperpigmented melanocytes

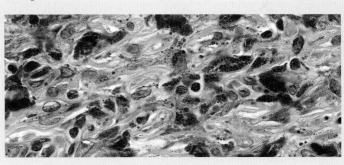

Variant: Cellular Deep Penetrating Blue Nevus (Neuro-Nevus)

Pattern of banal blue nevus on top, "dumb-bell pattern" of cellular nevus at the bottom

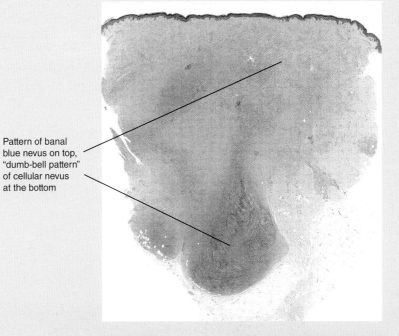

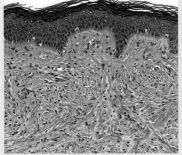

Subepidermal part

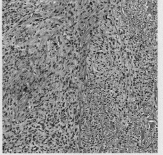

Deep dermal part

VARIANTS OF COMMON BLUE NEVUS

Variant: Cellular Blue Nevus, Hypopigmented

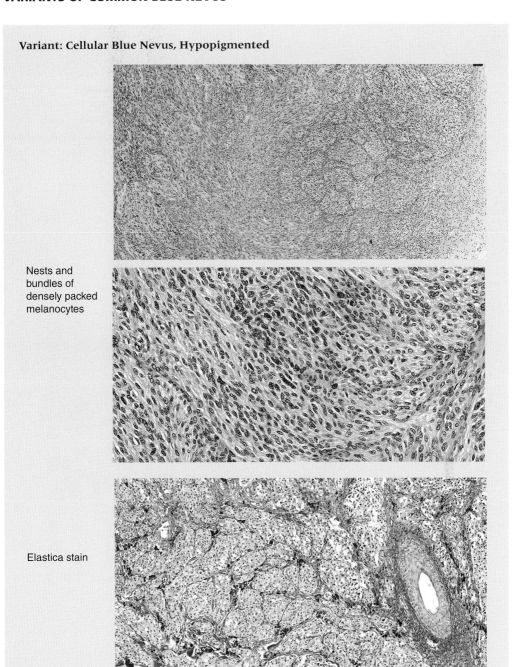

Nests and bundles of densely packed melanocytes

Elastica stain

VARIANTS OF COMMON BLUE NEVUS

Variant: Pigmented "Epithelioid" Blue Nevus

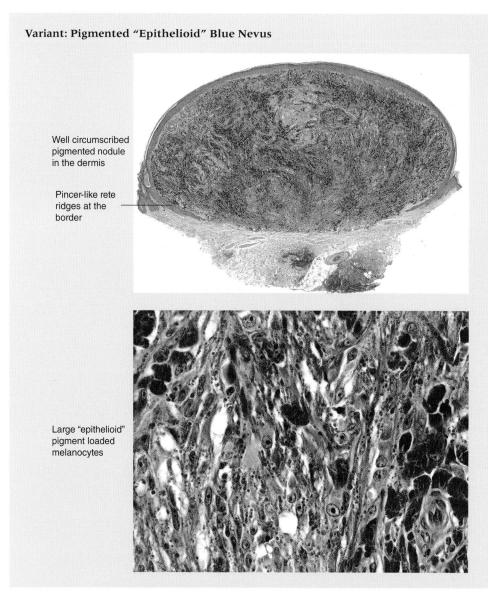

Well circumscribed pigmented nodule in the dermis

Pincer-like rete ridges at the border

Large "epithelioid" pigment loaded melanocytes

Cl: Features of common dermal nevus.

Hi:

- Symmetrical wedge-shaped or multi-wedge-shaped ("inverted pyramids") deep penetrating melanocytic proliferation, involving the entire dermis
- Pattern of banal blue nevus on top, dumb bell pattern of cellular nevus at the bottom
- Throughout the entire lesion, small nests composed of pigmented banal melanocytes and larger ("spitzoid") melanocytes with ample cytoplasm and vesicular nuclei showing various degrees of pigmentation
- Large melanophages, evenly distributed in a "net-like" pattern throughout the lesion
- No significant pleomorphism
- Very few mitoses (<2 per lesion)
- Multistep evolution into melanoma has been reported, with multiple mitoses as a significant indicator of transformation

DD: Malignant melanoma; pigmented epithelioid melanocytoma (PEM); Carney syndrome-associated nevus.

References

Almodovar-Real, A., Molina-Leyva, A., Aneiros-Fernandez, J., and Diaz-Martinez, M.A. (2017)

DERMAL MELANOCYTOSIS

Proliferative nodule in melanocytic nevi mimicking deep penetrating nevus. *An Bras Dermatol* **92**(2): 231–3.

Gupta, A., Srilatha, P.S., Suvarna, N., and Rao, L. (2011) Deep penetrating nevus: a distinct variant of melanocytic nevus. *Indian J Pathol Microbiol* **54**(1): 156–7.

Luzar, B and Calonje, E. (2011). Deep penetrating nevus: a review. *Arch Pathol Lab Med* **135**(3): 321–6.

Perez, O.G., Villoldo, M.S., Schroh, R., and Woscoff, A. (2009) Deep penetrating naevus. *J Eur Acad Dermatol Venereol* **23**(6): 703–4.

Ridha, H., Ahmed, S., Theaker, J.M., and Horlock, N. (2007) Malignant melanoma and deep penetrating naevus – difficulties in diagnosis in children. *J Plast Reconstr Aesthet Surg* **60**(11): 1252–5.

Robson, A., Morley-Quante, M., Hempel, H., McKee, P.H., and Calonje, E. (2003) Deep penetrating naevus: clinicopathological study of 31 cases with further delineation of histological features allowing distinction from other pigmented benign melanocytic lesions and melanoma. *Histopathology* **43**(6): 529–37.

Strazzula, L., Senna, M.M., Yasuda, M., and Belazarian, L. (2014) The deep penetrating nevus. *J Am Acad Dermatol* **71**(6): 1234–40.

Dermal Melanocytosis

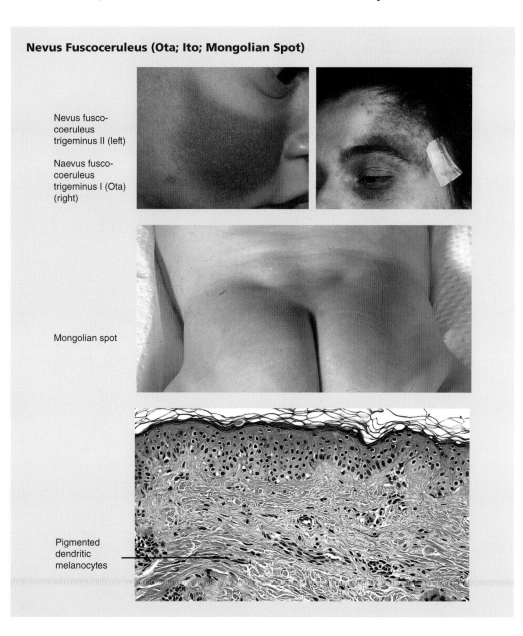

Nevus Fuscoceruleus (Ota; Ito; Mongolian Spot)

Nevus fusco-coeruleus trigeminus II (left)

Naevus fusco-coeruleus trigeminus I (Ota) (right)

Mongolian spot

Pigmented dendritic melanocytes

SPINDLE AND/OR EPITHELIOID CELL NEVUS

Dermal melanocytoses are macular variants of blue nevi in special localisations. Lesions are present from birth or appear in childhood.

Cl:

- Nevus Ota (nevus fuscoceruleus ophthalmomaxillaris) involving neural innervation domains of branch I or II of the trigeminal nerve (V. cranial nerve)
- Nevus Ito (acromiodeltoideus) involving the shoulder girdle
- Mongolian spot involving the sacral area

Hi: Remarkably, only a few dendritic melanocytes and scarce scattered pigment are found throughout the upper and mid dermis ("invisible dermatosis").

Immunohistochemistry: Melan A or S100 stains allow unequivocal diagnosis.

Spindle and/or Epithelioid Cell Nevus

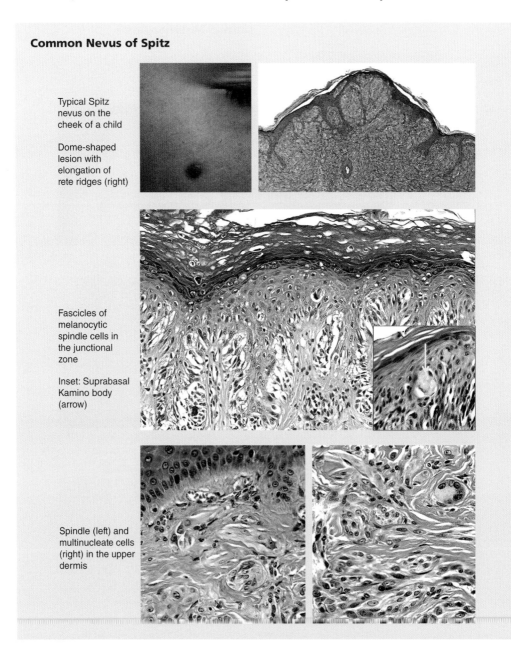

Common Nevus of Spitz

Typical Spitz nevus on the cheek of a child

Dome-shaped lesion with elongation of rete ridges (right)

Fascicles of melanocytic spindle cells in the junctional zone

Inset: Suprabasal Kamino body (arrow)

Spindle (left) and multinucleate cells (right) in the upper dermis

SPINDLE AND/OR EPITHELIOID CELL NEVUS

Cl: Pink or red-brown well-circumscribed papule with smooth surface, preferentially developing over several months in the face of children and young adults. Multiple, grouped or agminated lesions can occur.

Hi:

- Exophytic growth pattern
- The shape of the lesion is symmetrical, the bottom is usually flat or pyramid-like wedge shaped, lateral borders are sharp
- The hallmarks are nests of uniform large spindle-shaped and epithelioid melanocytes in the papillary dermis and between elongated rete ridges
  - Epithelioid cells with amphophilic eosinophilic cytoplasm, centrally located nucleus and relatively large nucleolus; fine dispersed chromatin
  - Fusiform spindle cells arranged as fascicles in vertical orientation
- Abundant "ground glass" cytoplasm of spindle cells and epithelioid cells
- Multinucleated cells may be present
- Clefts between the nests and the adjacent keratinocytes
- Eosinophilic amorphous pink globules of degenerative basement membrane material (Kamino bodies) in the lower part of the epidermis

- "Maturation" of the melanocytes from the top of the lesion with larger nests at the dermoepidermal junction to smaller nests and single cells in the deeper parts of the nevus
- Few mitoses in the upper dermal parts – minimal mitotic activity at the base
- Sometimes lymphocytic infiltrate
- Asymmetry, lack of maturation, and multiple mitoses at the base are criteria of severe atypia and presumed malignant transformation (AST: atypical spitzoid tumor)
- Comparative genomic hybridization can be helpful in separating benign lesions and spitzoid melanoma
- Frequent HRAS gene mutation

Variants of Spindle and Epithelioid Cell Nevus

- Junctional type
- Compound type
- Dermal type
- Desmoplastic forms with sclerotic stroma and interspersed single spitzoid melanocytes
- Balloon cell variant
- Pagetoid variant
- Intraoral nevus

Variant: Nevus Spitz, Junctional

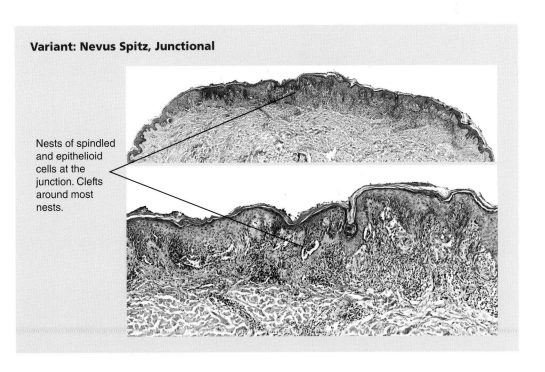

Nests of spindled and epithelioid cells at the junction. Clefts around most nests.

Variant: Nevus Spitz, Junctional

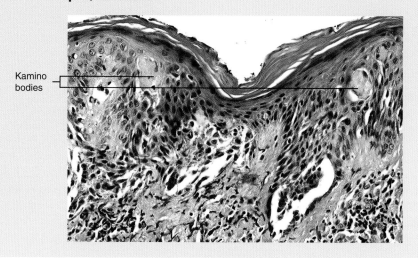

Kamino
bodies

Variant: Atypical (Desmoplastic sive Sclerosing Nevus Spitz)

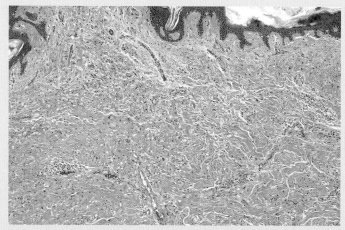

Large atypical melanocytes, solitary or grouped, in a background of thick collagen bundles

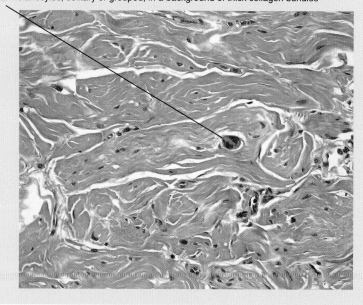

SPINDLE AND/OR EPITHELIOID CELL NEVUS

DD: Spitzoid melanoma; common melanocytic nevus; mastocytoma; juvenile xanthogranuloma; fibrohistiocytic proliferations (S100 negative).

References

Cavicchini, S., Nazzaro, G., Balice, Y., and Fiorani, R. (2015) Pigmented Spitz nevus simulating a solitary angiokeratoma. *J Am Acad Dermatol* **72**(4): e99–100.

Clarke, B., Essa, A., and Chetty, R. (2002) Plexiform spitz nevus. *Int J Surg Pathol* **10**(1): 69–73.

Dhouib, R.S., Sassi, S., Jbeli, A., et al. (2008) Desmoplastic spitz nevus: report of a case and review of the literature. *Pathologica* **100**(3): 181–4.

Fernandez-Flores, A., Saeb-Lima, M., and Rodriguez-Peralto, J.L. (2017) Polypoid Spitz nevus with a halo reaction. *Am J Dermatopathol* **39**(2): 130–3.

Ferrara, G., Gianotti, R., Cavicchini, S., Salviato, T., Zalaudek, I., and Argenziano, G. (2013) Spitz nevus, Spitz tumor, and spitzoid melanoma: a comprehensive clinicopathologic overview. *Dermatol Clin* **31**(4)) 589–98, viii.

Gill, M., Cohen, J., Renwick, N., Mones, J.M., Silvers, D.N., and Celebi, J.T. (2004) Genetic similarities between Spitz nevus and Spitzoid melanoma in children. *Cancer* **101**(11): 2636–40.

Han, M.H., Koh, K.J., Choi, J.H., Sung, K.J., Moon, K.C., and Koh, J.K. (2000) Pagetoid Spitz nevus: a variant of Spitz nevus. *Int J Dermatol* **39**(7): 555–7.

Hilliard, N.J., Krahl, D., and Sellheyer, K. (2009) p16 expression differentiates between desmoplastic Spitz nevus and desmoplastic melanoma. *J Cutan Pathol* **36**(7): 753–9.

Hoang, M.P. (2003) Myxoid Spitz nevus. *J Cutan Pathol* **30**(9): 566–8.

Isabel Zhu, Y. and Fitzpatrick, J.E. (2006) Expression of c-kit (CD117) in Spitz nevus and malignant melanoma. *J Cutan Pathol* **33**(1): 33–7.

Kamino, H., Misheloff, E., Ackerman, A.B., Flotte, T.J., and Greco, M.A. (1979) Eosinophilic globules in Spitz's nevi: new findings and a diagnostic sign. *Am J Dermatopathol* **1**(4): 323–4.

Kantrow, S., Kalemeris, G.C., and Prieto, V. (2008) Spitz nevus with rosette-like structures: a new histologic variant. *J Cutan Pathol* **35**(5): 510–12.

LeBoit, P. (2000) Spitz nevus: a look back and a look ahead. *Adv Dermatol* **16**: 81–109; discussion 110.

Lee, M.W., Choi, J.H., Sung, K.J., Moon, K.C., and Koh, J.K. (2000) Hyalinizing Spitz nevus. *J Dermatol* **27**(4): 273–5.

Li, C.C., Harrist, T.J., Noonan, V.L., and Woo, S.B. (2014) Intraoral Spitz nevus: case report and literature review. *Oral Surg Oral Med Oral Pathol Oral Radiol* **117**(4): e320–4.

Liu, J., Cohen, P.R., and Farhood, A. (2004) Hyalinizing Spitz nevus: spindle and epithelioid cell nevus with paucicellular collagenous stroma. *South Med J* **97**(1): 102–6.

Lyon, V.B. (2010) The spitz nevus: review and update. *Clin Plast Surg* **37**(1): 21–33.

Miteva, M. and Lazova, R. (2010) Spitz nevus and atypical spitzoid neoplasm. *Semin Cutan Med Surg* **29**(3): 165–73.

Mooi, W.J. (2002) Spitz nevus and its histologic simulators. *Adv Anat Pathol* **9**(4): 209–21.

Mooi, W. J. and Krausz, T. (2006) Spitz nevus versus spitzoid melanoma: diagnostic difficulties, conceptual controversies. *Adv Anat Pathol* **13**(4): 147–56.

Nojavan, H., Cribier, B., and Mehregan, D.R. (2009) [Desmoplastic *Spitz nevus: a histopathological review and comparison with desmoplastic melanoma]* Ann Dermatol Venereol **136**(10): 689–95.

Piepkorn, M. (2005).The Spitz nevus is melanoma. *Am J Dermatopathol* **27**(4): 367–9.

Requena, C., Botella, R., Nagore, E., et al. (2012) Characteristics of spitzoid melanoma and clues for differential diagnosis with spitz nevus. *Am J Dermatopathol* **34**(5): 478–86.

Requena, C., Requena, L., Kutzner, H., and Sanchez Yus, E. (2009) Spitz nevus: a clinicopathological study of 349 cases. *Am J Dermatopathol* **31**(2): 107–16.

Sabater Marco, V., Escutia Munoz, B., Morera Faet, A., Mata Roig, M., and Botella Estrada, R. (2013) Pseudogranulomatous Spitz nevus: a variant of Spitz nevus with heavy inflammatory infiltrate mimicking a granulomatous dermatitis. *J Cutan Pathol* **40**(3): 330–5.

Situm, M., Bolanca, Z., Buljan, M., Tomas, D., and Ivancic, M. (2008) Nevus Spitz – everlasting diagnostic difficulties – the review. *Coll Antropol* **32**(Suppl 2): 171–6.

Thakore, J., Guerriere-Kovach, P.M., and Brodell, R.T. (2002) Spitz nevus or malignant melanoma? Benign lesion often mistaken for deadly counterpart. *Postgrad Med* **112**(3): 115–18.

Valdivielso-Ramos, M., Burdaspal, A., Conde, E., and de la Cueva, P. (2016) Balloon-cell variant of the Spitz nevus. *J Eur Acad Dermatol Venereol* **30**(9): 1621–2.

Wititsuwannakul, J., Mason, A.R., Klump, V.R., and Lazova, R. (2013) Neuropilin-2 as a useful marker in the differentiation between Spitzoid malignant melanoma and Spitz nevus. *J Am Acad Dermatol* **68**(1): 129–37.

Yoradjian, A., Enokihara, M.M., and Paschoal, F.M. (2012) Spitz nevus and Reed nevus. *An Bras Dermatol* **87**(3): 349–57; quiz 358–9.

SPINDLE AND/OR EPITHELIOID CELL NEVUS

Variant: Pigmented Spindle Cell Nevus (Reed)

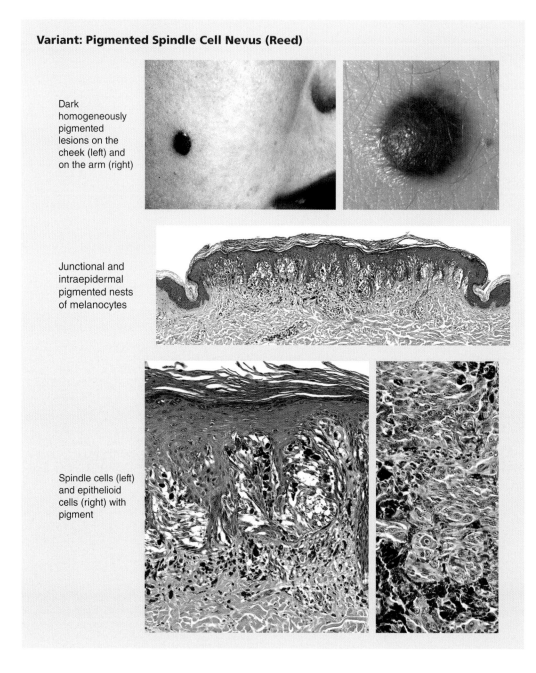

Dark homogeneously pigmented lesions on the cheek (left) and on the arm (right)

Junctional and intraepidermal pigmented nests of melanocytes

Spindle cells (left) and epithelioid cells (right) with pigment

The pigmented spindle cell nevus of Reed is considered a nevus entity of its own, always presenting as a heavily pigmented (black) circumscribed symmetrical nevus.

Cl: Heavily pigmented (jet black) symmetrical, sharply circumscribed macule or flat papule, preferentially on the trunk or extremities of adults.

Hi:
- Strikingly symmetrical and sharply circumscribed superficial melanocytic lesion
- Junctional or compound lesion with nests of heavily pigmented slender and spindled melanocytes

BENIGN MELANOCYTIC LESIONS WITH PECULIAR STRUCTURAL FEATURES

- Broad, horizontally arranged band of heavily pigmented melanophages underlying the lesion
- Fascicles of spindle cells in nest-like arrangement, mostly at the junction
- Evolving (intraepidermal) lesions with irregularly spaced spindles and slightly epithelioid melanocytes in the lower parts of the epidermis
- No mitoses
- Often overlying band of compact orthokeratosis with deposits of melanin granules

DD: Common pigmented nevus; malignant melanoma.

References

de Giorgi, V., Savarese, I., Rossari, S., et al. (2013) Clinical and dermoscopic features of small Reed nevus (<6 mm). *J Eur Acad Dermatol Venereol* **27**(7): 919–21.

Reed, R.J., Ichinose, H., Clark, W.H. Jr, and Mihm, M.C. Jr (1975) Common and uncommon melanocytic nevi and borderline melanomas. *Semin Oncol* **2**(2): 119–47.

Requena, C., Requena, L., Sanchez-Yus, E., et al. (2008) Hypopigmented Reed nevus. *J Cutan Pathol* **35**(Suppl 1): 87–9.

Yoradjian, A., Enokihara, M.M., and Paschoal, F.M. (2012) Spitz nevus and Reed nevus. *An Bras Dermatol* **87**(3): 349–57; quiz 358–9.

Benign Melanocytic Lesions with Peculiar Structural Features

Benign clonal expansions in melanocytic nevi are considered to be expressions of different *NRAS* mutations in conventional nevi.

Melanocytic Nevus with Clonal Proliferation

Dermal nevus (left) showing clones of HMB45-positive melanocytes (right)

HMB45

Clones of variably shaped melanocytes

BENIGN MELANOCYTIC LESIONS WITH PECULIAR STRUCTURAL FEATURES

Cl: Common melanocytic nevi.

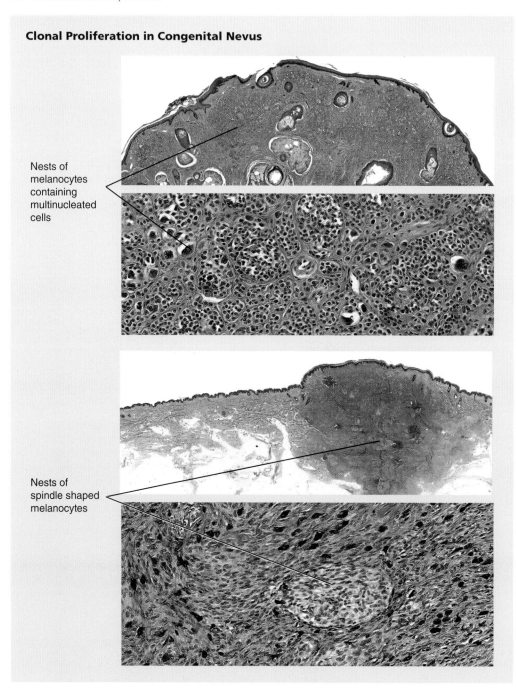

Clonal Proliferation in Congenital Nevus

Nests of melanocytes containing multinucleated cells

Nests of spindle shaped melanocytes

Hi: Within banal congenital dermal nevus there are circumscribed single or multiple nests of larger, roundish melanocytes and melanophages, without mitotic activity.

Immunohistochemistry: Distinct HMB45 expression.

BENIGN MELANOCYTIC LESIONS WITH PECULIAR STRUCTURAL FEATURES

Atypical (Dysplastic) Melanocytic (Clark's) Nevus (B-K Mole Syndrome)

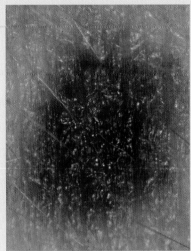 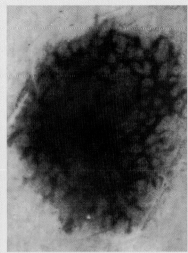

Atypical "dysplastic" nevus (left). Irregular net of pigment seen with the dermatoscope (right)

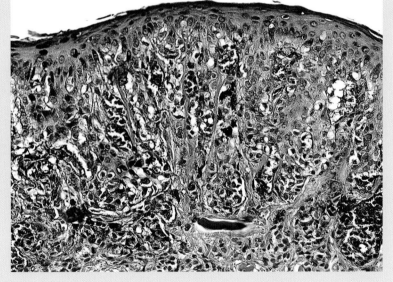

Lentiginous dysplastic nevus: junctional nevus with architectural disorder

When present as multiple lesions in the context of familial genetic predisposition (B-K mole syndrome, described by Clark and by Lynch), the diagnosis is straightforward. However, single lesions are difficult to identify histologically, because (1) the ABCD rule of melanoma may be fulfilled and (2) there is a great variety of melanocytic morphology and it is an issue of endless debates on what is typical, atypical or dysplastic. There is no specific histological feature and no consensus about histopathological definitions of atypia or dysplasia in melanocytic nevi.

The National Institutes of Health Consensus Conference recommended that the term *dysplastic nevus* be abandoned in favor of nevus with architectural disorder or cytologic atypia. Immunosuppression and UV exposure may play an etiological role. Dysplastic nevi may be precursors of melanoma or markers for melanoma susceptibility.

Cl: Usually flat or macular, pigmented lesion with ill-defined irregular borders and variable colors within the same lesion, varying from deep to light brown.

BENIGN MELANOCYTIC LESIONS WITH PECULIAR STRUCTURAL FEATURES

Hi: Mostly junctional melanocytic nevus with architectural disorder and cytological atypia.

- Banal dysplastic nevus (Clark's nevus): architecture of a conventional compound nevus with "active shoulders", i.e. small nests and groups of melanocytes tapering out towards the edges of the lesion
- Severely dysplastic nevus: features of a Clark's nevus in conjunction with high cytological atypia, albeit without mitoses and without atypical single melanocytes above the basal layer
- Bridging nests of melanocytes in the junctional zone in conjunction with lamellar fibroplasia
- Cytological features variable: spindle shaped or epithelioid melanocytes possible
- Nuclear pleomorphism (restricted to severely dysplastic nevus): large nuclei with prominent nucleoli

- Minimal mitotic activity (<2 mitoses/section)
- Lymphohistiocytic inflammatory infiltrate with melanophages

DD: Common melanocytic nevus; congenital melanocytic nevus; malignant melanoma.

References

Clark, W.H. Jr, Reimer, R.R., Greene, M., Ainsworth, A.M., and Mastrangelo, M.J. (1978) Origin of familial malignant melanomas from heritable melanocytic lesions. 'The B-K mole syndrome'. *Arch Dermatol* **114**(5): 732–8.

Lynch, H.T., Frichot, B.C. 3rd, and Lynch, J.F. (1978) Familial atypical multiple mole-melanoma syndrome. *J Med Genet* **15**(5): 352–6.

NIH Consensus Conference (1992) Diagnosis and treatment of early melanoma. *JAMA* **268**(10): 1314–19.

Congenital Nevi, Small and Medium-Sized (1.5–20 cm)

Small (left) and medium-sized (middle and right) congenital nevi

Compound congenital nevus

BENIGN MELANOCYTIC LESIONS WITH PECULIAR STRUCTURAL FEATURES

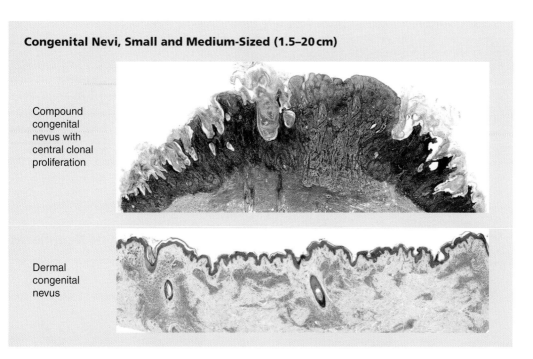

Congenital Nevi, Small and Medium-Sized (1.5–20 cm)

Compound congenital nevus with central clonal proliferation

Dermal congenital nevus

According to an NIH consensus conference (1984), small (0–1.5 cm) to medium-sized (1.5–20 cm) and large (>20 cm) congenital melanocytic nevi are differentiated, the latter showing high risk of CNS involvement and development of melanoma.

Cl: Brown macular lesions with irregular but sharp borders, with or without hairs. Usually lesions are present at birth and get darker over the first months or years of life. Lateral expansion of the nevus congruently with body growth.

Hi: The diagnosis is made clinically. However, histological evaluation of so-called proliferative nodule in congenital nevi is paramount in order to exclude melanoma.

- Features of common junctional (small congenital) and/or compound (large congenital) nevus; involvement of upper and mid dermis
- Nests of melanocytes at the dermal-epidermal junction and in the dermis respectively
- Architectural atypia (especially in young children and adolescents) with irregularly spaced ("dysplastic") melanocytic nests at the junction and single melanocytes
- Spread of melanocytes along the adnexal structures
- Deep parts may show neuroid differentiation
- Blue nevus-like clonal expansions amidst the nevus nests may be present

Immunohistochemistry: Nuclear H3K27me3 expression within the nodular melanocytes was shown to be a significant indicator of proliferative nodule (benign) versus malignant melanoma.

DD: Congenital nevus in the newborn may present with a melanoma-like scatter of single melanocytes throughout the epidermis, overlying a conventional dermal congenital nevus. Proliferative nodule in a congenital nevus (in a newborn or in an infant) is composed of isomorphic melanocytes that morphologically clearly differ from the adjacent nevus cells. The number of mitoses within the proliferative nodule may be increased. There may be a gradual blending of one melanocytic population into another, as well as a sharp circumscription between proliferative nodule and adjacent nevus.

References

Lee, N.R., Chung, H.C., Hong, H., Lee, J.W., and Ahn, S.K. (2015. Spontaneous involution of congenital melanocytic nevus with halo phenomenon. *Am J Dermatopathol* **37**(12): e137–9.

Machan, S., Molina-Ruiz, A.M., Fernandez-Acenero, M.J., et al. (2015) Metastatic melanoma in association with a giant congenital melanocytic nevus in an adult: controversial CGH findings. *Am J Dermatopathol* **37**(6): 487–94

Magana, M., Sanchez-Romero, E., Magana, P., Beck-Magana, A., and Magana-Lozano, M. (2015)

LENTIGO MALIGNA DUBREUILH (HUTCHINSON'S FRECKLE)

Congenital melanocytic nevus: two clinicopathological forms. *Am J Dermatopathol* **37**(1): 31–7.

Martinez-Barba, E., Polo-Garcia, L.A., Ferri-Niguez, B., Ruiz-Macia, J.A., Kutzner, H., and Requena, L. (2002) Congenital giant melanocytic nevus with pigmented epithelioid cells: a variant of epithelioid blue nevus. *Am J Dermatopathol* **24**(1): 30–5.

McGowan, J.W., Smith, M.K., Ryan, M., and Hood, A.F. (2006) Proliferative nodules with balloon-cell change in a large congenital melanocytic nevus. *J Cutan Pathol* **33**(3): 253–5.

Nguyen, T.L., Theos, A., Kelly, D.R., Busam, K., and Andea, A.A. (2013) Mitotically active proliferative nodule arising in a giant congenital melanocytic nevus: a diagnostic pitfall. *Am J Dermatopathol* **35**(1): e16–21.

NIH Consensus Panel Report (1984) Precursors to malignant melanoma. *Md State Med J* **33**(7): 532–5.

Rongioletti, F., Guadagno, A., Campisi, C., et al. (2015) Atypical Spitz tumor arising on a congenital linear plaque-type blue nevus: a case report with a review of the literature on plaque-type blue nevus. *Am J Dermatopathol* **37**(12): 915–19.

van Houten, A.H., van Dijk, M.C., and Schuttelaar, M.L. (2010) Proliferative nodules in a giant congenital melanocytic nevus-case report and review of the literature. *J Cutan Pathol* **37**(7): 764–76.

Wang, L., Wang, G., and Gao, T. (2013) Congenital melanocytic nevus with features of hybrid schwannoma/perineurioma. *J Cutan Pathol* **40**(5): 497–502.

Malignant Melanocytic Neoplasms

Lentigo Maligna Dubreuilh (Hutchinson's Freckle)

Irregular macular lesions on nose, cheek and neck

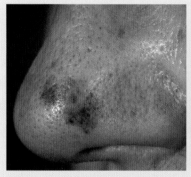
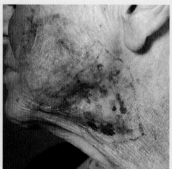

Atrophy of the epidermis, massive solar elastosis

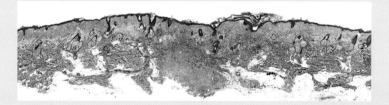

Increased number of melanocytes in the basal layer and within the adnexal epithelium

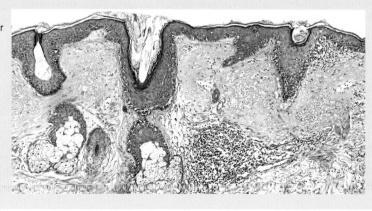

MALIGNANT MELANOMA

Most pathologists consider these lesions not as distinct entities but as melanoma *in situ*. However, there are many reasons to differentiate lentigo maligna from melanoma even though it may turn into lentigo maligna melanoma when not appropriately removed. Immunohistochemical investigation of cell markers (HMB45, S100) does not discriminate between lentigo maligna and melanoma.

Cl:

- Slowly growing (over years and decades) macular lesion in sun-exposed areas of elderly individuals
- Irregular fading borders
- Variable irregular pigmentation
- Slight atrophy
- Good prognosis

Hi:

- Atrophy of the epidermis and flattening of the papillary profile
- Increased number of single atypical large melanocytes in the basal epidermal layer
- No nests of atypical melanocytes in the dermis
- Atypical melanocytes extending down the follicular epithelia to the level of the infundibulum and down eccrine ducts
- Pigment in melanophages in the dermis
- Basement membrane intact; no junctional or basal melanocytic nests
- Horizontal growth
- Solar elastosis in the upper dermis
- There may be scarce lymphocytic infiltrate with scattered plasma cells (typical for the head and neck localisation) in the upper dermis

DD: Flat seborrheic keratosis; recurrent melanocytic nevus; lentigo maligna melanoma; superficial spreading melanoma; pigmented actinic keratosis.

References

Farrahi, F., Egbert, B.M., and Swetter, S.M. (2005) Histologic similarities between lentigo maligna and dysplastic nevus: importance of clinicopathologic distinction. *J Cutan Pathol* **32**(6): 405–12.

Feinmesser, M., Tsabari, C., Fichman, S., Hodak, E., Sulkes, J., and Okon, E. (2003) Differential expression of proliferation- and apoptosis-related markers in lentigo maligna and solar keratosis keratinocytes. *Am J Dermatopathol* **25**(4): 300–7.

Ribe, A. and McNutt, N.S. (2003) S100A protein expression in the distinction between lentigo maligna and pigmented actinic keratosis. *Am J Dermatopathol* **25**(2): 93–9.

Sethi, M., Craythorne, E., Al-Arashi, M.Y., Bhawan, J., and Stefanato, C.M. (2014) Macromelanosomes: their significantly greater presence in the margins of a lentigo maligna versus solar lentigo. *Am J Dermatopathol* **36**(6): 490–2.

Suchak, R., Hameed, O.A., and Robson, A. (2014) Evaluation of the role of routine melan-A immunohistochemistry for exclusion of microinvasion in 120 cases of lentigo maligna. *Am J Dermatopathol* **36**(5): 387–91.

Malignant Melanoma

Four major variants of malignant melanoma have to be differentiated, clinically and histologically.

- Superficial spreading melanoma (SSM): most common form of melanoma
- Lentigo maligna melanoma (LMM): evolves from lentigo maligna
- Nodular melanoma (NM): red, brown, black tumor, often ulcerating and/or bleeding
- Acral lentiginous melanoma (ALM): nails, fingers, palms, soles

Special clinical variants are melanoma of mucous membrane, conjunctiva, amelanotic melanoma, genital melanoma.

The ABCD rule (A – asymmetry, B – border, C – colour, D – diameter) serves the clinician in discriminating maligna melanoma from benign melanocytic or other simulators.

Comment: It has become the standard of care that for virtually all melanomas, testing for BRAF mutations and GNAQ/KRAS should be performed, indicating various morphological subtypes.

Reference

Bastian, B.C. (2014) The molecular pathology of melanoma: an integrated taxonomy of melanocytic neoplasia. *Annu Rev Pathol* **9**: 239–71.

MALIGNANT MELANOMA

Variant: Superficial Spreading Melanoma (SSM)

Superficial spreading melanoma with amelanotic tumor nodule in the center (left)

Superficial spreading melanoma with tumor regression in the center (right)

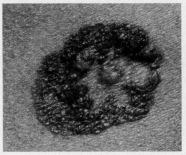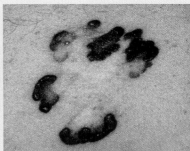

SSM, nests of tumor cells at the junction and in the upper dermis

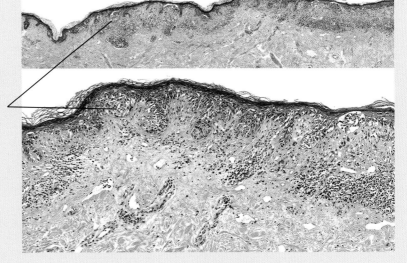

Transepidermal elimination of single melanocytes

Nests of atypical malanocytes

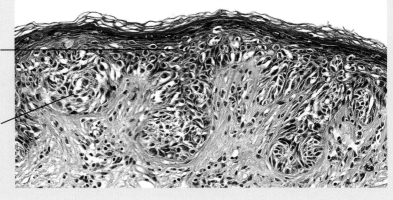

MALIGNANT MELANOMA

Cl: Preferentially on the legs of women but also at any other localisation. Round or oval, horizontally growing pigmented flat lesion with irregular sharp polycyclic borders. Tendency for central regression and sometimes resulting in an incomplete ring structure. Depigmentation in the middle of the lesion does not necessarily mean complete resolving of tumor cells in this area of immunological reaction. Over time, vertical growth can start. A variable spectrum of colors may be seen from white (regression zones) to red (inflammation), brown, and black.

Hi:

- Slightly acanthotic epidermis
- Spread of atypical melanocytes as single cells or in small clusters throughout all levels of the epidermis, featuring a pagetoid pattern
- Large tumor cells with abundant cytoplasm
- Nuclei are irregular, chromatin is clumped, nucleoli are prominent
- Balloon cell variants exist
- Some mitotic activity is usually present
- Involvement of adnexal epithelium
- Epidermal basement membrane effaced by proliferation of atypical melanocytes
- Infiltration of papillary dermis
- Irregular distribution of melanin preferentially on the bottom of the lesion and in dermal melanophages
- Fibrosis in the papillary dermis in areas of regression
- Scattered inflammatory infiltrate
- Vertical growth can arise after variable time of horizontal growth
  - Starting from one or several areas of the superficially spreading tumor
  - Invasion of mid and deeper parts of the dermis
  - May be associated with increased cellular atypia

DD: Solar lentigo; pigmented basal cell carcinoma; Bowen's disease; pigmented Paget's disease of the breast.

References

Auslender, S., Barzilai, A., Goldberg, I., Kopolovic, J., and Trau, H. (2002) Lentigo maligna and superficial spreading melanoma are different in their in situ phase: an immunohistochemical study. *Hum Pathol* **33**(10): 1001–5.

Carli, P., de Giorgi, V., Palli, D., et al. (2004) Patterns of detection of superficial spreading and nodular-type melanoma: a multicenter Italian study. *Dermatol Surg* **30**(11): 1371–5; discussion 1375–6.

D'Ath, P. and Thomson, P. (2012) Superficial spreading melanoma. *BMJ* **344**: e2319.

Greenwald, H.S., Friedman, E.B., and Osman, I. (2012) Superficial spreading and nodular melanoma are distinct biological entities: a challenge to the linear progression model. *Melanoma Res* **22**(1): 1–8.

Hasbun Acuna, P., Cullen Aravena, R., Maturana Donaire, C., Ares Mora, R., and Porras Kusmanic, N. (2016) Pigmented basal cell carcinoma mimicking a superficial spreading melanoma. *Medwave* **16**(11): e6805.

Helmbold, P., Altrichter, D., Klapperstuck, T., and Marsch, W. (2005) Intratumoral DNA stem-line heterogeneity in superficial spreading melanoma. *J Am Acad Dermatol* **52**(5): 803–9.

Hikawa, R.S., Kanehisa, E.S., Enokihara, M.M., Enokihara, M.Y., and Hirata, S.H. (2014) Polypoid melanoma and superficial spreading melanoma different subtypes in the same lesion. *An Bras Dermatol* **89**(4): 666–8.

Kutzner, H., Metzler, G., Argenyi, Z., et al. (2012) Histological and genetic evidence for a variant of superficial spreading melanoma composed predominantly of large nests. *Mod Pathol* **25**(6): 838–45.

Lang, J. and MacKie, R.M. (2005) Prevalence of exon 15 BRAF mutations in primary melanoma of the superficial spreading, nodular, acral, and lentigo maligna subtypes. *J Invest Dermatol* **125**(3): 575–9.

Napolitano, L. and Crowe, D. (2015) Pigmented mammary Paget disease mimicking superficial spreading melanoma in an elderly African-American female. *J Cutan Med Surg* **19**(3): 313–16.

Petkovic, M. and Jurakic Toncic, R. (2017) Nested melanoma, a new morphological variant of superficial spreading melanoma with characteristic dermoscopic features. *Acta Dermatovenerol Croat* **25**(1): 80–1.

Scope, A., Zalaudek, I., Ferrara, G., Argenziano, G., Braun, R.P., and Marghoob, A.A. (2008) Remodeling of the dermoepidermal junction in superficial spreading melanoma: insights gained from correlation of dermoscopy, reflectance confocal microscopy, and histopathologic analysis. *Arch Dermatol* **144**(12): 1644–9.

Singh, P., Kim, H.J., and Schwartz, R.A. (2016) Superficial spreading melanoma: an analysis of 97 702 cases using the SEER database. *Melanoma Res* **26**(4): 395–400.

MALIGNANT MELANOMA

Variant: Lentigo Maligna Melanoma (LMM)

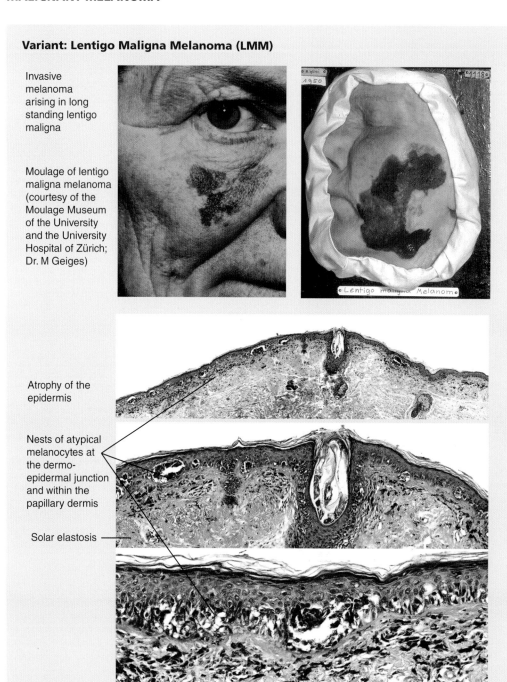

Invasive melanoma arising in long standing lentigo maligna

Moulage of lentigo maligna melanoma (courtesy of the Moulage Museum of the University and the University Hospital of Zürich; Dr. M Geiges)

Atrophy of the epidermis

Nests of atypical melanocytes at the dermo-epidermal junction and within the papillary dermis

Solar elastosis

Cl: Remnants of macules of lentigo maligna. After some years flat plaques or nodules arise due to the spread of tumor cells with invasive growth into the dermis.

Hi: Like lentigo maligna, but with invasion of malignant melanocytes beyond the epidermal basement membrane into the papillary dermis. Predominantly spindle-shaped dermal melanocytes in many cases, merging with desmoplastic melanomas.

MALIGNANT MELANOMA

Variant: Nodular Melanoma (NM)

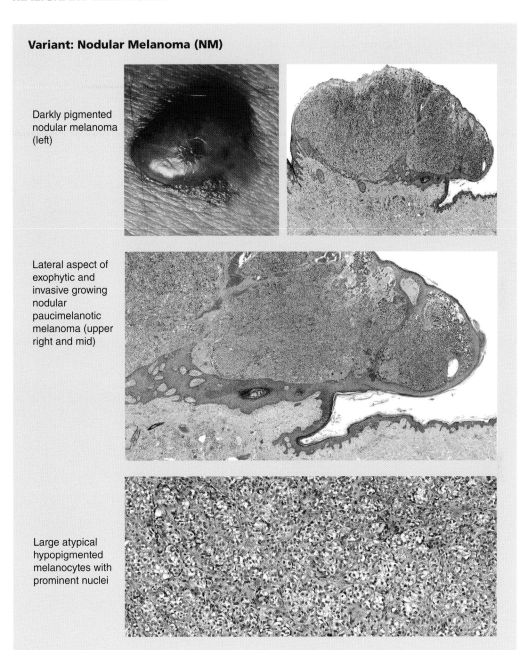

Darkly pigmented nodular melanoma (left)

Lateral aspect of exophytic and invasive growing nodular paucimelanotic melanoma (upper right and mid)

Large atypical hypopigmented melanocytes with prominent nuclei

Cl: Dark, rapidly growing nodule, usually arising on normal skin. Loss of skin tension lines and pilosebaceous follicles. The surface is smooth or ulcerated and crusty. The surrounding skin may show hyperpigmentation and small local satellites.

Hi:
- Exophytic tumor
- Large atypical melanocytes
- Variable cytomorphology, including spindle-shaped, epithelioid, clear cells and others
- Minimal epidermal but deep dermal invasion
- High mitotic activity

DD: Melanoma metastasis.

Reference

Gescheidt-Shoshany, H., Weltfriend, S., and Bergman, R. (2015) Nodular melanoma arising in a large segmental speckled lentiginous nevus. *Am J Dermatopathol* 37(8): 663–4.

MALIGNANT MELANOMA

Variant: Acral Lentiginous Melanoma (ALM)

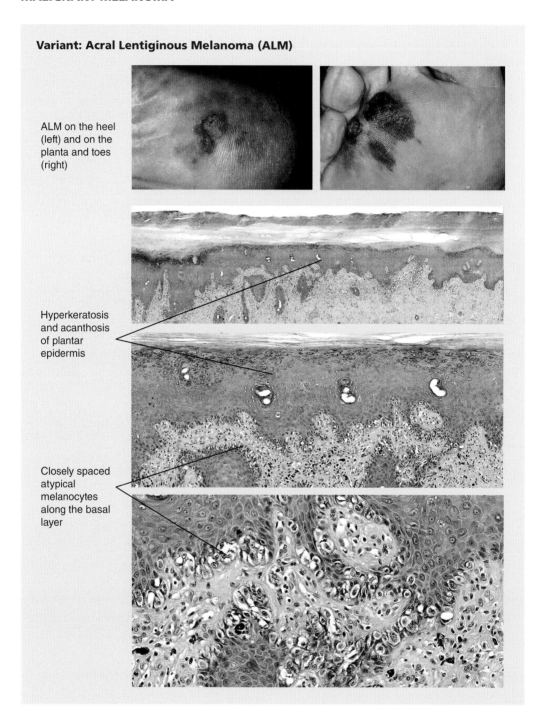

ALM on the heel (left) and on the planta and toes (right)

Hyperkeratosis and acanthosis of plantar epidermis

Closely spaced atypical melanocytes along the basal layer

Cl: Slowly growing, pigmented macule in acral localisation such as toes or fingers, starting from the nail matrix, nailbed or nailfold or on palms and soles, preferentially in black people. Loss of regular dermatoglyphs may give a diagnostic hint. Similar lesions can occur on mucous membranes.

Hi: Similar to lentigo maligna melanoma.
- Large, atypical melanocytes, initially distributed as single cells or in small clusters throughout the basal layer of the epidermis, later throughout the entire epidermis (pagetoid spread)

MALIGNANT MELANOMA

- Transepidermal elimination of pigment and single cells
- Fibrosis and scattered lymphocytic infiltrate in the upper dermis
- Migration of atypical cells into the papillary dermis
- The tumor spreads laterally
- Involvement of adnexal epithelium
- Frequent KIT gene mutation

DD: Intracorneal bleeding ("black heel"); superficial spreading melanoma; acral melanocytic nevus.

References

Donati, P., Paolino, G., Panetta, C., Donati, M., and Muscardin, L. (2015) Indolent subtype acral lentiginous melanoma with long radial growth phase: a dermatopathological pitfall. *Am J Dermatopathol* **37**(11): 873–4.

Fernandes, J.D., Hsieh, R., de Freitas, L.A., et al. (2015) MAP kinase pathways: molecular roads to primary acral lentiginous melanoma. *Am J Dermatopathol* **37**(12): 892–7.

Kim, J.Y., Choi, M., Jo, S.J., Min, H.S., and Cho, K.H. (2014) Acral lentiginous melanoma: indolent subtype with long radial growth phase. *Am J Dermatopathol* **36**(2): 142–7.

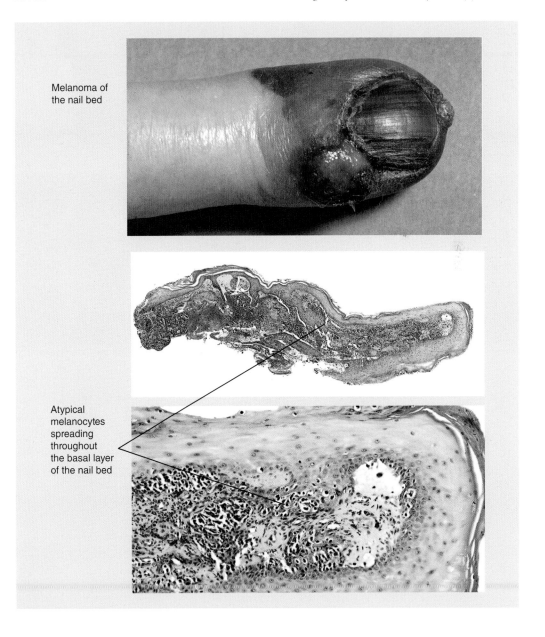

Melanoma of the nail bed

Atypical melanocytes spreading throughout the basal layer of the nail bed

MALIGNANT MELANOMA

Kwon, I.H., Lee, J.H., and Cho, K.H. (2004) Acral lentiginous melanoma in situ: a study of nine cases. *Am J Dermatopathol* **26**(4): 285–9.

Liau, J.Y., Tsai, J.H., Jeng, Y.M., Chu, C.Y., Kuo, K.T., and Liang, C.W. (2014) TERT promoter mutation is uncommon in acral lentiginous melanoma. *J Cutan Pathol* **41**(6): 504–8.

Ohata, C., Nakai, C., Kasugai, T., and Katayama, I. (2012) Consumption of the epidermis in acral lentiginous melanoma. *J Cutan Pathol* **39**(6): 577–81.

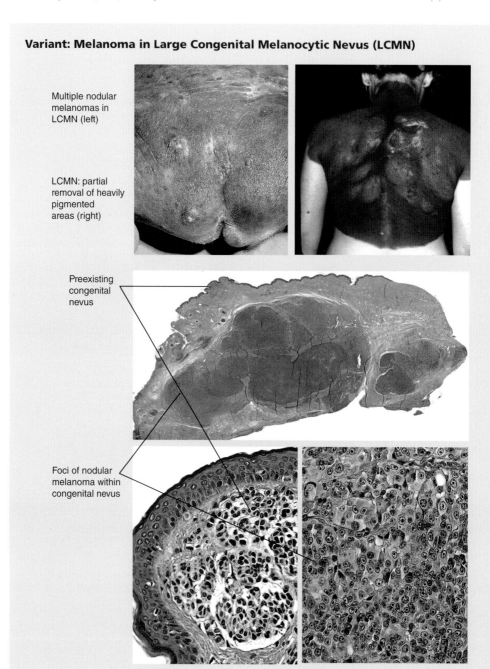

Variant: Melanoma in Large Congenital Melanocytic Nevus (LCMN)

Multiple nodular melanomas in LCMN (left)

LCMN: partial removal of heavily pigmented areas (right)

Preexisting congenital nevus

Foci of nodular melanoma within congenital nevus

MALIGNANT MELANOMA

Cl: In large congenital melanocytic nevi (>20 cm) especially areas with dark pigmentation bear a high risk for the development of melanoma.

Hi: Corresponds to the changes in common types of melanomas.

Variant: Cutaneous Metastasis of Melanoma

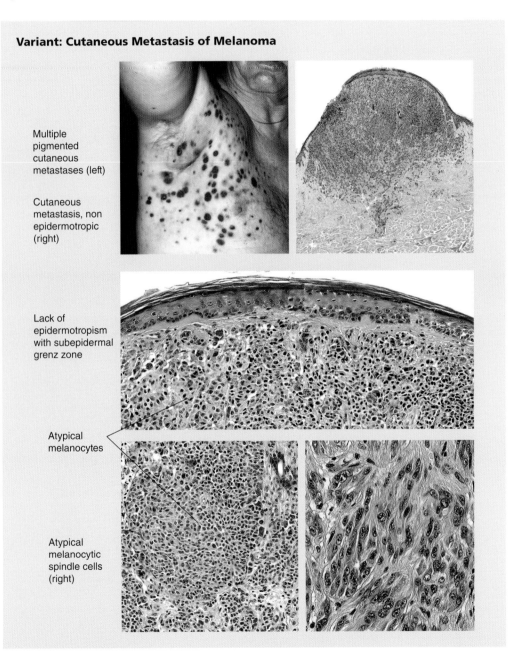

Multiple pigmented cutaneous metastases (left)

Cutaneous metastasis, non epidermotropic (right)

Lack of epidermotropism with subepidermal grenz zone

Atypical melanocytes

Atypical melanocytic spindle cells (right)

Cl: Pigmented or amelanotic skin-colored cutaneous and subcutaneous papules and nodules.

Hi:
• Atrophy of the epidermis

• Nodular proliferation of atypical melanocytes in the (upper) dermis
• Lacking or only focal epidermotropism of tumor cells

SPECIAL HISTOLOGICAL FEATURES OF MALIGNANT MELANOMA

- Variable shapes of tumor cells, including balloon cells and spitzoid spindle cells
- Mitotic activity and melanin production variable

DD: Common (dermal) nevus; dermal Spitz nevus; cellular blue nevus.

References

Murali, R., Zannino, D., Synnott, M., McCarthy, S.W., Thompson, J.F., and Scolyer, R.A. (2011) Clinical and pathological features of metastases of primary cutaneous desmoplastic melanoma. *Histopathology* **58**(6): 886–95.

Plaza, J.A., Torres-Cabala, C., Evans, H., Diwan, H.A., Suster, S., and Prieto, V.G. (2010) Cutaneous metastases of malignant melanoma: a clinicopathologic study of 192 cases with emphasis on the morphologic spectrum. *Am J Dermatopathol* **32**(2): 129–36.

Special Histological Features of Malignant Melanoma

- Minimal deviation melanoma
- Melanoma ex naevo
- Neurotropic melanoma
- Nevus-like (nested) melanoma

Neurotropic Melanoma

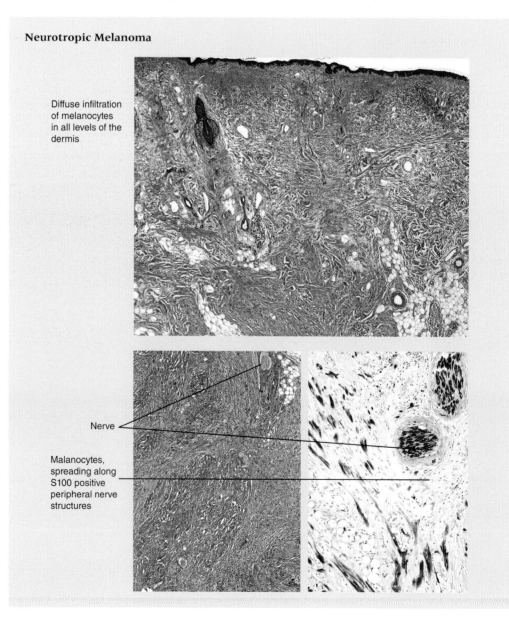

Diffuse infiltration of melanocytes in all levels of the dermis

Nerve

Malanocytes, spreading along S100 positive peripheral nerve structures

SPECIAL HISTOLOGICAL FEATURES OF MALIGNANT MELANOMA

Nevus-Like (Nested) Melanoma

Intraepidermal
nests of atypical
melanocytes
(top and bottom).
HMB45 positive
cells intraepidermal
single and in nests
(mid)

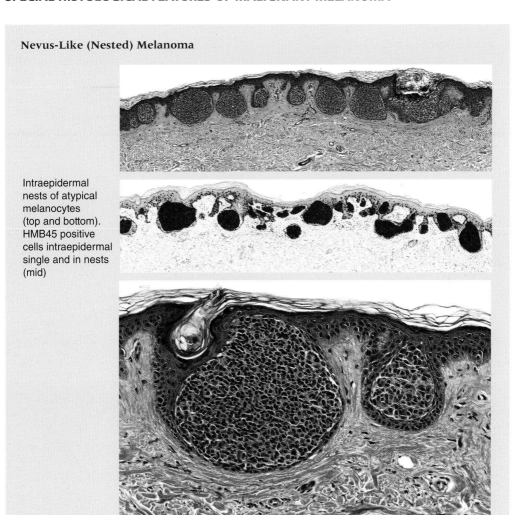

Variant: Balloon Cell Melanoma

Cl: Clinical features of this rare variant correspond to common melanomas.

Variant: Balloon Cell Melanoma

Large atypical
melanocytes with
abundant clear
cytoplasm
("balloon cells")
within the basal
layer, at the
junction and in
the papillary
dermis

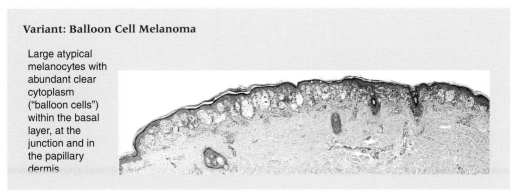

SPECIAL HISTOLOGICAL FEATURES OF MALIGNANT MELANOMA

Variant: Balloon Cell Melanoma

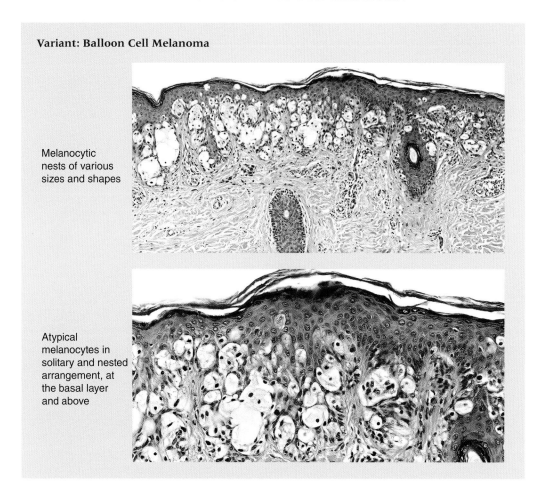

Melanocytic nests of various sizes and shapes

Atypical melanocytes in solitary and nested arrangement, at the basal layer and above

Hi: Large melanocytes with broad cytoplasm ("balloon cells") are the hallmark of this type of melanoma.

DD: Other clear cell tumors; xanthoma.

References

Chavez-Alvarez, S., Villarreal-Martinez, A., Miranda-Maldonado, I., Ocampo-Candiani, J., and Garza-Rodriguez, V. (2017) Balloon cell melanoma and its metastasis, a rare entity. *Am J Dermatopathol* **39**(5): 404–11.

Inskip, M., James, N., Magee, J., and Rosendahl, C. (2016) Pigmented primary cutaneous balloon cell melanoma demonstrating balloon cells in the dermoepidermal junction: a brief case report with dermatoscopy and histopathology. *Int J Dermatol* **55**(2): e110–12.

Han, J.S., Won, C.H., Chang, S.E., Lee, M.W., Choi, J.H., and Moon, K.C. (2014).Primary cutaneous balloon cell melanoma: a very rare variant. *Int J Dermatol* **53**(11): e535–6.

Northcutt, A.D. (2000) Epidermotropic xanthoma mimicking balloon cell melanoma. *Am J Dermatopathol* **22**(2): 176–8.

SPECIAL HISTOLOGICAL FEATURES OF MALIGNANT MELANOMA

Variant: Desmoplastic Malignant Melanoma (DMM)

Overlying LMM showing intraepidermal nests of atypical melanocytes

S100 stain (right)

Proliferation of spindle-shaped melanocytes (left and bottom)

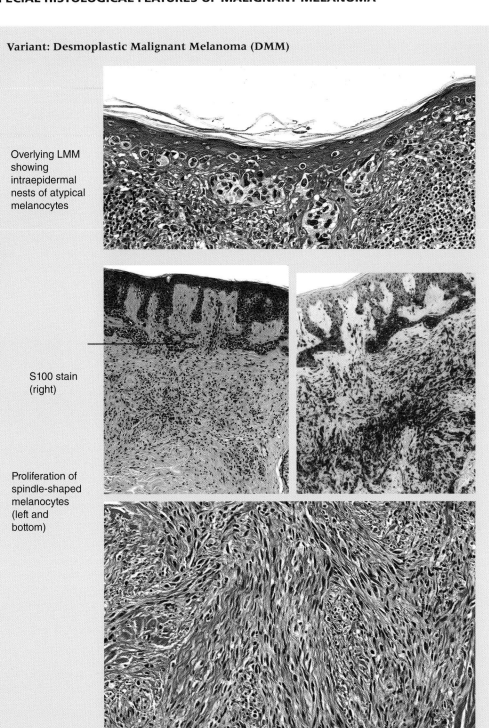

SPECIAL HISTOLOGICAL FEATURES OF MALIGNANT MELANOMA

Cl: Clinical features correspond to common melanomas. However, there are hypopigmented variants of DMM that simulate the morphology of a scar, basal cell carcinoma, or dermatofibroma. Association with lentigo maligna melanoma is not uncommon.

Hi:

- Regular epidermis or overlying lentigo maligna melanoma
- Scar-like fibrotic stroma often simulating dermatofibroma
- Hypocellular variants of DMM resemble scars, albeit with a stroma positive for p75, WT1, and alpha smooth muscle actin (stromal myofibroblasts)
- Diffuse proliferation of amelanotic spindled melanocytes, positive for S100 and SOX10
- Dermal melanocytes are negative for MiTF, HMB45, and Melan A
- Tumor cells of DMM are p53-positive in contrast to neurofibroma with p53-negative Schwann cells
- Focal pleomorphism, low mitotic activity
- Cellular variants showing overlap with spindle cell melanoma
- Neurotropism is a common feature

DD: Other spindle cell tumors; scar; desmoplastic nevus; neurofibroma; dermatofibroma; malignant peripheral nerve sheath tumor showing characteristic lack of nuclear expression of H3K27me3 (methylation marker); desmoplastic Spitz nevus.

References

Bernaba, B.N., Vogiatzis, P I., Binder, S.W., and Cassarino, D.S. (2011) Potentially useful markers for desmoplastic melanoma: an analysis of KBA.62, p-AKT, and ezrin. *Am J Dermatopathol* **33**(4): 333–7; quiz 338–40.

Blokhin, E., Pulitzer, M., and Busam, K.J. (2013) Immunohistochemical expression of p16 in desmoplastic melanoma. *J Cutan Pathol* **40**(9): 796–800.

Chorny, J.A. and Barr, R.J. (2002) S100-positive spindle cells in scars: a diagnostic pitfall in the re-excision of desmoplastic melanoma. *Am J Dermatopathol* **24**(4): 309–12.

de Almeida, L.S., Requena, L., Rutten, A., et al. (2008) Desmoplastic malignant melanoma: a clinicopathologic analysis of 113 cases. *Am J Dermatopathol* **30**(3): 207–15.

Eng, W. and Tschen, J.A. (2000) Comparison of S-100 versus hematoxylin and eosin staining for evaluating dermal invasion and peripheral margins by desmoplastic malignant melanoma. *Am J Dermatopathol* **22**(1): 26–9.

Garrido, M.C., Requena, L., Kutzner, H., Ortiz, P., Perez-Gomez, B., and Rodriguez-Peralto, J.L. (2014) Desmoplastic melanoma: expression of epithelial-mesenchymal transition-related proteins. *Am J Dermatopathol* **36**(3): 238–42.

Hilliard, N.J., Krahl, D., and Sellheyer, K (2009) p16 expression differentiates between desmoplastic Spitz nevus and desmoplastic melanoma. *J Cutan Pathol* **36**(7): 753–9.

Hoang, M.P., Selim, M.A., Bentley, R.C., Burchette, J.L., and Shea, C.R. (2001) CD34 expression in desmoplastic melanoma. *J Cutan Pathol* **28**(10): 508–12.

Husain, S. and Silvers, D.N. (2013) Fingerprint CD34 immunopositivity to distinguish neurofibroma from an early/paucicellular desmoplastic melanoma can be misleading. *J Cutan Pathol* **40**(11): 985–7.

Kanner, W.A., Brill, L.B. 2nd, Patterson, J.W., and Wick, M.R. (2010) CD10, p63 and CD99 expression in the differential diagnosis of atypical fibroxanthoma, spindle cell squamous cell carcinoma and desmoplastic melanoma. *J Cutan Pathol* **37**(7): 744–50.

Kucher, C., Zhang, P.J., Pasha, T., et al. (2004) Expression of Melan-A and Ki-67 in desmoplastic melanoma and desmoplastic nevi. *Am J Dermatopathol* **26**(6): 452–7.

Machado, I., Llombart, B., Cruz, J., et al. (2017) Desmoplastic melanoma may mimic a cutaneous peripheral nerve sheath tumor: report of 3 challenging cases. *J Cutan Pathol* Apr 12. doi: 10.1111/cup.12949 [epub ahead of print].

North, J. (2011) CD117 (c-KIT) staining in desmoplastic melanoma. *J Cutan Pathol* **38**(9): 753–5.

Palla, B., Su, A., Binder, S., and Dry, S. (2013) SOX10 expression distinguishes desmoplastic melanoma from its histologic mimics. *Am J Dermatopathol* **35**(5): 576–81.

Plaza, J.A., Bonneau, P., Prieto, V., et al. (2016) Desmoplastic melanoma: an updated immunohistochemical analysis of 40 cases with a proposal for an additional panel of stains for diagnosis. *J Cutan Pathol* **43**(4): 313–23.

Ramos-Herberth, F.I., Karamchandani, J., Kim, J., and Dadras, S.S. (2010) SOX10 immunostaining distinguishes desmoplastic melanoma from excision scar. *J Cutan Pathol* **37**(9): 944–52.

Robson, A., Allen, P., and Hollowood, K. (2001) S100 expression in cutaneous scars: a potential diagnostic pitfall in the diagnosis of desmoplastic melanoma. *Histopathology* **38**(2): 135–40.

Sidiropoulos, M., Sholl, L.M., Obregon, R., Guitart, J., and Gerami, P. (2014) Desmoplastic nevus of chronically sun-damaged skin: an entity to be distinguished from desmoplastic melanoma. *Am J Dermatopathol* **36**(8): 629–34.

Yeh, I. and McCalmont, T.H. (2011) Distinguishing neurofibroma from desmoplastic melanoma: the value of the CD34 fingerprint. *J Cutan Pathol* **38**(8): 625–30.

SPECIAL HISTOLOGICAL FEATURES OF MALIGNANT MELANOMA

Differential Diagnosis: Clear Cell Sarcoma (Melanoma of Soft Parts)

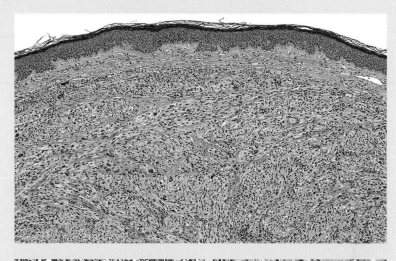

Dermal clear cell infiltrate, non epidermotropic fascicles and multinucleate giant cells.

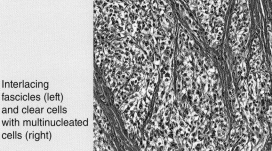
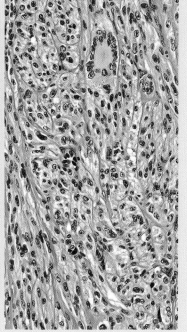

Interlacing fascicles (left) and clear cells with multinucleated cells (right)

This rare tumor nosologically is considered to be a clinicopathological entity originating from soft tissue in association with tendons and aponeuroses.

Cl: Deep, slowly growing tumor, preferentially involving the foot. Local recurrences and distal metastases occur.

Hi:
- Well-circumscribed dermal tumor
- Nests of tumor cells with eosinophilic granular cytoplasm
- Fibrous septae between tumor nests
- Multinucleated giant cells
- Melanin may be present

SPECIAL LOCALISATIONS OF MALIGNANT MELANOMA

Immunohistochemistry: Vimentin, S-100 protein, HMB45, MART-1 are expressed in most tumor cells.

DD: Metastatic melanoma; spindle cell melanoma; Spitz nevus; cellular blue nevus; fibrosarcoma; nerve sheath tumor.

References

Falconieri, G., Bacchi, C.E., and Luzar, B. (2012) Cutaneous clear cell sarcoma: report of three cases of a potentially underestimated mimicker of spindle cell melanoma. *Am J Dermatopathol* **34**(6): 619–25.

Feasel, P.C., Cheah, A.L., Fritchie, K., Winn, B., Piliang, M., and Billings, S.D. (2016) Primary clear cell sarcoma of the head and neck: a case series with review of the literature. *J Cutan Pathol* **43**(10): 838–46.

Kiuru, M., Hameed, M., and Busam, K.J. (2013) Compound clear cell sarcoma misdiagnosed as a Spitz nevus. *J Cutan Pathol* **40**(11): 950–4.

Mooi, W.J., Deenik, W., Peterse, J.L., and Hogendoorn, P.C. (1995) Keratin immunoreactivity in melanoma of soft parts (clear cell sarcoma). *Histopathology* **27**(1): 61–5.

Warner, T.F., Hafez, G.R., Padmalatha, C., and Lange, T.A. (1983) Acral lentiginous melanoma simulating "clear cell sarcoma of tendon and aponeuroses". *J Cutan Pathol* **10**(3): 193–200.

Special Localisations of Malignant Melanoma

- Conjunctiva
- Male genitalia; orificium urethrae
- Oral mucous membrane and palate

Special Localisations of Malignant Melanoma

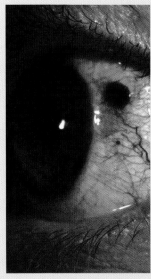 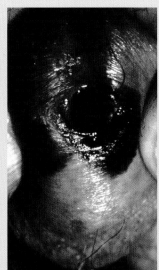 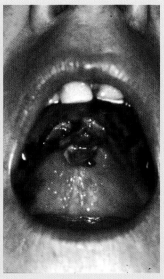

| Conjunctiva | Orificium urethrae | Oral palate |

MALIGNANT MELANOMA

Tumor Thickness and Levels

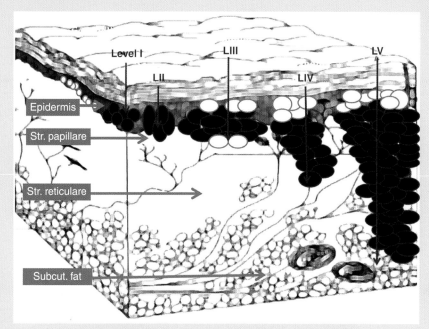

Level I Tumor cells in epidermis; Level II Tumor cells in papillary dermis;
Level III Tumor cells filling papillary dermis; Level IV Tumor cells in reticular dermis;
Level V Tumor cells in subcutaneous fat

The major independent risk factor in malignant melanoma is tumor thickness, measured with an ocular micrometer as distance from the stratum corneum to the deepest tumor cell at the base of the tumor, and given in mm Breslow depth.

As a rule of thumb, there is an almost linear correlation between the measured Breslow depth and the tumor level, which is also reflected in the AJCC staging classification (pT1 < 1 mm; pT2 up to 2 mm; pT3 up to 4 mm; pT4 > 4 mm).

- Level I Tumor cells in the epidermis
- Level II Tumor cells in the papillary dermis
- Level III Tumor cells filling the papillary dermis
- Level IV Tumor cells in the reticular dermis
- Level V Tumor cells in the subcutis

References

Balch, C.M., Gershenwald, JE., Soong, S. J., et al. (2009) Final version of 2009 AJCC melanoma staging and classification. *J Clin Oncol* **27**(36): 6199–206.

Breslow, A. (1970) Thickness, cross-sectional areas and depth of invasion in the prognosis of cutaneous melanoma. *Ann Surg* **172**(5): 902–8.

Rose, C. (2017) Diagnostics of malignant melanoma of the skin: recommendations of the current S3 guidelines on histology and molecular pathology. *Pathologe* **38**(1): 49–61.

Common Clinical Differential Diagnoses of Malignant Melanoma

- Post-traumatic intracorneal thrombi ("black heel")
- Pigmented basal cell carcinoma, pigmented Bowen's disease
- Pigmented seborrheic keratosis (melano-acanthoma)
- Subungual hematoma
- Angioma or hematoma of the oral mucosa
- Angiokeratoma (see Chapter 6)

MALIGNANT MELANOMA

Common Clinical Differential Diagnoses of Malignant Melanoma

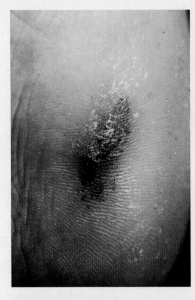
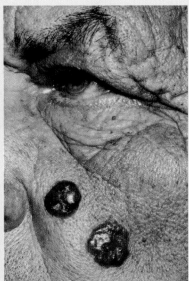

Black heel (left)

Pigmented BCC (right)

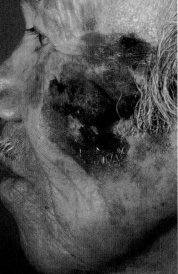
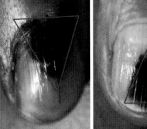
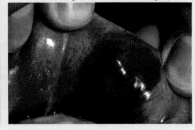

Seborrheic keratosis (left)

Acrolentiginous melanoma (left) and Subungual hematoma (right)

Angioma of the oral mucosa (bottom right)

CHAPTER 5
Connective Tissue

Atlas of Dermatopathology: Tumors, Nevi, and Cysts, First Edition. Günter Burg, Heinz Kutzner,
Werner Kempf, Josef Feit, and Bruce R. Smoller.
© 2019 John Wiley & Sons Ltd. Published 2019 by John Wiley & Sons Ltd.

Nevi

Connective Tissue Nevus (Shagreen Patch; Cobblestone Nevus; Nevus Collagenicus)

Multiple coalescent soft nodules on the buttock

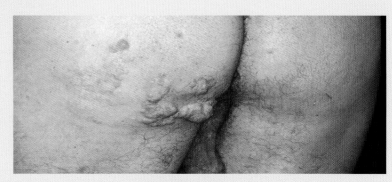

Normal epidermis; broad dermis

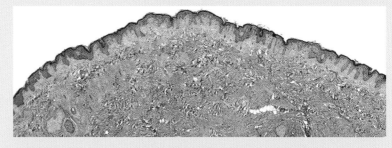

Densely packed collagenous fibres without parallel arrangement

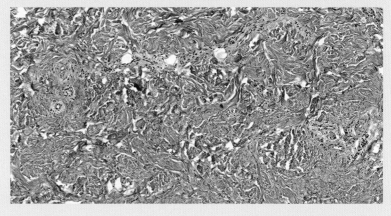

These lesions are frequently associated with syndromes, such as tuberous sclerosis or Buschke–Ollendorff syndrome.

Cl: Skin-colored solitary or multiple coalescent soft plaques or nodules in linear or zosteriform arrangement at birth or later in life, preferentially localized in the lumbosacral region.

Hi: This type of nevus is a simulator of "normal skin."

- Normal epidermis
- Paucicellular thickening of the dermis
- Homogeneous interwoven thickened and densely packed bundles of collagen
- No proliferation of fibroblasts
- Variable amount of elastic fibers
- No parallel arrangement of fascicles as seen in scar tissue or keloids

DD: Normal skin; dermatofibroma; pseudoxanthoma elasticum; scar tissue; dermatofibrosis lenticularis disseminata (Buschke–Ollendorff).

References

Chu, D.H., Goldbach, H., Wanat, K.A., Rubin, A.I., Yan, A.C., and Treat, J.R. (2015) A new variant of connective tissue nevus with elastorrhexis and predilection for the upper chest. *Pediatr Dermatol* **32**(4): 518–21.

de Feraudy, S. and Fletcher, C.D. (2012) Fibroblastic connective tissue nevus: a rare cutaneous lesion analyzed in a series of 25 cases. *Am J Surg Pathol* **36**(10): 1509–15.

Furfaro, T. (2006) Connective tissue nevus. *Dermatol Nurs* **18**(2): 165.

Velez, M.J., Billings, S.D., and Weaver, J.A. (2016) Fibroblastic connective tissue nevus. *J Cutan Pathol* **43**(1): 75–9.

Fibrous Neoplasms

Soft Fibroma (Skin Tag; Acrochordon)

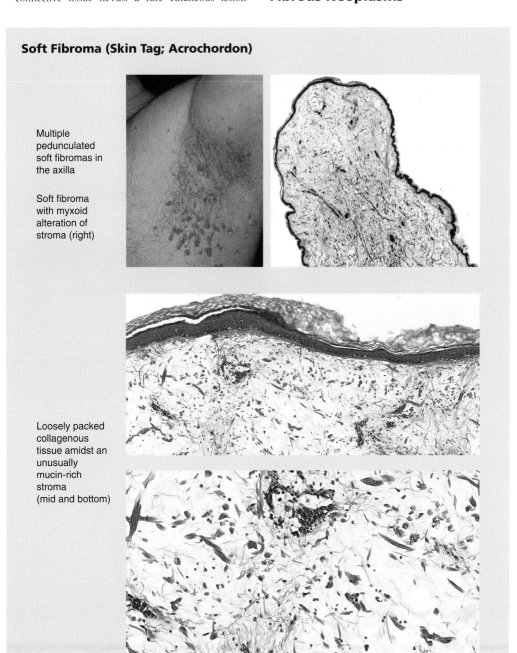

Multiple pedunculated soft fibromas in the axilla

Soft fibroma with myxoid alteration of stroma (right)

Loosely packed collagenous tissue amidst an unusually mucin-rich stroma (mid and bottom)

Cl: Common lesion in middle-aged or elderly individuals, preferentially in large skinfolds but also at any other localisation. Skin-colored or variably pigmented polypous or papular soft lesions, sometimes pedunculated. When the shaft of the lesion is twisted, infarction with necrosis and black discoloration can occur.

Hi:

- Exophytic polypous lesion
- Epidermis acanthotic papillomatous, normal or flattened
- Stroma composed of collagen tissue showing variable texture, loosely to densely packed
- Variable amount of fat tissue and small vessels
- Elastic fibers may be reduced

DD: Fibrolipoma (variant); fibroepithelial polyp; seborrheic keratosis; nevus lipomatosus; angiofibroma; involuted melanocytic nevus

References

Paredes, B.E. and Mentzel, T. (2011) Atypical lipomatous tumor/"well-differentiated liposarcoma" of the skin clinically presenting as a skin tag: clinicopathologic, immunohistochemical, and molecular analysis of 2 cases. *Am J Dermatopathol* **33**(6): 603–7.

Tan, O., Atik, B., and Bayram, I. (2005) Skin tag. *Dermatology* **210**(1): 82–3.

Perifollicular Fibroma (Fibrofolliculoma; Trichodiscoma)

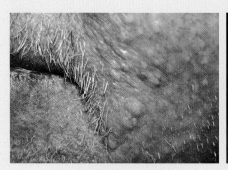
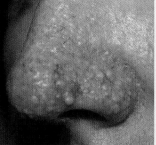

Papular lesions on cheek (left) and nose (right)

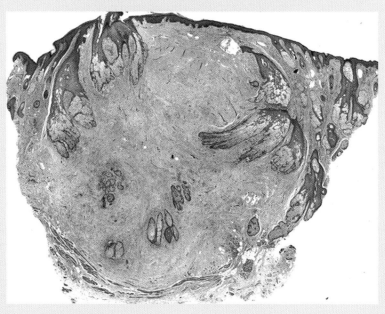

Downward proliferation of fibrous tissue including central pilosebaceous structures

Perifollicular Fibroma (Fibrofolliculoma; Trichodiscoma)

Horizontal cut through spindle cell predominant trichodiscoma. H&E (left) and CD34 (right)

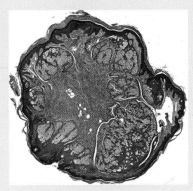 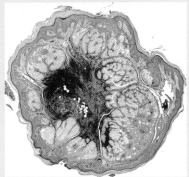

Cl: Perifollicular papules, solitary or multiple. Lesions are related to, if not identical with, trichodiscoma. Association with Birt–Hogg–Dubé syndrome, presenting as multiple flat white papules in the face.

Hi:

- Protuberant symmetrical papular tumor
- CD34-positive fibroblasts in the center, arranged in fascicles and strands
- Mucinous stroma
- Hyperplastic ("mitt-like") sebaceous glands on both sides of the tumor
- Ostiofollicular vestiges may be present in the center
- Focal entrapment of adipocytes

DD: Angiofibroma.

References

Nam, J.H., Min, J.H., Lee, G.Y., and Kim, W.S. (2011) A case of perifollicular fibroma. *Ann Dermatol* **23**(2): 236–8.

Misago, N., Kimura, T., and Narisawa, Y. (2009) Fibrofolliculoma/trichodiscoma and fibrous papule (perifollicular fibroma/angiofibroma): a revaluation of the histopathological and immunohistochemical features. *J Cutan Pathol* **36**(9): 943–51.

Shvartsbeyn, M., Mason, A.R., Bosenberg, M.W., and Ko, C.J. (2012) Perifollicular fibroma in Birt-Hogg-Dube syndrome: an association revisited. *J Cutan Pathol* **39**(7): 675–9.

Variant: Sclerotic Fibroma (Plywood Fibroma; Storiform Collagenoma)

Dermal nodule with paucicellular fibrosis

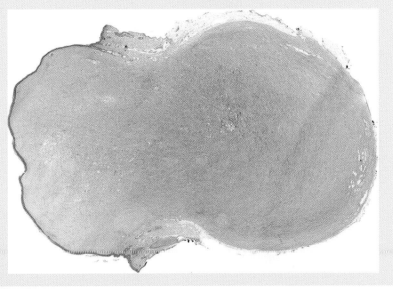

Variant: Sclerotic Fibroma (Plywood Fibroma; Storiform Collagenoma)

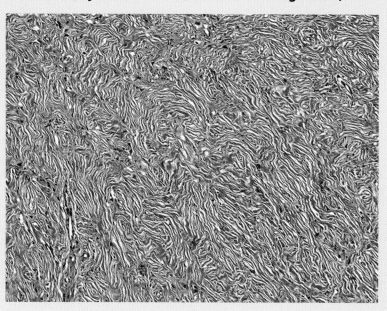

Characteristic "fingerprint" or "plywood" pattern

Cl: Solitary lesion. Multiple lesions may occur in association with Cowden's disease.

Hi: Symmetrical protuberant nodule with paucicellular CD34-positive fibroblastic proliferation embedded in a sclerotic whirl-like stroma (so-called "fingerprint" or "plywood" pattern).

Variant: Fibrous Papule of the Nose

Cl: Skin-colored dome-shaped papule.

Hi: Connective tissue with some larger, stellate, spindle or bizarre cells. Often ectatic blood vessels.

Variant: Pleomorphic Sclerosing Fibroma with Multinucleated Cells

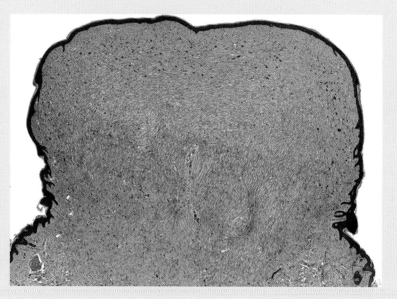

Dermal nodule of fibrous tissue

Variant: Pleomorphic Sclerosing Fibroma with Multinucleated Cells

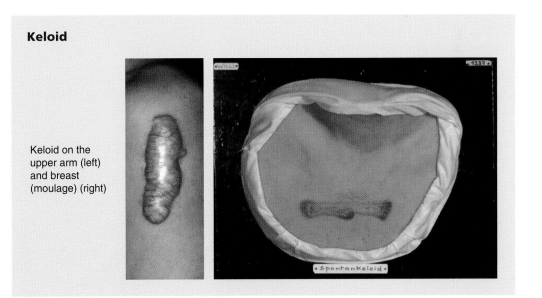

Pleomorphic cells in a fibrous background

Cl: polypous nodule, resembling skin tag.
Hi: Pleomorphic stellate fibroblastic cells, negative for both CD34 and alpha smooth muscle actin.

Keloid

Keloid on the upper arm (left) and breast (moulage) (right)

Keloid

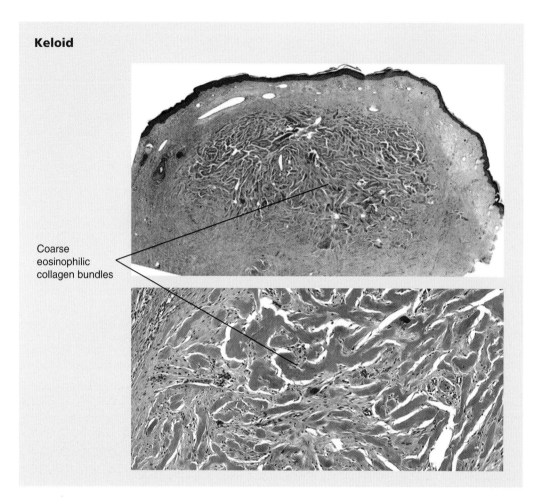

Coarse eosinophilic collagen bundles

Cl: In contrast to hypertrophic scars, keloids are well-circumscribed, slowly growing benign tumors, proliferating beyond margins of earlier tissue injury, burning, inflammatory condition, acne or surgery. Predilection for the head and neck, upper chest, and shoulder region of black individuals. The pruritic red firm tumors show a smooth surface.

Hi:
- Epidermis normal or atrophic
- Broad hyalinized and sclerotic collagen bundles and fibroblasts
- Scarce inflammatory infiltrate

DD: Hypertrophic scar.

Infantile Digital Fibromatosis (Inclusion Body Fibromatosis; Recurring Digital Fibrous Tumor of Children; Reye's Tumor)

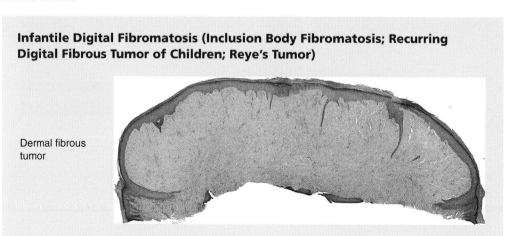

Dermal fibrous tumor

Infantile Digital Fibromatosis (Inclusion Body Fibromatosis; Recurring Digital Fibrous Tumor of Children; Reye's Tumor)

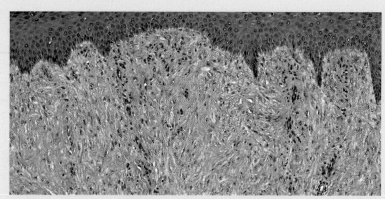

Spindle shaped fibroblasts and myofibroblasts

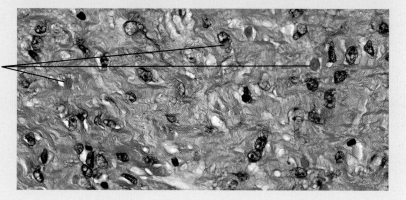

Eosinophilic inclusion bodies

CI: Solitary, rarely multiple soft tumorous swelling on the fingers or toes, rarely in other localisations. Usually present at birth or shortly thereafter but occurrence in adults has been reported. Tendency to spontaneous regression.

Hi:
- Poorly circumscribed dermal tumor, extending into the subcutis
- Interlacing bundles of spindle-shaped fibroblasts and myofibroblasts, positive for actin and vimentin
- The eosinophilic inclusion bodies (accumulation of actin) within the cytoplasm of fibroblasts may be as large as erythrocytes

DD: Dermatofibroma.

References

Choi, K.C., Hashimoto, K., Setoyama, M., Kagetsu, N., Tronnier, M., and Sturman, S. (1990) Infantile digital fibromatosis. Immunohistochemical and immunoelectron microscopic studies. *J Cutan Pathol* **17**(4): 225–32.

Henderson, H., Peng, Y.J., and Salter, D.M. (2014) Anti-calponin 1 antibodies highlight intracytoplasmic inclusions of infantile digital fibromatosis. *Histopathology* **64**(5): 752–5.

Kaya, A., Yuca, S.A., Karaman, K., et al. (2013) Infantile digital fibromatosis (inclusion body fibromatosis) observed in a baby without finger involvement. *Indian J Dermatol* **58**(2): 160.

Pettinato, G., Manivel, J.C., Gould, E.W., and Albores-Saavedra, J. (1994) Inclusion body fibromatosis of the breast. Two cases with immunohistochemical and ultrastructural findings. *Am J Clin Pathol* **101**(6): 714–18.

Suryawanshi, P., Rekhi, B., and Jambhekar, N.A. (2010) Morphological spectrum of inclusion body fibromatosis: a rare case report. *Indian J Pathol Microbiol* **53**(4): 827–28.

Viale, G., Doglioni, C., Iuzzolino, P., et al. (1988) Infantile digital fibromatosis-like tumour (inclusion body fibromatosis) of adulthood: report of two cases with ultrastructural and immunocytochemical findings. *Histopathology* **12**(4): 415–24.

Zardawi, I.M. and Earley, M.J. (1982) Inclusion body fibromatosis. *J Pathol* **137**(2): 99–107.

Malformations with Supernumerary Tissue Elements

Supernumerary Digit (Rudimentary Digit; Rudimentary Polydactyly)

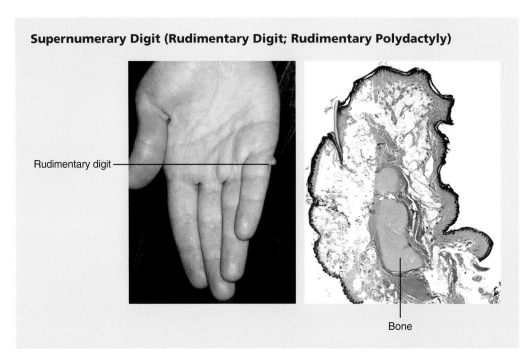

Rudimentary digit

Bone

Cl: These are congenital supernumerary rudimentary fingers, potentially composed of all elements of normal fingers, including bone, cartilage, nerves, and nail. Preferential localisation is the lateral side of the fifth digit, most frequently in black people.

Hi:

- Digital outgrowth
- Fibrous stroma
- Hypertrophic nerves
- Association with mature cartilage or bone

DD: Post-traumatic neuroma, digital fibrokeratoma; skin tag; pedunculated wart; fibroma; neurofibroma.

Reference

Kim, J., Zambrano, E.V., and McNiff, J.M. (2007) Congenital panfollicular nevus associated with polydactyly. *J Cutan Pathol* **34**(Suppl 1): 14–17.

Differential Diagnosis: Acral Acquired Fibrokeratoma

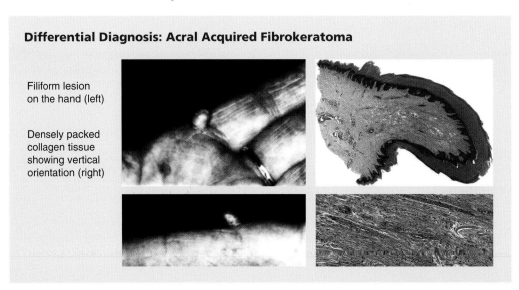

Filiform lesion on the hand (left)

Densely packed collagen tissue showing vertical orientation (right)

Cl: Solitary exophytic fibroma-like hyperkeratotic, narrow-based lesion, preferentially localized on the lateral side of the hands, sometimes also feet, fingers or toes. Preceding trauma may play an etiological role.

Hi:

• Exophytic filiform lesion
• Acanthosis and hyperkeratosis
• Proliferation of densely packed, hyalinized fibrous tissue with parallel orientation along the vertical axis
• No bone or cartilage

DD: Supernumerary digit; pedunculated wart; soft fibroma; dermatofibroma (histiocytoma); angiofibroma; periungual fibroma (Koenen tumor, associated with tuberous sclerosis); superficial acral fibromyxoma (positive for CD34 and nestin).

References

Bode, U. and Burg, G. (1978) [The acquired digital fibrokeratoma] *Hautarzt* **29**(12): 659–60.

Kint, A. and Baran, R. (1988) Histopathologic study of Koenen tumors. Are they different from acquired digital fibrokeratoma? *J Am Acad Dermatol* **18**: 369–72.

Accessory Tragus (Preauricular Tag)

Preauricular polypous papule (left)

Cartilage   Vellus hair follicles

Cl: Inborn preauricular pedunculated, polypous skin-colored nodule or papule. Association with various syndromes.

Hi:
- Normal epidermis

- Cartilage in the dermis and subcutaneous tissue
- Many vellus hair follicles

DD: Regular tragus; fibroepithelial lesion; hair follicle nevus.

Accessory Nipple (Ectopic Breast; Polythelia)

Bundles of smooth muscle (right top) around tubular structures with apocrine secretion (right bottom)

Pigmented papule with central dell (left)

Cl: Solitary or multiple inborn reddish-brown papules with central dell, preferentially on the ventral trunk along the milk line.

Hi:
- Vertically oriented collagenous fibers
- Central follicle or dilated duct
- Bundles of smooth muscle

- Tubules with two-layered ductal apocrine epithelium
- Intraepidermal splaying of solitary CK7-positive Toker cells

DD: Dermal nevus; neurofibroma; leiomyoma.

Fibrohistiocytic Neoplasms

Dermatofibroma (Benign Fibrous Histiocytoma; Fibroma Durum; Sclerosing Hemangioma)

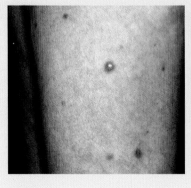
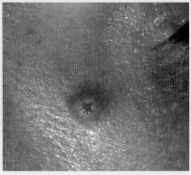

Dermatofibromas on the leg and in the face

Dermatofibroma (Benign Fibrous Histiocytoma; Fibroma Durum; Sclerosing Hemangioma)

Acanthosis and papillomatosis on top of underlying mesenchymal proliferation

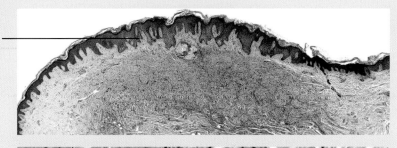

Diffuse proliferation of fibroblasts and histiocytes in the dermis

Broad "entrapped" collagen fibres: Radial spread of fibroblasts between collagen bundles

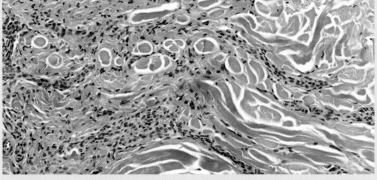

Proliferation of fibroblasts and histiocytes

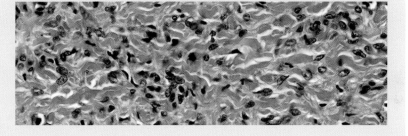

Cl: Common lesion preferentially on the extremities, presumably following insect bites or banal trauma. Solitary or multiple firm broad-based papules or nodules, which are red in the begin-ning and turn skin colored or brownish after some time. Evolution into a slightly depressed scarring pigmented lesion. Several clinical variants of dermatofibroma exist.

VARIANTS

Sclerosing Hemangioma (Hemosiderotic Dermatofibroma)

Nodular dermatofibroma on the arm (left)

Dense proliferation of fibroblasts and histiocytes with pseudo-vascular spaces (mid) and siderophages (right)

Prussian blue staining of siderophages (right)

Pseudo-vascular (sinusoidal) spaces and sheets of siderophages

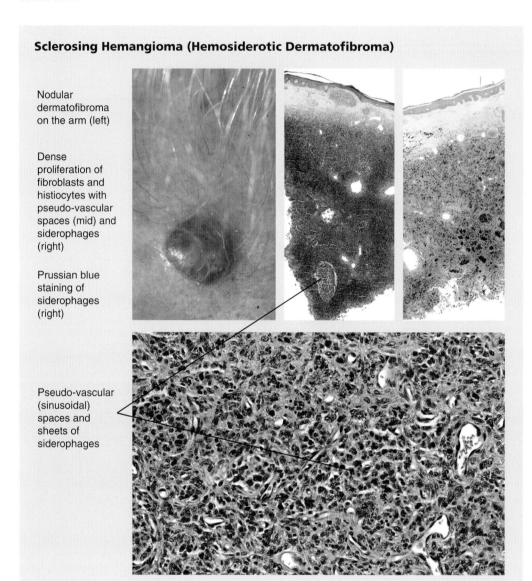

VARIANTS

Dermatofibroma (Histiocytoma) with Basaloid Proliferation of the Epidermis

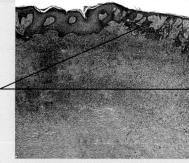
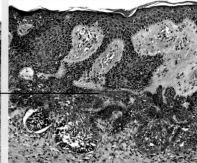

Induction of basaloid proliferation imitating BCC

Paucicellular Dermatofibroma

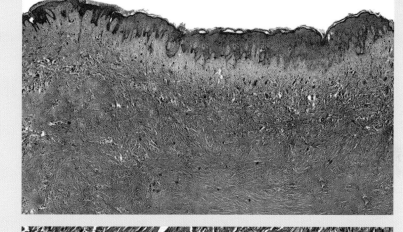

Hyperplastic epidermis

Paucicellular fibrosis with few embedded fibroblasts and histiocytes (mid and bottom)

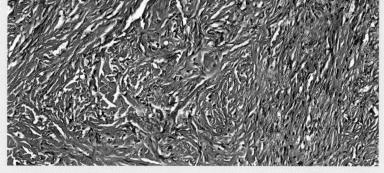

VARIANTS

Clear Cell Dermatofibroma

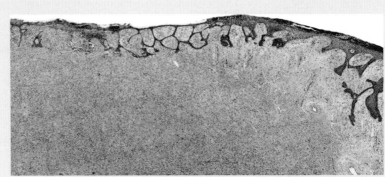

Branching epithelial proliferation (top and mid)

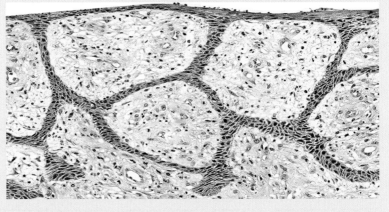

Proliferation of large histiocytic cells with ample clear cytoplasm (mid and bottom)

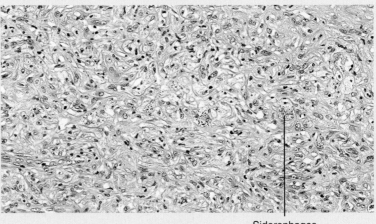

Siderophages

VARIANTS

Dermatofibroma with Monster Cells

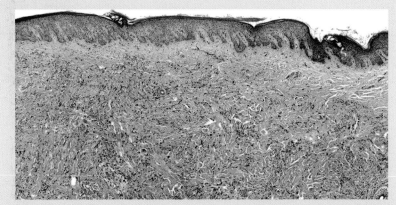

Large atypical cells amidst regular fibroblasts and histiocytes. Very few mitoses (top and mid)

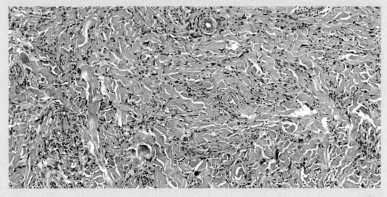

Marked hyperchromasia and pleomorphism of "monster cells"

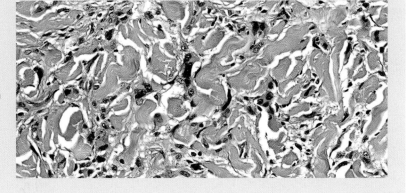

VARIANTS

Mucinous Dermatofibroma

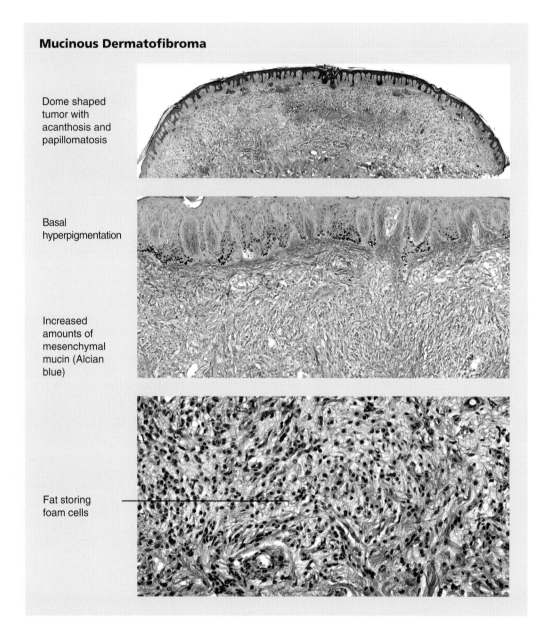

Dome shaped tumor with acanthosis and papillomatosis

Basal hyperpigmentation

Increased amounts of mesenchymal mucin (Alcian blue)

Fat storing foam cells

VARIANTS

Aneurysmatic Dermatofibroma

Circumscribed
dermal
infiltrate (left)

Thrombosed
pseudovascular
spaces (right)

Granulation
tissue in
pseudovascular
spaces (left)
with CD68
positive
cells (right)

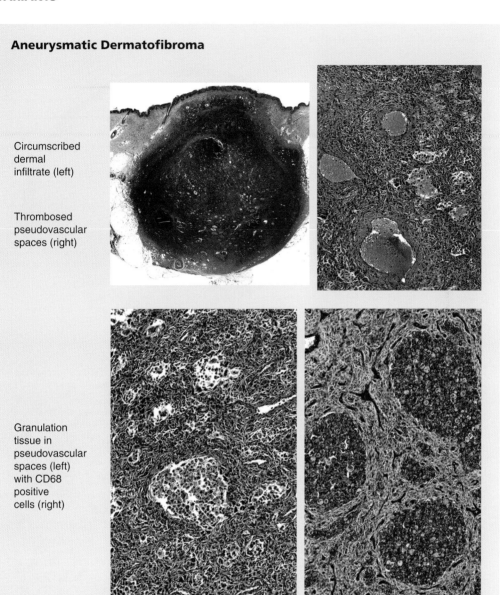

VARIANTS

Epithelioid Dermatofibroma

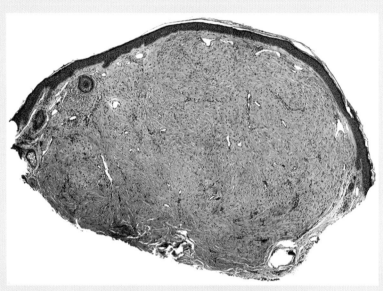

Richly vascularized well circumscribed dermal tumor

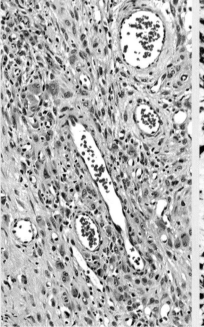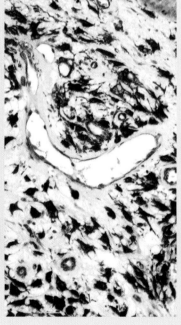

Epithelioid ALK-positive (right) histiocytes with ample eosinophilic cytoplasm. Many interspersed vessels (left)

Hi:
- Circumscribed acanthosis and papillomatosis
- Occasional basaloid buds extending from the acanthotic epidermis. They represent follicular induction resembling basal cell carcinoma
- In the dermis, proliferation of spindle cell fibroblasts with variable amount of newly formed collagen
- Lesions are circumscribed with irregular borders, which in the periphery show radial Indian file-like spread of fibroblasts between collagen bundles ("entrapped" broadened collagen bundles)
- Inflammatory infiltrate in the surrounding stroma, occasionally containing many plasma cells and eosinophils

- Initial lesions may have strong vascularization with extravasation of erythrocytes
- Later lesions may show xanthomatous changes with foamy histiocytes and macrophages
- Atrophy of the epidermis and paucicellular dense fibrous scarring tissue in the epidermis in resolving atrophic dermatofibromas
- Variants of common histiocytoma include cellular or large cellular histiocytomas with "monster cells," paucicellular, aneurysmatic, clear cell, mucinous, xanthomatous, and epithelioid forms

DD: Melanocytic nevus; Spitz nevus; juvenile xanthogranuloma; nodular basal cell carcinoma; mastocytoma.

References

Agarwal, A., Gopinath, A., Tetzlaff, M.T., and Prieto, V.G. (2017) Phosphohistone-H3 and Ki67: useful markers in differentiating dermatofibroma from dermatofibrosarcoma protuberans and atypical fibrohistiocytic lesions. *Am J Dermatopathol* **39**(7): 504–7.

Calonje, E. (2000) Is cutaneous benign fibrous histiocytoma (dermatofibroma) a reactive inflammatory process or a neoplasm? *Histopathology* **37**(3): 278–80.

Calonje, E. (2001) Dermatofibroma (fibrous histiocytoma): an inflammatory or neoplastic disorder? *Histopathology* **39**(2): 213.

Chen, T.C., Kuo, T., and Chan, H.L. (2000) Dermatofibroma is a clonal proliferative disease. *J Cutan Pathol* **27**(1): 36–9.

Davis, T.T., Calilao, G., and Fretzin, D. (2006) Sebaceous hyperplasia overlying a dermatofibroma. *Am J Dermatopathol* **28**(2): 155–7.

Garrido-Ruiz, M.C., Carrillo, R., Enguita, A.B., and Peralto, J.L. (2009) Signet-ring cell dermatofibroma. *Am J Dermatopathol* **31**(1): 84–7.

Goodman, W.T., Bang, R.H., and Padilla, R.S. (2002) Giant dermatofibroma with monster cells. *Am J Dermatopathol* **24**(1): 36–8.

Kazlouskaya, V., Malhotra, S., Kabigting, F.D., Lal, K., and Elston, D.M. (2014) CD99 expression in dermatofibrosarcoma protuberans and dermatofibroma. *Am J Dermatopathol* **36**(5): 392–6.

Kiyohara, T., Kumakiri, M., Kobayashi, H., Ohkawara, A., and Lao, L.M. (2000) Atrophic dermatofibroma. Elastophagocytosis by the tumor cells. *J Cutan Pathol* **27**(6): 312–15.

Labonte, S., Hanna, W., and Bandarchi-Chamkhaleh, B. (2007) A study of CD117 expression in dermatofibrosarcoma protuberans and cellular dermatofibroma. *J Cutan Pathol* **34**(11): 857–60.

Li, N., McNiff, J., Hui, P., Manfioletti, G., and Tallini, G. (2004) Differential expression of HMGA1 and HMGA2 in dermatofibroma and dermatofibrosarcoma protuberans: potential diagnostic applications, and comparison with histologic findings, CD34, and factor XIIIa immunoreactivity. *Am J Dermatopathol* **26**(4): 267–72.

Mentzel, T., Kutzner, H., Rutten, A., and Hugel, H. (2001) Benign fibrous histiocytoma (dermatofibroma) of the face: clinicopathologic and immunohistochemical study of 34 cases associated with an aggressive clinical course. *Am J Dermatopathol* **23**(5): 419–26.

Nestle, F.O., Nickoloff, B.J., and Burg, G. (1995) Dermatofibroma: an abortive immunoreactive process mediated by dermal dendritic cells? *Dermatology* **190**(4): 265–8.

Sachdev, R. and Sundram, U. (2006) Expression of CD163 in dermatofibroma, cellular fibrous histiocytoma, and dermatofibrosarcoma protuberans: comparison with CD68, CD34, and Factor XIIIa. *J Cutan Pathol* **33**(5): 353–60.

Shuweiter, M. and Boer, A. (2009) Spectrum of follicular and sebaceous differentiation induced by dermatofibroma. *Am J Dermatopathol* **31**(8): 778–85.

Spaun, E. and Zelger, B. (2009) Dermatofibroma with intracytoplasmic eosinophilic globules: an unusual phenomenon. *J Cutan Pathol* **36**(7): 796–8.

Tran, T.A., Hayner-Buchan, A., Jones, D.M., McRorie, D., and Carlson, J.A. (2007) Cutaneous balloon cell dermatofibroma (fibrous histiocytoma). *Am J Dermatopathol* **29**(2): 197–200.

Yan, X., Takahara, M., Xie, L., Tu, Y., and Furue, M. (2010) Cathepsin K expression: a useful marker for the differential diagnosis of dermatofibroma and dermatofibrosarcoma protuberans. *Histopathology* **57**(3): 486–8.

Zelger, B. (2002) It's a dermatofibroma, CD34 is irrelevant! *Am J Dermatopathol* **24**(5): 453–4.

Zelger, B. (2004) Pigmented atypical fibroxanthoma, a dermatofibroma variant? *Am J Dermatopathol* **26**(1): 84–6; author reply 86–7.

Zelger, B.G. and Zelger, B. (2001) Dermatofibroma (fibrous histiocytoma): an inflammatory or neoplastic disorder? *Histopathology* **38**(4): 379–81.

Dermatofibrosarcoma Protuberans

Cl: Upper trunk, shoulder, head of young or middle-aged individuals are the most common localisations of this initially slowly growing, firm tumor with cutaneous and subcutaneous multiple confluent nodules. The overlying skin is red-brown with telangiectasias and shows a smooth surface without ulceration. Due to the mostly underestimated spread beyond clinically visible borders, removal is often incomplete and recurrences and final metastases occur frequently, occasionally with transformation into fibrosarcoma.

Dermatofibrosarcoma Protuberans

Large tumor composed of confluent plaques and nodules

Proliferation of monomorphous spindle cells, and characteristic "entrapped" fat cells – producing a sieve-like pattern (right top and mid)

Monomorphous spindle cells (left)

CD34-positive tumor cells (right)

Hi:

- Epidermal hyperplasia with hyperpigmentation of the stratum basale
- Dermal and subcutaneous tumor with poorly defined borders
- Sparing of the papillary dermis
- Monomorphous spindle cells with prominent nuclei
- Storiform, honeycomb- or cartwheel-like growth pattern
- Fascicles spreading between collagen bundles and along septae of subcutaneous fat tissue with entrapment of fat lobules, resulting in a sieve-like appearance
- Mitoses are rare, but number may be increased, when transformation to sarcomatous growth occurs
- Variants include sclerosing, giant cell, myxoid, granular cell and fibrosarcomatous forms
- The pigmented Bednar tumor is a DFSP variant which is rich in melanocytes

Dermatofibrosarcoma Protuberans, Storiform Pattern

Storiform pattern

CD34

Immunohistochemistry: diffusely positive for CD34. Specific translocation t(17;22) and fusion gene may be shown by FISH or RT-PCR respectively.

DD: Keloid; dermatofibroma (usually factor XIIIa positive and CD34 negative).

References

Abdaljaleel, M.Y. and North, J.P. (2017) Sclerosing dermatofibrosarcoma protuberans shows significant overlap with sclerotic fibroma in both routine and immunohistochemical analysis: a potential diagnostic pitfall. *Am J Dermatopathol* **39**(2): 83–8.

Agarwal, A., Gopinath, A., Tetzlaff, M.T., and Prieto, V.G. (2017) Phosphohistone-H3 and Ki67: useful markers in differentiating dermatofibroma from dermatofibrosarcoma protuberans and atypical fibrohistiocytic lesions. *Am J Dermatopathol* **39**(7): 504–7.

Bague, S. and Folpe, A.L. (2008) Dermatofibrosarcoma protuberans presenting as a subcutaneous mass: a clinicopathological study of 15 cases with exclusive or near-exclusive subcutaneous involvement. *Am J Dermatopathol* **30**(4): 327–32.

Calikoglu, E., Augsburger, E., Chavaz, P., Saurat, J.H., and Kaya, G. (2003) CD44 and hyaluronate in the differential diagnosis of dermatofibroma and dermatofibrosarcoma protuberans. *J Cutan Pathol* **30**(3): 185–9.

Kazlouskaya, V., Malhotra, S., Kabigting, F.D., Lal, K., and Elston, D.M. (2014) CD99 expression in dermatofibrosarcoma protuberans and dermatofibroma. *Am J Dermatopathol* **36**(5): 392–6.

Labonte, S., Hanna, W., and Bandarchi-Chamkhaleh, B. (2007) A study of CD117 expression in dermatofibrosarcoma protuberans and cellular dermatofibroma. *J Cutan Pathol* **34**(11): 857–60.

Li, N., McNiff, J., Hui, P., Manfioletti, G., and Tallini, G. (2004) Differential expression of HMGA1 and HMGA2 in dermatofibroma and dermatofibrosarcoma protuberans: potential diagnostic applications, and comparison with histologic findings, CD34, and factor XIIIa immunoreactivity. *Am J Dermatopathol* **26**(4) L 267–72.

Mentzel, T., Scharer, L., Kazakov, D.V., and Michal, M. (2007) Myxoid dermatofibrosarcoma protuberans: clinicopathologic, immunohistochemical, and molecular analysis of eight cases. *Am J Dermatopathol* **29**(5): 443–8.

Park, H.J., Nguyen, J.V., Miller, C.J., Klein, W.M., Rubin, A.I., and Elenitsas, R. (2014) Follicular induction overlying a dermatofibrosarcoma protuberans. *Am J Dermatopathol* **36**(2): 186–8.

Sachdev, R. and Sundram, U. (2006) Expression of CD163 in dermatofibroma, cellular fibrous histiocytoma, and dermatofibrosarcoma protuberans: comparison with CD68, CD34, and Factor XIIIa. *J Cutan Pathol* **33**(5): 353–60.

Santos-Briz, A., Riveiro-Falkenbach, E., Roman-Curto, C., Mir-Bonafe, J.M., Acquadro, F., and Mentzel, T. (2014) Braided pattern in a dermatofibrosarcoma protuberans: a potential mimicker of neural neoplasms. *Am J Dermatopathol* **36**(11): 920–4.

Swaby, M.G., Evans, H.L., Fletcher, C.D., et al. (2011) Dermatofibrosarcoma protuberans with unusual sarcomatous transformation: a series of 4 cases with molecular confirmation. *Am J Dermatopathol* **33**(4): 354–60.

Wood, L., Fountaine, T.J., Rosamilia, L., Helm, K.F., and Clarke, L.E. (2010) Cutaneous CD34+ spindle cell neoplasms: histopathologic features distinguish spindle cell lipoma, solitary fibrous tumor, and dermatofibrosarcoma protuberans. *Am J Dermatopathol* **32**(8): 764–8.

Yan, X., Takahara, M., Xie, L., Tu, Y., and Furue, M. (2010) Cathepsin K expression: a useful marker for the differential diagnosis of dermatofibroma and dermatofibrosarcoma protuberans. *Histopathology* **57**(3): 486–8.

Variant: Pigmented Dermatofibrosarcoma Protuberans (Bednar's Tumor)

Interspersed pigmented dendritic melanocytes

Cl: Clinical features are the same as found in dermatofibrosarcoma protuberans.

Hi:

- Typical features of dermatofibrosarcoma protuberans
- Diffuse splaying of intratumoral solitary melanocytes (Melan A positive)

References

Bednar, B. (1957) Storiform neurofibromas of the skin, pigmented and nonpigmented. *Cancer* **10**(2): 368–76.

Goncharuk, V., Mulvaney, M., and Carlson, J.A. (2003) Bednar tumor associated with dermal melanocytosis: melanocytic colonization or neuroectodermal multidirectional differentiation? *J Cutan Pathol* **30**(2): 147–51.

McAllister, J.C., Recht, B., Hoffman, T.E., and Sundram, U.N. (2008) CD34+ pigmented fibrous proliferations: the morphologic overlap between pigmented dermatofibromas and Bednar tumors. *Am J Dermatopathol* **30**(5): 484–7.

Variant: Giant Cell Fibroblastoma

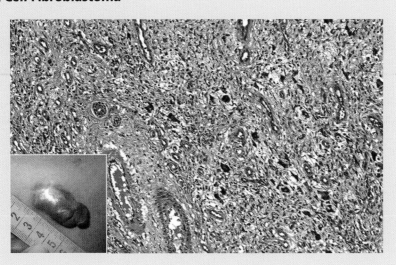

Fibrous stroma with stellate and dendritic giant cells. Nodular lesion on the trunk (inset)

Cl: Rare variant of dermatofibrosarcoma protuberans occuring on the chest wall, back, and thigh of children as a poorly circumscribed tumor.

Hi:
- Dermatofibrosarcomatous structures
- Multinuclear stellate or dendritic CD34-positive giant cells
- Myxoid pseudovascular pseudocysts

Reference

Shmookler, B.M., Enzinger, F.M., and Weiss, S.W. (1989) Giant cell fibroblastoma. A juvenile form of dermatofibrosarcoma protuberans. *Cancer* **64**(10): 2154–61.

Pleomorphic Dermal Sarcoma (PDS)

Storiform growth pattern with marked pleomorphism and hyperchromasia (left)

Large atypical cells (right)

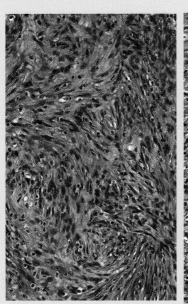
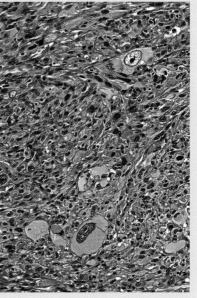

Pleomorphic Dermal Sarcoma (PDS)

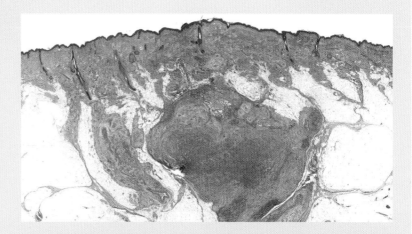

Subcutaneous
tumor

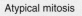

Atypical mitosis

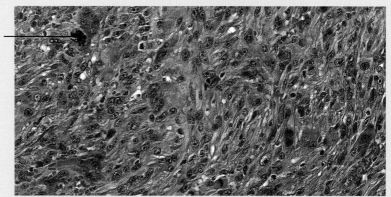

Pleomorphic
hyperchromatic
cells
(mid and bottom)

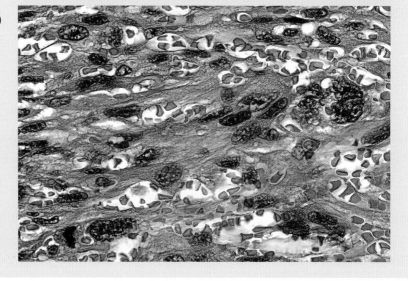

The term "malignant fibrous histiocytoma" (MFH) is outdated and was used to designate a heterogeneous group of sarcomas with markedly anaplastic or pleomorphic features. This obsolete term has been replaced by atypical fibroxanthoma (AFX) for the nodular exophytic form and pleomorphic dermal sarcoma (PDS) for the infiltrative deep variant. Advances in immunohistochemistry and molecular pathology have made it possible to diagnose most of the tumors formerly subsumed under the waste-basket diagnosis of MFH with greater precision.

Cl: The superficial form of "MFH" (AFX) is a nodular, locally aggressive tumor in sun-exposed areas of adults, preferentially in the head and neck, or dorsa of the hands. In the deeper form of "MFH" (PDS), the skin is affected usually as a part of deep involvement of a more aggressive soft tissue tumor, arising most probably from vessels or perivascular myoid cells. Ulceration and necroses are common features in both.

Hi:

- Growth pattern:
  - AFX: strictly symmetrical, exophytic, and superficial, not infiltrative
  - PDS: infiltrative growth with poorly defined margins, reaching the subcutaneous fat
- The common denominators of AFX and PDS are:
  - Spindle-shaped cells, sometimes in storiform pattern
  - Admixture of large, pleomorphic cells with nuclear atypia
  - Variable number of foam cells and giant cells
  - Mitotic activity and necrosis
- Inflammatory, myxoid, angiomatoid, clear cell, pigmented, granular and non-pleomorphic, keloidal, and sclerotic variants have been reported

DD: Spindle cell carcinoma (keratin markers); amelanotic malignant melanoma (melanoma markers).

References

Beer, T.W., Drury, P., and Heenan, P.J. (2010) Atypical fibroxanthoma: a histological and immunohistochemical review of 171 cases. *Am J Dermatopathol* **32**(6): 533–40.

Bruecks, A.K., Medlicott, S.A., and Trotter, M.J. (2003) Atypical fibroxanthoma with prominent sclerosis. *J Cutan Pathol* **30**(5): 336–9.

Calonje, E., Wadden, C., Wilson-Jones, E., and Fletcher, C.D. (1993) Spindle-cell non-pleomorphic atypical fibroxanthoma: analysis of a series and delineation of a distinctive variant. *Histopathology* **22**(3): 247–54.

Crowson, A.N., Carlson-Sweet, K., Macinnis, C., et al. (2002) Clear cell atypical fibroxanthoma: a clinicopathologic study. *J Cutan Pathol* **29**(6): 374–81.

Diaz-Cascajo, C., Borghi, S., and Bonczkowitz, M. (1998) Pigmented atypical fibroxanthoma. *Histopathology* **33**(6): 537–41.

Diaz-Cascajo, C., Bernd, R., Teresa, M., Fernandez, F., and Borghi, S. (2002) Malignant fibrous histiocytoma of the skin with marked inflammatory infiltrate: a sarcoma mimicking malignant lymphoma. *Am J Dermatopathol* **24**(3): 251–6.

Diaz-Cascajo, C., Weyers, W., and Borghi, S. (2003) Pigmented atypical fibroxanthoma: a tumor that may be easily mistaken for malignant melanoma. *Am J Dermatopathol* **25**(1): 1–5.

Gulmann, C., Egan, B., Cottell, D., Keane, F.B., and Jeffers, M.D. (2002) Aberrant S100 expression in cutaneous malignant fibrous histiocytoma: a potential pitfall in diagnosis. *Histopathology* **41**(4): 363–4.

Harding-Jackson, N., Sangueza, M., Mackinnon, A., Suster, S., and Plaza, J.A. (2015) Spindle cell atypical fibroxanthoma: myofibroblastic differentiation represents a diagnostic pitfall in this variant of AFX. *Am J Dermatopathol* **37**(7): 509–14; quiz 515–16.

Hartel, P.H., Jackson, J., Ducatman, B.S., and Zhang, P. (2006) CD99 immunoreactivity in atypical fibroxanthoma and pleomorphic malignant fibrous histiocytoma: a useful diagnostic marker. *J Cutan Pathol* **33**(Suppl 2): 24–8.

Kim, J. and McNiff, J.M. (2009) Keloidal atypical fibroxanthoma: a case series. *J Cutan Pathol* **36**(5): 535–9.

Lahat, G., Zhang, P., Zhu, Q.S., et al. (2011) The expression of c-Met pathway components in unclassified pleomorphic sarcoma/malignant fibrous histiocytoma (UPS/MFH): a tissue microarray study. *Histopathology* **59**(3): 556–61.

Luzar, B. and Calonje, E. (2010) Morphological and immunohistochemical characteristics of atypical fibroxanthoma with a special emphasis on potential diagnostic pitfalls: a review. *J Cutan Pathol* **37**(3): 301–9.

McCalmont, T.H. (2012) Correction and clarification regarding AFX and pleomorphic dermal sarcoma. *J Cutan Pathol* **39**(1): 8.

Morgan, M.B., Pitha, J., Johnson, S., Dunn, B., and Everett, M.A. (1997) Angiomatoid malignant fibrous histiocytoma revisited. An immunohistochemical and DNA ploidy analysis. *Am J Dermatopathol* **19**(3): 223–7.

Murali, R. and Palfreeman, S. (2006) Clear cell atypical fibroxanthoma – report of a case with review of the literature. *J Cutan Pathol* **33**(5): 343–8.

Nguyen, C.M., Chong, K., and Cassarino, D. (2016) Clear cell atypical fibroxanthoma: a case report and review of the literature. *J Cutan Pathol* **43**(6): 538–42.

Osio, A., Vignon-Pennamen, M.D., Pedeutour, F., et al. (2017) PDGFRa amplification in multiple skin lesions of undifferentiated pleomorphic sarcoma: a clue for intimal sarcoma metastases. *J Cutan Pathol* **44**(5): 477–9.

Patton, A., Page, R., Googe, P.B., and King, R. (2009) Myxoid atypical fibroxanthoma: a previously undescribed variant. *J Cutan Pathol* **36**(11): 1177–84.

Requena, L., Sangueza, O.P., Sanchez Yus, E., and Furio, V. (1997) Clear-cell atypical fibroxanthoma: an uncommon histopathologic variant of atypical fibroxanthoma. *J Cutan Pathol* **24**(3): 176–82.

Rudisaile, S.N., Hurt, M.A., and Santa Cruz, D.J. (2005) Granular cell atypical fibroxanthoma. *J Cutan Pathol* **32**(4): 314–17.

Stephen, M.R. and Morton, R. (1998) Myxoid malignant fibrous histiocytoma mimicking papular mucinosis. *Am J Dermatopathol* **20**(3): 290–5.

Tardio, J.C., Pinedo, F., Aramburu, J.A., et al. (2016) Clear cell atypical fibroxanthoma: clinicopathological study of 6 cases and review of the literature with special emphasis on the differential diagnosis. *Am J Dermatopathol* **38**(8): 586–92.

Tardio, J.C., Pinedo, F., Aramburu, J.A., et al. (2016) Pleomorphic dermal sarcoma: a more aggressive neoplasm than previously estimated. *J Cutan Pathol* **43**(2): 101–12.

Thum, C., Hollowood, K., Birch, J., Goodlad, J.R., and Brenn, T. (2011) Aberrant Melan-A expression in atypical fibroxanthoma and undifferentiated pleomorphic sarcoma of the skin. *J Cutan Pathol* **38**(12): 954–60.

Toll, A., Gimeno, J., Baro, T., Hernandez-Munoz, M.I., and Pujol, R.M. (2016) Study of epithelial to mesenchymal transition in atypical fibroxanthoma and undifferentiated pleomorphic sarcoma to discern an epithelial origin. *Am J Dermatopathol* **38**(4): 270–7.

Wilk, M. and Zelger, B. (2010) Atypical fibroxanthoma – what is it, what it is not. *J Cutan Pathol* **37**(10): 1119–20.

Wright, N.A., Thomas, C.G., Calame, A., and Cockerell, C.J. (2010) Granular cell atypical fibroxanthoma: case report and review of the literature. *J Cutan Pathol* **37**(3): 380–5.

Zheng, R., Ma, L., Bichakjian, C.K., Lowe, L., and Fullen, D.R. (2011) Atypical fibroxanthoma with lymphomatoid reaction. *J Cutan Pathol* **38**(1): 8–13.

Miscellaneous Tumors

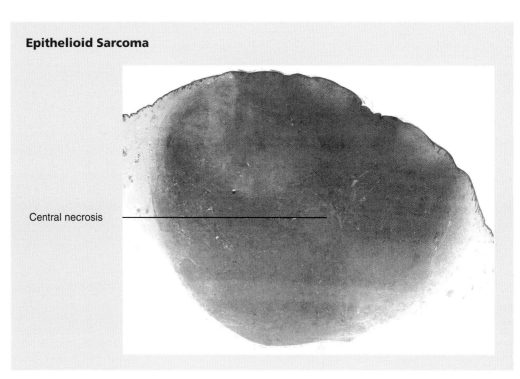

Epithelioid Sarcoma

Central necrosis

Epithelioid Sarcoma

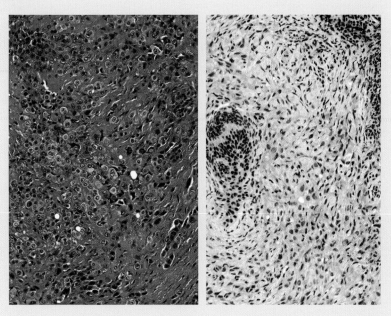

Polygonal cells with abundant eosinophilic cytoplasm (left)

Tumor cells are INI1 negative (right)

Cl: Subcutaneous, slowly growing malignant tumor preferentially on the distal extremities of young adults (distal type of epithelioid sarcoma) or at the pelvis and shoulder girdle (proximal type of epithelioid angiosarcoma). Ulceration may occur. Tendency to early multifocal spread and to local recurrences after incomplete excision.

Hi:

- Superficial biopsy may show pseudogranulomatous inflammation, imitating granuloma annulare
- The tumor presents as a poorly defined nodule in the deep dermis, extending into the fat, occasionally multifocal
- Plexiform and diffuse infiltrative growth pattern along the fascia and tendons
- Central necrosis, surrounded by tumor cells in palisade arrangement ("geographical necrosis"), simulating a deep granulomatous process with central necrobiosis
- Polygonal spindle cells with abundant eosinophilic cytoplasm and nuclear atypia

Immunohistochemistry: Tumor cells are positive for vimentin, keratin-markers, EMA, and CD34 while macrophage markers are negative. Tumor suppressor gene *INI1* (*SMARCB1*) shows conspicuous lack of nuclear expression. INI1 negativity is taken as a hallmark of epithelioid sarcoma.

DD: Deep granuloma annulare; necrobiosis lipoidica; rheumatoid nodule; granulomatous infection; giant cell tumor of tendon sheath; epithelioid angiosarcoma; epithelioid hemangioendothelioma.

References

Enzinger, F.M. (1970) Epitheloid sarcoma. A sarcoma simulating a granuloma or a carcinoma. *Cancer* **26**(5): 1029–41.

Flucke, U., Hulsebos, T.J., van Krieken, J.H., and Mentzel, T. (2010) Myxoid epithelioid sarcoma: a diagnostic challenge. A report on six cases. *Histopathology* **57**(5): 753–9.

Humble, S.D., Prieto, V.G., and Horenstein, M.G. (2003) Cytokeratin 7 and 20 expression in epithelioid sarcoma. *J Cutan Pathol* **30**(4): 242–6.

Kaddu, S., Wolf, I., Horn, M., and Kerl, H. (2008) Epithelioid sarcoma with angiomatoid features: report of an unusual case arising in an elderly patient within a burn scar. *J Cutan Pathol* **35**(3): 324–8.

Lin, L., Skacel, M., Sigel, J.E., et al. (2003) Epithelioid sarcoma: an immunohistochemical analysis evaluating the utility of cytokeratin 5/6 in distinguishing superficial epithelioid sarcoma from spindled squamous cell carcinoma. *J Cutan Pathol* **30**(2): 114–17.

Orrock, J.M., Abbott, J.J., Gibson, L.E., and Folpe, A.L. (2009) INI1 and GLUT-1 expression in epithelioid sarcoma and its cutaneous neoplastic and nonneoplastic mimics. *Am J Dermatopathol* **31**(2): 152–6.

Stuart, L.N., Gardner, J.M., Lauer, S.R., Monson, D.K., Parker, D.C., and Edgar, M.A. (2013) Epithelioid sarcoma-like (pseudomyogenic) hemangioendothelioma, clinically mimicking dermatofibroma, diagnosed by skin biopsy in a 30-year-old man. *J Cutan Pathol* **40**(10): 909–13.

Dermatomyofibroma

Tumorous plaque on the abdomen

Dermal tumor of horizontally arranged myofibroblasts. Adnexal structures are preserved (right)

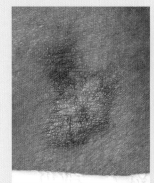
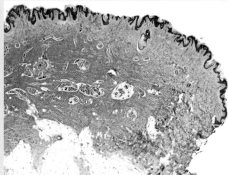

Slender fascicles of spindled myofibroblasts

Inset: partial expression of smooth muscle actin (ASMA)

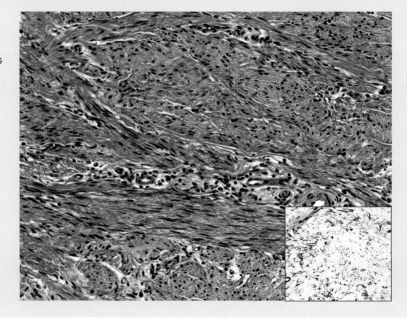

Cl: Benign, plaque-like tumor in young adults and adolescents. Predilection sites are the major skinfolds. Lesions clinically imitate flat dermatofibroma or neurofibroma. The tumor is considered to be an acquired benign myofibroblastic proliferation.

Hi:

- Flat, poorly circumscribed spindle cell proliferation involving the entire dermis
- Horizontally arranged intermingling fascicles of spindled myofibroblasts
- Adnexal structures and elastic fibers are preserved
- No polymorphism or mitotic activity

Immunohistochemistry: Incipient lesions show myofibroblastic expression of alpha smooth muscle actin (ASMA) while advanced lesions are both ASMA and desmin negative.

DD: Piloleiomyoma; dermatofibroma; fibroblastic connective tissue nevus.

References

Mentzel, T. and Kutzner, H. (2003) Haemorrhagic dermatomyofibroma (plaque-like dermal fibromatosis): clinicopathological and immunohistochemical analysis of three cases resembling plaque-stage Kaposi's sarcoma. *Histopathology* **42**(6): 594–8.

Mentzel, T. and Kutzner, H. (2009) Dermatomyofibroma: clinicopathologic and immunohistochemical analysis of 56 cases and reappraisal of a rare and distinct cutaneous neoplasm. *Am J Dermatopathol* **31**(1): 44–9.

CHAPTER 6

Vessels

CHAPTER MENU

Hamartomas, Nevi, and Malformations
  Phacomatosis Pigmentovascularis
  Eccrine Angiomatous Hamartoma
  Nevus Anemicus
Capillary Malformations
  Nevus Flammeus (Port-Wine Stain)
  Nevus Araneus (Spider Angioma)
  Cutis Marmorata Telangiectatica (van Lohuizen) (Nevus
    Vascularis Reticularis)
  Congenital Telangiectatic Erythema (Bloom's
    Syndrome)
Venous Malformations
  Blue Rubber Bleb Nevus Syndrome (Familial Venous
    Malformation)
  Hereditary Hemorrhagic Telangiectasia (Osler–Weber–
    Rendu)
  Angioma Serpiginosum
  Venular Aneurysm (Venous Lake)
  Cavernous Hemangioma (in Maffucci Syndrome)
  Sinusoidal Hemangioma
  Spindle Cell Hemangioma (Formerly Spindle Cell
    Hemangioendothelioma)
Arteriovenous Malformations
  Acral Arteriovenous Hemangioma (Cirsoid Aneurysm)
  Glomuvenular Malformation ("Glomangioma")
Lymphatic Malformations
  Superficial Lymphatic Malformation (Superficial
    Lymphangioma)
  Cystic Lymphatic Malformation (Cystic Hygroma)
  Targetoid Hemosiderotic (Hobnail) Hemangioma
  Progressive Lymphangioma
    (Benign Lymphangioendothelioma)
  Lymphangiomatosis
Angiokeratomas
  Verrucous Hemangioma (Venous Malformation)
  Variant: Solitary Angiokeratoma
  Variant: Angiokeratoma Circumscriptum Naeviformis
  Variant: Fordyce Angiokeratoma
  Variant: Angiokeratoma Acroasphycticum Digitorum
    (Mibelli)
  Variant: Multiple "Pinpoint" Angiokeratomas
    (Angiokeratoma Corporis Diffusum; Fabry's
    Disease)
  Variant: Acral Pseudolymphomatous Angiokeratoma
    of Children (APACHE)

Hyperplasias
  Granuloma Pyogenicum (Lobular Capillary
    Hemangioma; Botryomykoma)
  Differential Diagnosis: Pyogenic Granuloma-Like
    Granulation Tissue
  Bacillary Angiomatosis
  Verruga Peruana
  Intravascular Papillary Endothelial Hyperplasia (Masson)
  Acroangiodermatitis Mali (Pseudo-Kaposi's Sarcoma)
Benign Vascular Neoplasms
  Epithelioid Hemangioma (Angiolymphoid Hyperplasia
    with Eosinophilia, ALHE)
  Endothelial Differentiation
  Pericytic Differentiation
  Glomoid and Myoid Differentiation
  Recently Described Benign Vascular Tumors
Vascular Neoplasms of Intermediate Malignant Potential
  Kaposi's Sarcoma (KS)
  Retiform Hemangioendothelioma
  Composite Hemangioendothelioma
  Papillary Intralymphatic
    Angioendothelioma (PILA)
    (Malignant Endovascular Papillary
    Angioendothelioma (Dabska Tumor); Endovascular
    Papillary Hemangioendothelioma)
  Radiation-Induced Atypical Vascular Lesion (AVL)
    (Benign Lymphangiomatous Papule (BLAP))
Vascular Neoplasms with High Malignant Potential
  Cutaneous Angiosarcoma
  Radiation-Induced (Postradiation) Angiosarcoma
  Epithelioid Hemangioendothelioma
  Epithelioid Angiosarcoma
  Differential Diagnosis: Acantholytic (Angiosarcoma-Like)
    Squamous Cell Carcinoma
  Glomangiosarcoma (Malignant Glomus Tumor)
Other Neoplasms with Significant Vascular Component
  Multinucleate Angiohistiocytoma
  Angiofibroma (Adenoma Sebaceum Associated
    with Pringle–Bourneville Disease)
  Angiolipoma
  Angiolipoleiomyoma (Angiomyolipoma)
  Angiomyxoma
  Intralymphatic Histiocytosis
  Kimura's Disease

Atlas of Dermatopathology: Tumors, Nevi, and Cysts, First Edition. Günter Burg, Heinz Kutzner,
Werner Kempf, Josef Feit, and Bruce R. Smoller.
© 2019 John Wiley & Sons Ltd. Published 2019 by John Wiley & Sons Ltd.

Hamartomas, Nevi, and Malformations

Phacomatosis Pigmentovascularis

Nevus flammeus (trunk) and nevus pigmentosus (buttocks) in a baby

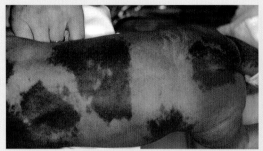
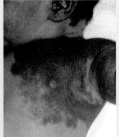

Dilated capillaries in the papillary dermis

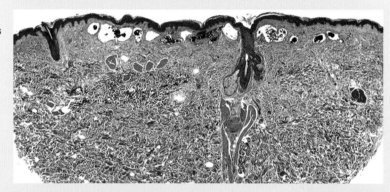

Pigment-loaded dendritic cells in the dermis

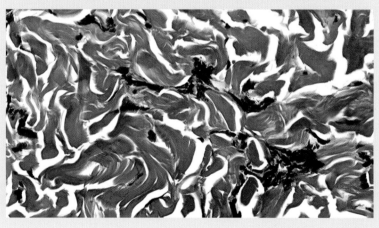

Variants:
- Type I: Nevus flammeus and nevus pigmentosus verrucosus
- Type II: Nevus flammeus and Mongolian spot (dermal melanocytosis)
- Type III: Nevus flammeus and nevus spilus
- Type IV: Nevus flammeus and nevus spilus and Mongolian spot and/or nevus anemicus

Eccrine Angiomatous Hamartoma

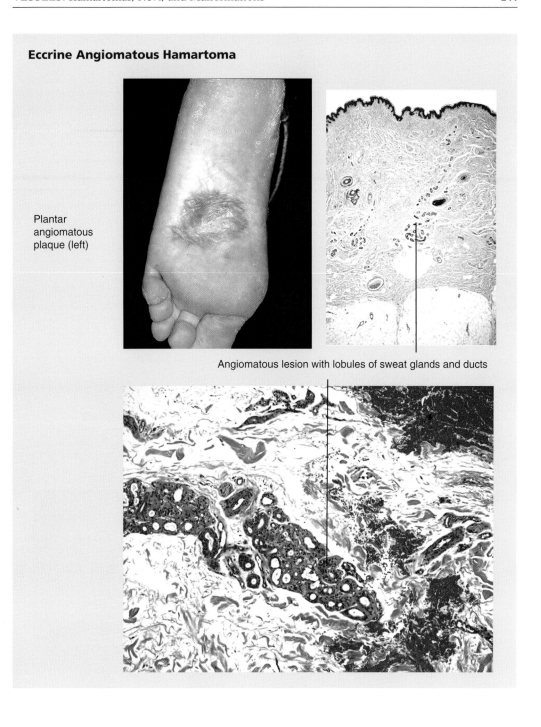

Plantar angiomatous plaque (left)

Angiomatous lesion with lobules of sweat glands and ducts

Cl: Red hyperhidrotic plaques, preferentially on palms and soles.

Hi: Increased number of lobularly grouped sweat glands and ducts in close proximity to dilated small blood vessels.

DD: Vascular malformations.

References

Hyman, A.B., Harris, H., and Brownstein, M.H. (1968) Eccrine angiomatous hamartoma. *N Y State J Med* **68**(21): 2803–6.

Requena, L. and Sangueza, O.P. (1997) Cutaneous vascular anomalies. Part I. Hamartomas, malformations, and dilation of preexisting vessels. *J Am Acad Dermatol* **37**(4): 523–49; quiz 549–52.

Sanmartin, O., Botella, R., Alegre, V., Martinez, A., and Aliaga, A. (1992) Congenital eccrine angiomatous hamartoma. *Am J Dermatopathol* **14**(2): 161–4.

Nevus Anemicus

This congenital lesion has a functional (vasoconstriction) rather than anatomical (decreased number of capillaries) background. Using reflectance confocal microscopy, there is no difference compared with normal skin. Association with neurofibromatosis type 1 and other syndromes is common.

Cl: Pale macules, especially when surrounding skin is irritated.

Hi: The skin histologically appears normal.

DD (clinical): Vitiligo; nevus depigmentosus.

References

Ahkami, R.N. and Schwartz, R.A. (1999) Nevus anemicus. *Dermatology* **198**(4): 327–9.

Errichetti, E. and Piccirillo, A. (2016) Co-occurrence of nevus anemicus and Becker nevus: a possible instance of pseudodidymosis? *Int J Dermatol* **55**(4): e219–20.

Lai, L.G. and Xu, A.E. (2011) In vivo reflectance confocal microscopy imaging of vitiligo, nevus depigmentosus and nevus anemicus. *Skin Res Technol* **17**(4): 404–10.

Ma, H., Liao, M., Qiu, S., Luo, R., Lu, R., and Lu, C. (2015) The case of a boy with nevus of Ota, extensive Mongolian spot, nevus flammeus, nevus anemicus and cutis marmorata telangiectatica congenita: a unique instance of phacomatosis pigmentovascularis. *An Bras Dermatol* **90**(3 Suppl 1): 10–12.

Mizutani, H., Ohyanagi, S., Umeda, Y., Shimizu, M., and Kupper, T.S. (1997) Loss of cutaneous delayed hypersensitivity reactions in nevus anemicus. Evidence for close concordance of cutaneous delayed hypersensitivity and endothelial E-selectin expression. *Arch Dermatol* **133**(5): 617–20.

Sachs, C. and Lipsker, D. (2016) Nevus anemicus and Bier spots in tuberous sclerosis complex. *JAMA Dermatol* **152**(2): 217–18.

Salvini, C., Fabroni, C., Francalanci, S., Massi, D., and Difonzo, E.M. (2007) Generalized nevus anaemicus in an adult. *J Eur Acad Dermatol Venereol* **21**(8): 1142–4.

Vaassen, P. and Rosenbaum, T. (2016) Nevus anemicus as an additional diagnostic marker of neurofibromatosis type 1 in childhood. *Neuropediatrics* **47**(3): 190–3.

Capillary Malformations

Nevus Flammeus (Port-Wine Stain)

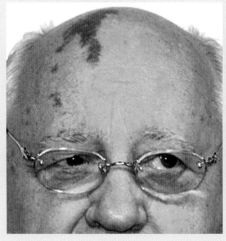
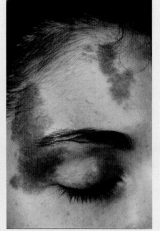

Nevus flammeus

Cl: Congenital pink or red-wine colored patch, which proportionally enlarges with body growth. No regression. Nodular or plaque-like hypertrophy in higher age. Association with several syndromes: Sturge–Weber (congenital, but not familial angiomatosis affecting the skin of the face, leptomeninges, and brain), Klippel–Trénaunay (nevus flammeus, congenital AV fistulae and hypertrophy of the bones and soft tissues in affected area).

Nevus Flammeus (Port-Wine Stain)

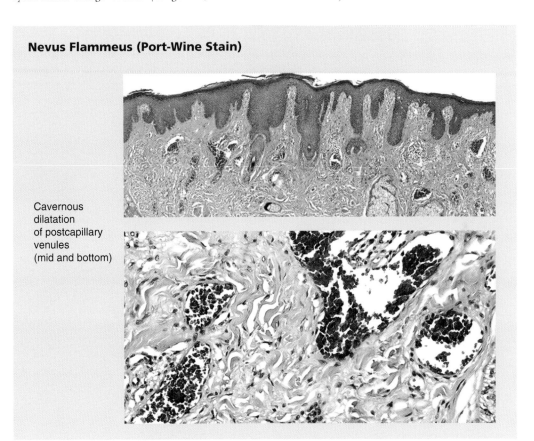

Cavernous dilatation of postcapillary venules (mid and bottom)

Hi: In early lesions, the histological picture is often inconspicuous and difficult to evaluate.
- Slightly increased number and dilation of postcapillary venules of the upper vascular plexus
- Later, variably dilated blood vessels appear
- In adults, there are usually many cavernous vascular spaces, vascular proliferations, and fibrosis

Immunohistochemistry: Distinct endothelial negativity for WT1 (immunohistochemical hallmark of malformative endothelia).

References

Finley, J.L., Noe, J.M., Arndt, K.A., and Rosen, S. (1984) Port-wine stains. Morphologic variations and developmental lesions. *Arch Dermatol* **120**(11): 1453–5.

Holloway, K.B., Ramos-Caro, F.A., Brownlee, R.E. Jr, and Flowers, F.P. (1994) Giant proliferative hemangiomas arising in a port-wine stain. *J Am Acad Dermatol* **31**(4): 675–6.

Rosen, S. and Smoller, B.R. (1987) Port-wine stains: a new hypothesis. *J Am Acad Dermatol* **17**(1): 164–6.

Nevus Araneus (Spider Angioma)

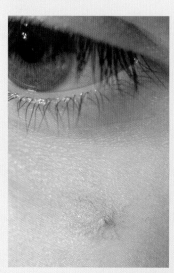

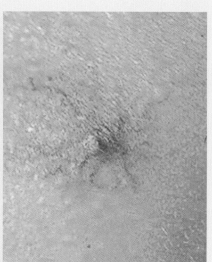

Central angioma
with radial
spreading
capillaries

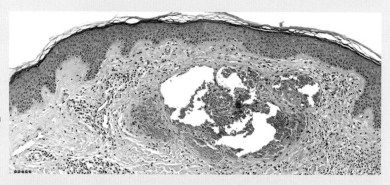

Dilated vascular
spaces with
thrombi. Dilatation
of vessels in the
periphery

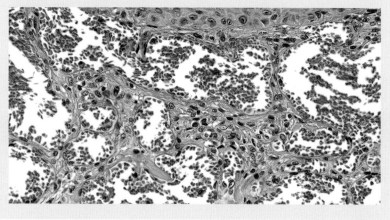

Dilated vascular
spaces

Cl: Tiny angiomatous lesion, pulsating, blanching, and refilling under diascopy. Array of tiny capillaries spread in the periphery of the lesion in a spider web fashion. Spontaneous spider angiomas are seen on the face of young individuals. Multiple symptomatic spider angiomas occur in systemic sclerosis, pregnancy, and hepatic cirrhosis.

Hi:

- In serial sections: central arteriole in the superficial dermis
- Small anastomosing venules in the periphery

DD: Telangiectases.

Reference

Bean, W.B. (1958) *Vascular Spider and Related Lesions of the Skin*. Springfield: Thomas.

Cutis Marmorata Telangiectatica (van Lohuizen) (Nevus Vascularis Reticularis)

Blue-red vascular mottling of the skin in a child

Cl: Congenital reticular or netlike vascular mottling of the skin, simulating livedo reticularis or racemosa and spreading mostly unilaterally over a large area of extremities or trunk. Superficial ulceration can occur in rare cases. Improvement of the condition with age.

Cutis Marmorata Telangiectatica (van Lohuizen) (Nevus Vascularis Reticularis)

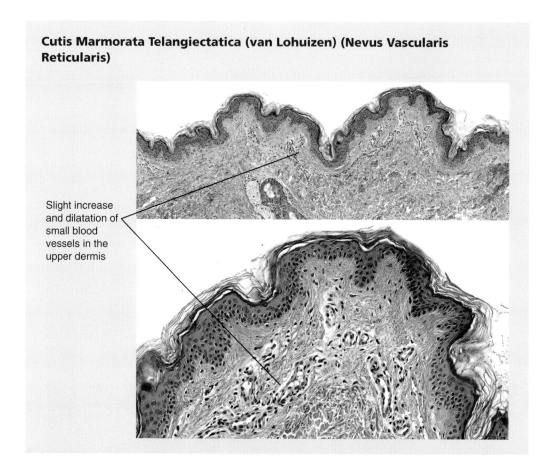

Slight increase and dilatation of small blood vessels in the upper dermis

Hi: Inconspicuous areas with increased and dilated thin-walled blood vessels. The histology is usually not diagnostic and clinical correlation is required. However, hemangiomatous histological features may be seen.

DD: Functional cutis marmorata; livedo reticularis; vascular malformations; lupus erythematosus.

Reference

Fujita, M., Darmstadt, G.L., and Dinulos, J.G. (2003) Cutis marmorata telangiectatica congenita with hemangiomatous histopathologic features. *J Am Acad Dermatol* **48**(6): 950–4.

Congenital Telangiectatic Erythema (Bloom's Syndrome)

Telangiectatic erythema of the cheeks in a young boy

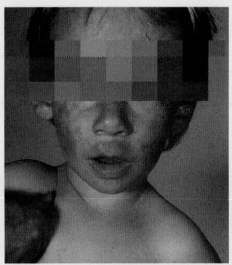
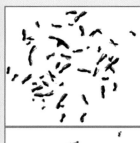
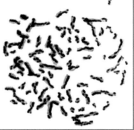

Various degrees of sister chromatid exchanges (BrdU-labelling) in a disease-free proband (above) and in a proband with Bloom syndrome (below)

Acanthosis, papillomatosis, lichenoid lymphocytic Infiltrate and telangiectasias

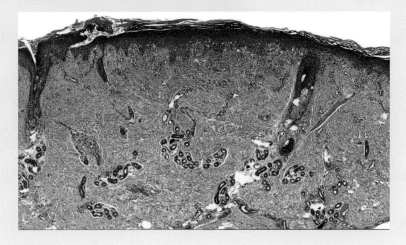

Diagnosis has to be confirmed by demonstration of increased sister chromatid exchange.

Cl: Inherited disease showing essential telangiectasia of the cheeks and photosensitivity, which lead to lupus erythematosus or lichen planus-like symptoms and finally result in a poikilodermatous picture. Growth retardation, triangular face; hypo- and hyperpigmentations. Patients are prone to develop malignancies and have a reduced life expectancy.

Hi:

- Acanthosis, papillomatosis, hypergranulosis, and elongation of rete ridges
- Dense epidermotropic lymphocytic infiltrate in the upper dermis, simulating lichen planus or cutaneous T-cell lymphoma
- Increased number and dilation of small blood vessels in the upper dermis resulting in telangiectatic erythema

DD: Syndromes with poikiloderma; lupus erythematosus; lichen planus; cutaneous T-cell lymphoma (see pseudo-mycosis fungoides); telangiectatic erythemas.

References

Bloom, D. (1954) Congenital telangiectatic erythema resembling lupus erythematosus in dwarfs; probably a syndrome entity. *AMA Am J Dis Child* **88**(6): 754–8.

Grob, M., Wyss, M., Spycher, M.A., et al. (1998) Histopathologic and ultrastructural study of lupus-like skin lesions in a patient with Bloom syndrome. *J Cutan Pathol* **25**(5): 275–8.

McGowan, J., Maize, J., and Cook, J. (2009) Lupus-like histopathology in bloom syndrome: reexamining the clinical and histologic implications of photosensitivity. *Am J Dermatopathol* **31**(8): 786–91.

Venous Malformations

Blue Rubber Bleb Nevus Syndrome (Familial Venous Malformation)

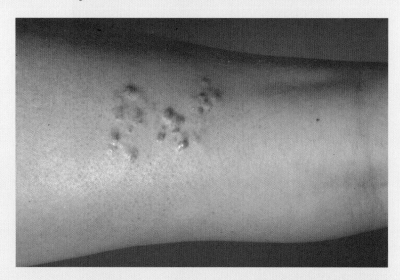

Soft blue cutaneous and subcutaneous nodules

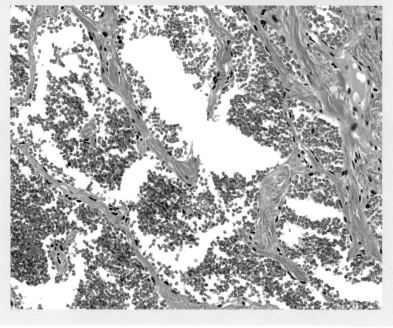

Dilated capillary spaces

Cl: Autosomal dominant venous malformations. Variant of cavernous malformation ("venous hemangioma") accompanied by similar lesions in the gastrointestinal tract and in other visceral organs. Sometimes accompanied by hyperhidrosis.

Hi:

- Deep dermis and subcutis

- Dilated thin-walled vascular channels with WT1-negative endothelia
- Thickened vessel walls with caliber variation

DD: Lymphatic and glomuvenous malformations (glomangioma); portwine stain; arteriovenous malformations; juvenile capillary hemangioma.

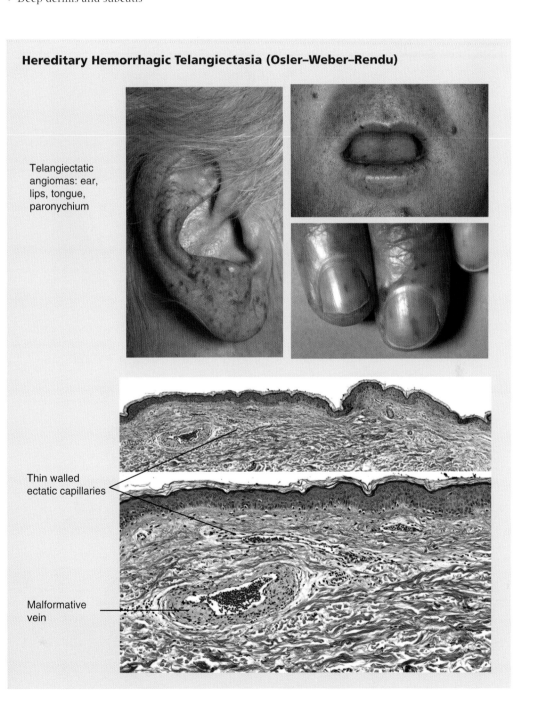

Hereditary Hemorrhagic Telangiectasia (Osler–Weber–Rendu)

Telangiectatic angiomas: ear, lips, tongue, paronychium

Thin walled ectatic capillaries

Malformative vein

Cl: Rare autosomal dominant disorder with small mucocutaneous telangiectatic angiomas and arteriovenous fistulae, especially on the lips, nose, ears, and large visceral organs, which tend to bleed, causing anemia.

Hi:

- Dilated thin-walled ectatic venules in the upper dermis

- Aberrant, thick-walled arteries in the deeper dermis

DD: Multiple spider nevi; multiple cherry angiomas; diseases associated with multiple angiokeratomas.

Angioma Serpiginosum

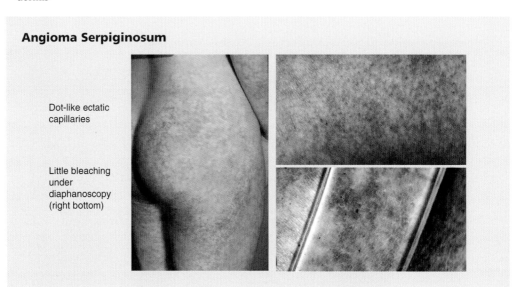

Dot-like ectatic capillaries

Little bleaching under diaphanoscopy (right bottom)

Cl: This microvenular malformation starts early in childhood and affects almost exclusively girls; some cases are familial. The buttocks, thighs or arms are the preferential localisation for grouped, dot-like ectatic capillaries. Peripheral growth and central regression result in a serpiginous pattern. There may be a Blaschko line distribution.

Angioma Serpiginosum

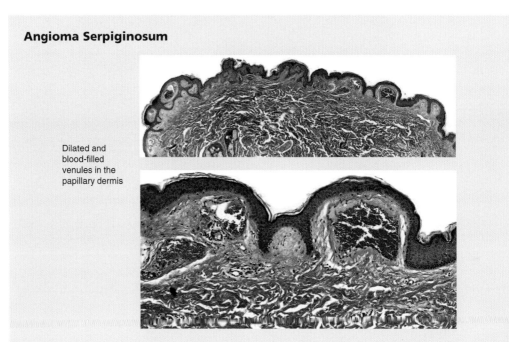

Dilated and blood-filled venules in the papillary dermis

Hi: Dilated small vessels in the papillary dermis.

DD: Purpura; hereditary hemorrhagic telangiectasia; multiple angiokeratomas.

References

Bayramgurler, D., Filinte, D., and Kiran, R. (2008) Angioma serpiginosum with sole involvement. *Eur J Dermatol* **18**(6): 708–9.

Chen, W., Liu, T.J., Yang, Y.C., and Happle, R. (2006) Angioma serpiginosum arranged in a systematized segmental pattern suggesting mosaicism. *Dermatology* **213**(3): 236–8.

Cox, N.H. and Paterson, W.D. (1991) Angioma serpiginosum: a simulator of purpura. *Postgrad Med J* **67**(794): 1065–6.

Das, D., Nayak, C.S., and Tambe, S.A. (2016) Blaschko-linear angioma serpiginosum. *Indian J Dermatol Venereol Leprol* **82**(3): 335–7.

Sancheti, K., Das, A., Podder, I., and Gharami, R.C. (2016) Angioma serpiginosum in a patchy and blaschkoid distribution: a rare condition with an unconventional presentation. *Indian J Dermatol* **61**(5): 570–2.

Venular Aneurysm (Venous Lake)

Multiple blue-black soft papules on the cheek (left)

Thin-walled angiomatous space with thrombus (right)

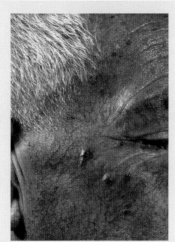
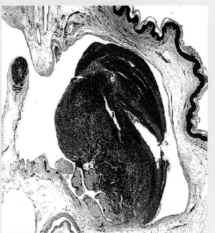

Cl: Solitary or multiple blue-black soft angiomatous papules, preferentially on the lips, in older people, simulating a melanocytic lesion.

Hi: Large ectatic thin-walled thrombosed vascular space(s) in the upper dermis.

DD: Telangiectases; glomangioma; blue rubber bleb nevus and other venous malformations.

Reference

Singh, S., Khanna, N., Ramam, M., and Singh, M. (2013) Solitary glomangioma mimicking a venous lake at an unusual site. *Int J Dermatol* **52**(11): 1409–11.

Cavernous Hemangioma (in Maffucci Syndrome)

Large cavernous venous malformation, showing subcutaneous and exophytic growth

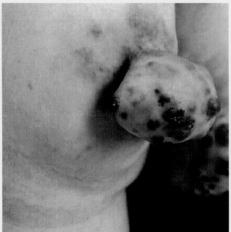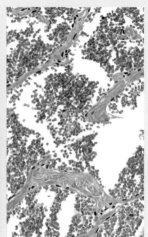

Cl: Inherited venous malformation, in which large and deep cavernous hemangiomas are associated with dyschondroplasia of the hands and feet and other symptoms. No spontaneous regression.

Hi: Variety of mostly large, cavernous vascular spaces, lined by endothelium; thrombi, calcifications. Areas corresponding to capillary hemangioma may be found.

Reference

Pansuriya, T.C., van Eijk, R., d'Adamo, P., et al. (2011) Somatic mosaic IDH1 and IDH2 mutations are associated with enchondroma and spindle cell hemangioma in Ollier disease and Maffucci syndrome. *Nat Genet* **43**(12): 1256–61.

Sinusoidal Hemangioma

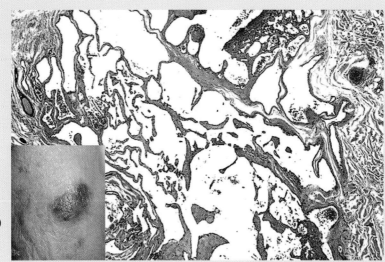

Bruise-like hemangioma on the arm (inset)

Labyrinthian pattern of anastomosing vascular channels with septa and folds of regular endothelia (top and bottom)

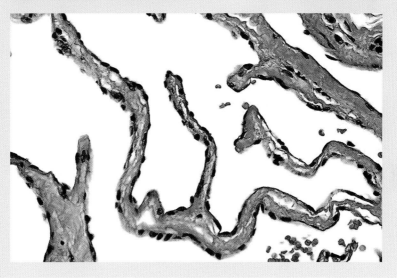

Cl: Variant of cavernous venous malformations, presenting as a solitary cutaneous-subcutaneous violaceous nodule. Important differential diagnosis for well-differentiated angiosarcoma of the female breast parenchyma.

Hi:

- Lobular tumor in the deep dermis and subcutis
- Thin-walled anastomosing and interconnected lacunar vascular spaces
- Pseudopapillary projections, septa, and endothelial folds reaching into the lumina
- Malformative venous vessels with WT1-negative endothelia

DD: Well-differentiated angiosarcoma (of the female breast parenchyma).

References

Ban, M., Kamiya, H., and Kitajima, Y. (2010) Giant sinusoidal hemangioma revealing diffuse ancient change: hyalinization and organized thrombi. *Int J Dermatol* **49**(5): 589–90.

Calonje, E. and Fletcher, C.D. (1991) Sinusoidal hemangioma. A distinctive benign vascular neoplasm within the group of cavernous hemangiomas. *Am J Surg Pathol* **15**(12): 1130–5.

Ciurea, M., Ciurea, R., Popa, D., Parvanescu, H., Marinescu, D., and Vrabete, M. (2011) Sinusoidal hemangioma of the arm: case report and review of literature. *Rom J Morphol Embryol* **52**(3): 915–18.

Pique-Duran, E., Paredes, B.E., and Palacios-Llopis, S. (2010) [Sinusoidal hemangioma: Immunohistochemical analysis with glucose transporter 1 (GLUT1) and williams tumor protein 1 (WT1)] *Actas Dermosifiliogr* **101**(4): 364–6.

Salemis, N.S. (2017) Sinusoidal hemangioma of the breast: diagnostic evaluation management and literature review. *Gland Surg* **6**(1): 105–9.

Spindle Cell Hemangioma (Formerly Spindle Cell Hemangioendothelioma)

Blue-red cutaneous nodule on the planta (left)

Cavernous vascular spaces with thrombi (right)

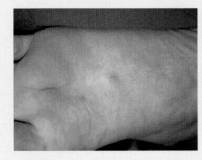
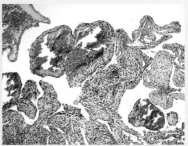

Cl: Arteriovenous-lymphatic malformation, presenting as solitary or multiple blue or blue-red, sometimes painful nodules, mostly in adults, preferentially on the extremities. Association with Maffucci syndrome and Klippel–Trenaunay syndrome. Does not metastasize. Reported pseudo-recurrences (in >50% of excised lesions) are typical persistences of incompletely excised vascular malformations with a multicentric vascular growth pattern, which is highly characteristic of spindle cell hemangioma.

Spindle Cell Hemangioma (Formerly Spindle Cell Hemangioendothelioma)

Fascicles composed of spindle cells (pericytes) and epithelioid endothelial cells with vacuoles ("pseudo-fat cells")

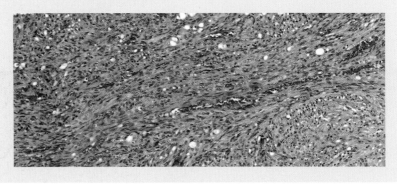

Hi:

- Biphasic vascular tumor composed of solid "kaposiform" zones and richly vascularized cavernous areas
  - Solid cellular (kaposiform) zones contain alpha smooth muscle actin-positive pericytes and CD31-positive endothelia in a compact layered arrangement ("lasagne pattern"). Pericytes are spindled, while the endothelia are cuboidal or roundish, sometimes with intracytoplasmic vacuoles ("pseudo-fat cells")
  - Vascular zones are composed of lacuna-like dilated thin-walled venous spaces with thin endothelial septa and folds ("Roman bridges"). There may be thrombi and phleboliths
- Importantly, there are foci of podoplanin positivity as an indicator of the malformative nature of the lesion. Endothelia are negative for HHV8 and MYC
- Accompanying thick-walled malformative vessels are often present

Spindle Cell Hemangioma (Formerly Spindle Cell Hemangioendothelioma)

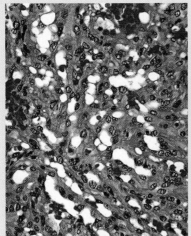 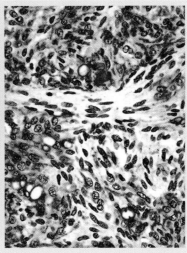

Epithelioid endothelial cells with vacuoles (left), CD31 + (right)

DD: Kaposi's sarcoma; kaposiform hemangioendothelioma; tufted hemangioma.

References

Chan, J. (1997) Vascular tumours with a prominent spindle cell component. *Curr Diagn Pathol* **4**: 76–90.

Ding, J., Hashimoto, H., Imayama, S., Tsuneyoshi, M., and Enjoji, M. (1992) Spindle cell haemangioendothelioma: probably a benign vascular lesion not a low-grade angiosarcoma. A clinicopathological, ultrastructural and immunohistochemical study. *Virchows Arch A Pathol Anat Histopathol* **420**(1): 77–85.

Fletcher, C.D., Beham, A., and Schmid, C. (1991) Spindle cell haemangioendothelioma: a clinicopathological and immunohistochemical study indicative of a nonneoplastic lesion. *Histopathology* **18**(4): 291–301.

Imayama, S., Murakamai, Y., Hashimoto, H., and Hori, Y. (1992) Spindle cell hemangioendothelioma exhibits the ultrastructural features of reactive vascular proliferation rather than of angiosarcoma. *Am J Clin Pathol* **97**(2): 279–87.

Pellegrini, A.E., Drake, R.D., and Qualman, S.J. (1995) Spindle cell hemangioendothelioma: a neoplasm associated with Maffucci's syndrome. *J Cutan Pathol* **22**(2): 173–6.

Tronnier, M., Vogelbruch, M., and Kutzner, H. (2006) Spindle cell hemangioma and epithelioid hemangioendothelioma arising in an area of lymphedema. *Am J Dermatopathol* **28**(3): 223–7.

Weiss, S.W. and Enzinger, F.M. (1986) Spindle cell hemangioendothelioma. A low-grade angiosarcoma resembling a cavernous hemangioma and Kaposi's sarcoma. *Am J Surg Pathol* **10**(8): 521–30.

Arteriovenous Malformations

Arteriovenous malformations (arteriovenous hemangioma) are vascular lesions, composed of capillaries, veins, and arteries.

Acral Arteriovenous Hemangioma (Cirsoid Aneurysm)

Angiomatous lesions on the cheek (top left) and the temple (mid left)

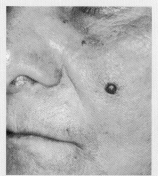
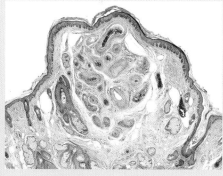

Exophytic aneurysmatic aggregation of vessels of variable calibers (top and mid right)

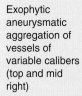
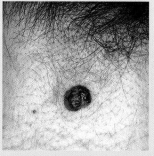
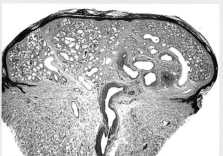

Thick-walled vessels juxtaposed to dilated venular spaces

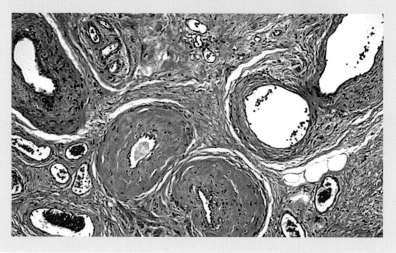

Cl: Solitary red-blue nodule, preferentially in the head and neck area of adults. The nosological classification of cirsoid aneurysm (aneurysm, arteriovenous shunt, venous hemangioma, malformation or hamartoma) is still a matter of debate.

Hi:

- Aggregation of small venous or arterial vessels
- Thick fibromuscular vessel walls with elastic fibers
- Lumina show variable diameter with marked caliber variation of all vessels throughout the lesion
- Single layer of endothelial cells
- Fibrous, sometimes myxoid stroma

- WT1-positive endothelia (which militates against the malformation hypothesis)

References

Connelly, M.G. and Winkelmann, R.K. (1985) Acral arteriovenous tumor. A clinicopathologic review. *Am J Surg Pathol* **9**(1): 15–21.

Girard, C., Graham, J.H., and Johnson, W.C. (1974) Arteriovenous hemangioma (arteriovenous shunt). A clinicopathological and histochemical study. *J Cutan Pathol* **1**(2): 73–87.

Neumann, R.A., Knobler, R.M., Schuller-Petrovic, S., Lindmaier, A., and Gebhart, W. (1989) Giant arteriovenous hemangioma (cirsoid aneurysm) of the nose. *J Dermatol Surg Oncol* **15**(7): 739–42.

Glomuvenular Malformation ("Glomangioma")

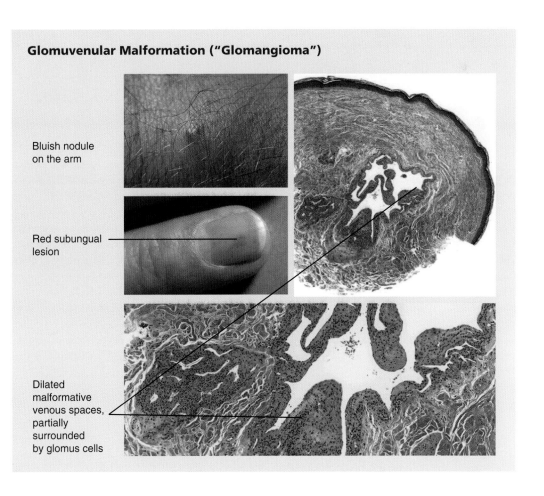

Bluish nodule on the arm

Red subungual lesion

Dilated malformative venous spaces, partially surrounded by glomus cells

Glomuvenular Malformation ("Glomangioma")

Glomus cells showing typical cuboidal shapes

ASMA-positive glomus cells

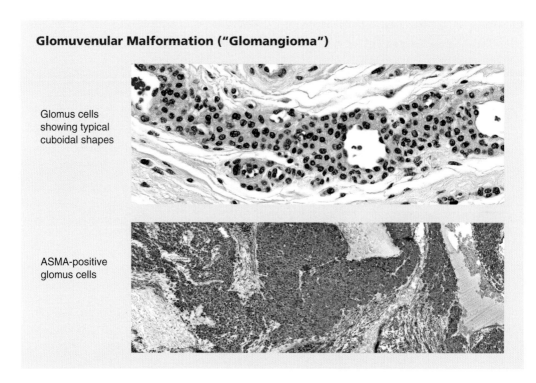

Glomus tumor originates from modified smooth muscle cells of the outer vascular wall while glomuvenular malformation ("glomangioma") represents a classic venular vascular malformation with focal masses of glomus cells in the outer vessel wall. The common denominator of both entities is the glomus cell, a small cuboid myoid cell that is characteristically enveloped by a collagen IV-positive outer sheath.

Cl: Glomuvenular malformation presents as blue-violet nodules, painful spontaneously or upon pressure, as in glomus tumor. Large anastomosing venular malformative vessels in deeper layers of the skin and subcutis are the characteristic feature.

Hi:

- Histopathologically, the glomus cell proliferations are divided into three morphological subtypes:
  - Glomuvenular malformation ("glomangioma"), showing large dilated venules and veins with WT1-negative endothelia and broad rims of aggregated glomus cells in the outer vessel wall
  - Solid glomus tumor is composed of densely packed sheets of isomorphic cuboid glomus cells, with minimal accompanying vascularization

- Glomangiomyoma is a morphological variant which contains glomus cells of various shapes; usually, there is a gradual blending of sheets of conventional glomus cells into areas with glomoid spindle cell variation
- Immunophenotypically, glomus cells express alpha smooth muscle actin and are individually enveloped by collagen IV-positive fibers. Myxoid variants express CD34
- Plaque-like telangiectatic lesions are rare. They are variants of the glomuvenular malformation

DD: Blue rubber bleb nevus syndrome; cavernous hemangioma; blue nevus; melanoma; nodular hidradenoma.

References

Acebo, E., Val-Bernal, J.F., and Arce, F. (1997) Giant intravenous glomus tumor. *J Cutan Pathol* **24**(6): 384–9.

Calonje, E. and Fletcher, C.D. (1995) Cutaneous intraneural glomus tumor. *Am J Dermatopathol* **17**(4): 395–8.

Dervan, P.A., Tobbia, I.N., Casey, M., O'Loughlin, J., and O'Brien, M. (1989) Glomus tumours: an immunohistochemical profile of 11 cases. *Histopathology* **14**(5): 483–91.

Haupt, H.M., Stern, J.B., and Berlin, S.J. (1992). Immunohistochemistry in the differential diagnosis of nodular hidradenoma and glomus tumor. *Am J Dermatopathol* **14**(4): 310–14.

Herbst, W.M., Nakayama, K., and Hornstein, O.P. (1991) Glomus tumours of the skin: an immunohistochemical investigation of the expression of marker proteins. *Br J Dermatol* **124**(2): 172–6.

Landthaler, M., Braun-Falco, O., Eckert, F., Stolz, W., Dorn, M., and Wolff, H.H. (1990) Congenital multiple plaquelike glomus tumors. *Arch Dermatol* **126**(9): 1203–7.

Requena, L., Galvan, C., Sanchez Yus, E., Sangueza, O., Kutzner, H., and Furio, V. (1998) Solitary plaque-like telangiectatic glomangioma. *Br J Dermatol* **139**(5): 902–5.

Lymphatic Malformations

Superficial Lymphatic Malformation (Superficial Lymphangioma)

Aggregates of small cystic papules (left)

Diascopy (right)

Subepidermal malformative lymphatic vessels

In the past, vascular lesions with a lymphatic vessel wall were uniformly classified as lymphangiomas. This classification has changed dramatically with the advent of new diagnostic imaging techniques and immunohistochemical methods. Presently, there is a tendency to subsume all lymphatic vascular growths under the heading of lymphatic vascular malformations.

- Superficial lymphatic malformations (lymphangioma; lymphangioma circumscriptum cysticum)
- Deep lymphatic malformations (lymphangioma; cavernous lymphangioma; cystic hygroma)
- Lymphangiomatosis – as a specific malformative variant with diffuse involvement of large body planes
- Clinical variants of superficial lymphatic malformations: targetoid hemosiderotic hemangioma (hobnail hemangioma); progressive lymphangioma (benign lymphangioendothelioma)

Cystic Lymphatic Malformation (Cystic Hygroma)

Cavernous
lymphatic
spaces

Cl:

- *Superficial types*: mostly grouped or aggregated red or clear small vesicular papules ("frog spawn") on the extremities, tongue or mucous membranes. The surface may be verrucous. Some lesions may be hemorrhagic ("hematolymphangioma")
- *Deep types*: soft skin-colored indurations and swellings
- *Lymphangiomatosis*: diffuse swelling of a limb; later stages show dark brownish skin

Hi:

- In the upper dermis: dilated thin-walled lymphatic vessels, some containing erythrocytes. No myoid/pericytic vessel wall. Accompanying hemosiderosis
- Deeper forms show lymphatic vessels with myoid vessel walls. Remarkably, there are caliber variations within the same malformative vessel ("thin-thick vessel wall")
- Common denominators are endothelial WT1 negativity (indicator of malformative endothelia) and expression of podoplanin

DD: Secondary lymphangiectases following surgery or radiation therapy; angiokeratoma; verrucous hemangioma; herpes virus infections; Kaposi's sarcoma.

References

Calonje, E. and Fletcher, C. (1995) Tumors of blood vessels and lymphatics. In: Diagnostic Histopathology of Tumors, vol. **1**, pp. 43–77 (ed. Fletcher, C.). Edinburgh: Churchill Livingstone.

Lymboussaki, A., Partanen, T.A., Olofsson, B., et al. (1998) Expression of the vascular endothelial growth factor C receptor VEGFR-3 in lymphatic endothelium of the skin and in vascular tumors. *Am J Pathol* **153**(2): 395–403.

Peachey, R.D., Lim, C.C., and Whimster, I.W. (1970) Lymphangioma of skin. A review of 65 cases. *Br J Dermatol* **83**(5): 519–27.

Rao, M.V., Thappa, D.M., and Ratnakar, C. (1998) Lymphangioma circumscriptum of the skin and tongue associated with cystic hygroma. *Indian J Otolaryngol Head Neck Surg* **50**(3): 266–8.

Targetoid Hemosiderotic (Hobnail) Hemangioma

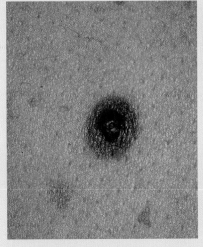

Targetoid pigmented lesion (left)

Superficial part showing dilated lymphatic vessels (right)

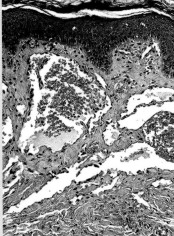

Dilated vessel with protrusions of isomorphic "lymphocyte-like" lymphatic endothelial cells ("hobnails") (left);

CD31-positive endothelia (right)

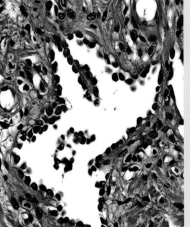

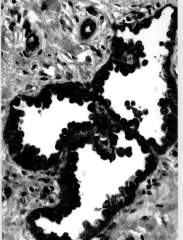

Cl: Solitary superficial lymphatic vascular malformation. Flat angiomatous patch, often of targetoid appearance: rusty colored papule in the middle, surrounded by paler erythematous ring and by darker area with ecchymoses in the periphery. Lesions characteristically imitate pigmented nevi.

Hi: Hobnail hemangioma presents with a characteristic zonation pattern.

- *Upper dermis*: dilated bizarre vessels with plump, isomorphic ("lymphocyte-like") endothelia ("hobnails") protruding into the lumina

- *Deep dermis*: collapsed lymphatic vessels with very narrow lumina amidst a fibrous stroma containing many sideropahages

Immunohistochemistry: Endothelial cells express the lymphatic marker podoplanin and are negative for WT1. An outer myoid vessel wall (alpha smooth muscle actin) does not exist.

DD: Kaposi's sarcoma; benign (progressive) lymphangioendothelioma; melanocytic nevus.

References

Guillou, L., Calonje, E., Speight, P., Rosai, J., and Fletcher, C.D. (1999) Hobnail hemangioma: a pseudomalignant vascular lesion with a reappraisal of targetoid hemosiderotic hemangioma. *Am J Surg Pathol* **23**(1): 97–105.

Lymboussaki, A., Partanen, T.A., Olofsson, B., et al. (1998) Expression of the vascular endothelial growth factor C receptor VEGFR-3 in lymphatic endothelium of the skin and in vascular tumors. *Am J Pathol* **153**(2): 395–403.

Mentzel, T., Partanen, T.A., and Kutzner, H. (1999) Hobnail hemangioma ("targetoid hemosiderotic hemangioma"): clinicopathologic and immunohistochemical analysis of 62 cases. *J Cutan Pathol* **26**(6): 279–86.

Santa Cruz, D.J. and Aronberg, J. (1988) Targetoid hemosiderotic hemangioma. *J Am Acad Dermatol* **19**(3): 550–8.

Progressive Lymphangioma (Benign Lymphangioendothelioma)

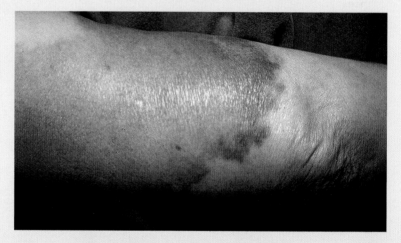

Typical brownish centrifugally progressing plaque

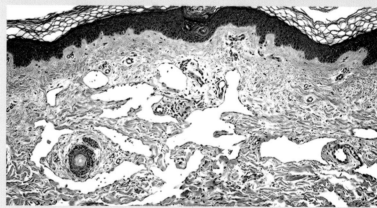

Bizarre anastomizing dilated thin walled lymphatic vessels with regular endothelia

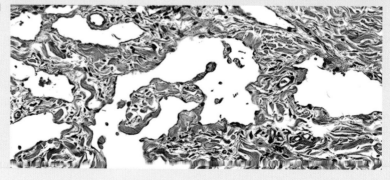

Cl: Rare single, brown, slowly expanding macular lymphatic malformation, resembling a large lentigo or even evolving early Kaposi's sarcoma.

Hi: Dilated superficial thin-walled bizarrely anastomosing lymphatic spaces spreading between collagen bundles. The lack of cellular atypia allows for differentiation from angiosarcoma. Endothelial cells are negative for HHV8 (DD: Kaposi's sarcoma) and MYC, Ki67 (DD: angiosarcoma).

DD: Kaposi's sarcoma.

References

Guillou, L. and Fletcher, C.D. (2000) Benign lymphangioendothelioma (acquired progressive lymphangioma): a lesion not to be confused with well-differentiated angiosarcoma and patch stage Kaposi's sarcoma: clinicopathologic analysis of a series. *Am J Surg Pathol* **24**(8): 1047–57.

Leshin, B., Whitaker, D.C., and Foucar, E. (1986) Lymphangioma circumscriptum following mastectomy and radiation therapy. *J Am Acad Dermatol* **15**(5 Pt 2): 1117–19.

Messeguer, F., Sanmartin, O., Martorell-Calatayud, A., Nagore, E., Requena, C., and Guillen-Barona, C. (2010) [Acquired progressive lymphangioma (benign lymphangioendothelioma)] *Actas Dermosifiliogr* **101**(9): 792–7.

Mizuno, K. and Okamoto, H. (2015) Benign lymphangioendothelioma on a vascular birthmark following examination of a cardiac catheter. *Int J Dermatol* **54**(7): e273–4.

Revelles, J.M., Diaz, J.L., Angulo, J., Santonja, C., Kutzner, H., and Requena, L. (2012) Giant benign lymphangioendothelioma. *J Cutan Pathol* **39**(10): 950 6.

Sevila, A., Botella-Estrada, R., Sanmartin, O., et al. (2000) Benign lymphangioendothelioma of the thigh simulating a low-grade angiosarcoma. *Am J Dermatopathol* **22**(2): 151–4.

Wang, L., Chen, L., Yang, X., Gao, T., and Wang, G. (2013) Benign lymphangioendothelioma: a clinical, histopathologic and immunohistochemical analysis of four cases. *J Cutan Pathol* **40**(11): 945–9.

Yamada, S., Yamada, Y., Kobayashi, M., et al. (2014) Post-mastectomy benign lymphangioendothelioma of the skin following chronic lymphedema for breast carcinoma: a teaching case mimicking low-grade angiosarcoma and masquerading as Stewart-Treves syndrome. *Diagn Pathol* **9**: 197.

Lymphangiomatosis

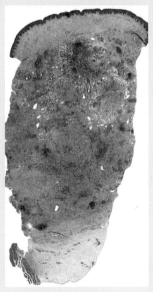
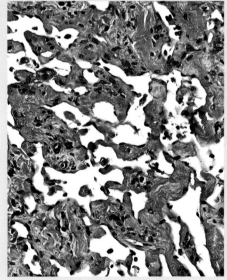

Dermal lesion, showing anastomosing lymphatic slits (right)

Lymphangiomatosis

Hair blower
pattern (left)

Podoplanin
positive
lymphatic
vessels (right)

Cl: Swelling mostly of lower limbs since birth or starting early in life, produced by benign proliferation and dilation of lymph vessels. Apart from cutaneous manifestation, involvement of deep structures, bone, and viscera is possible.

Hi: Sponge-like features by anastomosing bizarre and jagged lymphatic slits and cavernous spaces in superficial and deep tissue layers without cellular anomalies. Stunning morphological similarities with tumor pattern of diffusely invasive angiosarcoma, albeit with marked lack of endothelial atypia. Importantly, endothelia of lymphangiomatosis are negative for MYC (DD: angiosarcoma) and HHV8 (DD: Kaposi's sarcoma).

DD: Angiosarcoma, Kaposi's sarcoma.

References

Gomez, C.S., Calonje, E., Ferrar, D.W., Browse, N.L., and Fletcher, C.D. (1995) Lymphangiomatosis of the limbs. Clinicopathologic analysis of a series with a good prognosis. *Am J Surg Pathol* **19**(2): 125–33.

Ramani, P. and Shah, A. (1993) Lymphangiomatosis. Histologic and immunohistochemical analysis of four cases. *Am J Surg Pathol* **17**(4): 329–35.

Angiokeratomas

Angiokeratomas are red-blue or red-black malformations of small vessels in conjunction with massive acanthosis and hyperkeratosis at later stages of evolution. There are several variants, which differ in their clinical presentation and histomorphological correlation. Angiokeratoma is the smaller variant with exclusively subepidermally and upper dermal layer-localized thin-walled vessels, while verrucous hemangioma, as the deeper variant, shows involvement also of the deep dermis and subcutis. Remarkably, angiokeratomas of all types are vascular malformations, and as such do not regress.

Verrucous Hemangioma (Venous Malformation)

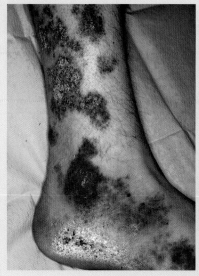 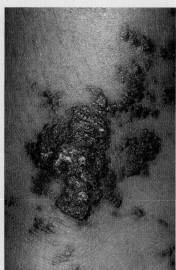

Hyperkeratotic angiomatous plaques with satellite lesions (right)

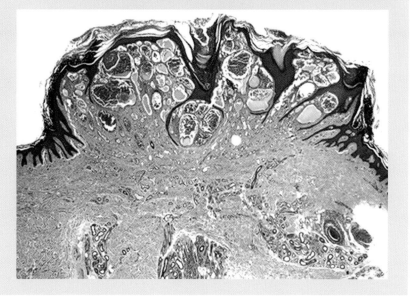

Compact hyperkeratosis, acanthosis, papillomatosis and convolutes of capillary and cavernous structures in the upper dermis

Cl: Vascular malformation involving capillary and cavernous (venous) elements in superficial and deep layers of the dermis and subcutis. Hemorrhagic red plaques or papules, occasionally in linear formation, developing in early life without alterations of the epidermis. Later, during proportionate enlargement resulting in tumorous lesions with satellites, reactive epidermal hyperplasia and verrucous hyperkeratosis occur. The legs are the preferential localisation. No tendency for spontaneous regression, in contrast to cherry angiomas.

Hi:
- Acanthosis and verrucous hyperkeratosis
- Malformative thin-walled venular vessels at all levels of the dermis, and of the subcutis
- Mid dermis may be spared: "mid-dermal grenz zone"
- Convolution of dilated venules and venous cavernous spaces
- No endothelial atypia
- Endothelia negative for WT1

DD: Angiokeratoma; capillary hemangioma; cherry angioma; verrucous melanoma.

References

Brown, A., Warren, S., Losken, H.W., and Morrell, D.S. (2008) Verrucous lymphovascular malformation versus verrucous hemangioma: controversial nomenclature. *Cutis* **81**(5): 390–6.

Chan, J., Tsang, W., Calonje, E., and Fletcher, C.D.M. (1995) Verrucous hemangioma. A distinct but neglected variant of cutaneous hemangioma. *Int J Surg Pathol* **2**: 171–6.

Clairwood, M.Q., Bruckner, A.L., and Dadras, S.S. (2011) Verrucous hemangioma: a report of two cases and review of the literature. *J Cutan Pathol* **38**(9): 740–6.

Del Pozo, J., Tellado, M., and Lopez-Gutierrez, J.C. (2009) [Verrucous hemangioma versus microcystic lymphatic malformation] *Actas Dermosifiliogr* **100**(5): 437; author reply 438–9.

Garrido-Rios, A.A., Sanchez-Velicia, L., Marino-Harrison, J.M., Torrero-Anton, M.V., and Miranda-Romero, A. (2008) [A histopathologic and imaging study of verrucous hemangioma] *Actas Dermosifiliogr* **99**(9): 723–6.

Imperial, R. and Helwig, E.B. (1967) Verrucous hemangioma. A clinicopathologic study of 21 cases. *Arch Dermatol* **96**(3): 247–53.

Jain, V.K., Aggarwal, K., and Jain, S. (2008) Linear verrucous hemangioma on the leg. *Indian J Dermatol Venereol Leprol* **74**(6): 656–8.

Knopfel, N. and Hoeger, P.H. (2016) Verrucous hemangioma or verrucous venous malformation? Towards a classification based on genetic analysis. *Actas Dermosifiliogr*, **107**(5): 427–8.

Laing, E.L., Brasch, H.D., Steel, R., et al. (2013) Verrucous hemangioma expresses primitive markers. *J Cutan Pathol* **40**(4): 391–6.

Pavithra, S., Mallya, H., Kini, H., and Pai, G.S. (2011) Verrucous hemangioma or angiokeratoma? A missed diagnosis. *Indian J Dermatol* **56**(5): 599–600.

Puig, L., Llistosella, E., Moreno, A., and de Moragas, J.M. (1987) Verrucous hemangioma. *J Dermatol Surg Oncol* **13**(10): 1089–92.

Rossi, A., Bozzi, M., and Barra, E. (1989) Verrucous hemangioma and angiokeratoma circumscriptum: clinical and histologic differential characteristics. *J Dermatol Surg Oncol* **15**(1): 88–91.

Wang, L., Gao, T., and Wang, G. (2014) Verrucous hemangioma: a clinicopathological and immunohistochemical analysis of 74 cases. *J Cutan Pathol* **41**(11): 823–30.

Watanabe, T., Wada, H., Hotta, A., Okudela, K., and Aihara, M. (2016) Case of adult-onset verrucous hemangioma developed after repeated trauma. *J Dermatol* **43**(3): 348–9.

Wentscher, U. and Happle, R. (2000) Linear verrucous hemangioma. *J Am Acad Dermatol* **42**(3): 516–18.

Yasar, A., Ermertcan, A.T., Bilac, C., Bilac, D.B., Temiz, P., and Ozturkcan, S. (2009) Verrucous hemangioma. *Indian J Dermatol Venereol Leprol* **75**(5): 528–30.

Clinical Variants of Angiokeratoma

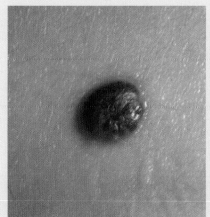

Solitary angiokeratoma

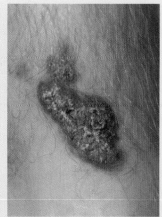

Angiokeratoma
circumscriptum naeviforme

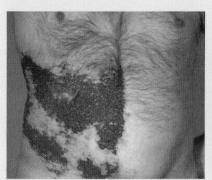

Segmental angiokeratoma
circumscriptum naeviforme

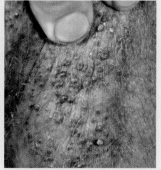

Fordyce angiokeratoma of
the scrotum

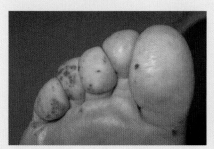

Angiokeratoma acroasphycticum
digitorum (Mibelli)

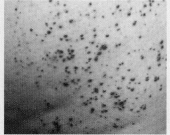

Angiokeratoma corporis
diffusum Fabry

VARIANTS

Variant: Solitary Angiokeratoma

Acanthosis and papillomatosis with hyperkeratosis

Thin-walled vascular spaces in the papillary dermis

Intracytoplasmatic PAS-positive granules in endothelial cells of Fabry's disease (inset)

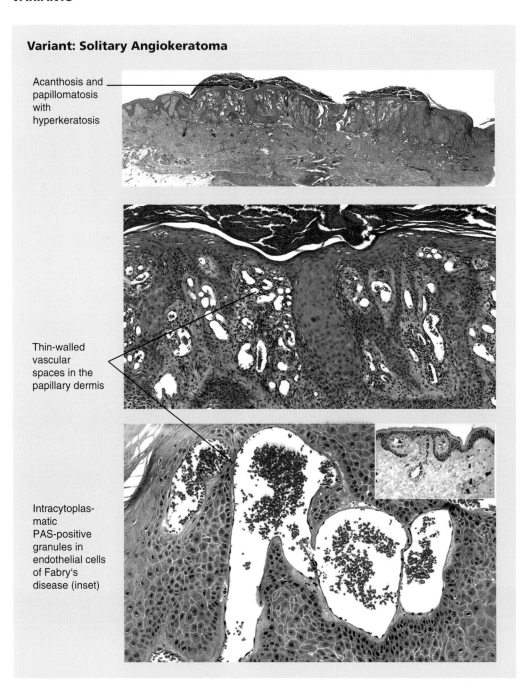

Cl: Solitary red-brown plaque with hyperkeratosis, preferentially on the lower extremities. There may be a history of trauma.

Hi: Epidermal hyperplasia with hyperkeratosis and dilated thin-walled vascular lacunae in the papillary dermis.

VARIANTS

Variant: Angiokeratoma Circumscriptum Naeviformis

Cl: Blue-red hyperkeratotic plaque since birth, occasionally covering a larger segmental area of the body, or following Blaschko lines.

Hi: Comparable with solitary angiokeratoma. When deeper parts of the dermis are involved, differentiation from verrucous hemangioma may be impossible.

Variant: Fordyce Angiokeratoma

Cl: Multiple small red papules on the scrotum, penis or labia major of the vulva, simulating cherry angiomas.

Hi: Comparable with solitary angiokeratoma.

Variant: Angiokeratoma Acroasphycticum Digitorum (Mibelli)

Cl: Tiny red-black hyperkeratotic spots on toes or fingers.

Hi: Comparable with solitary angiokeratoma.

Variant: Multiple "Pinpoint" Angiokeratomas (Angiokeratoma Corporis Diffusum; Fabry's Disease)

Cl: Multiple tiny red papules distributed widely over the trunk. In this particular context, angiokeratoma is a misnomer: these lesions are exclusively composed of dilated subepidermal venules in association with underlying metabolic disorders (deficiencies of galactosidase, fucosidase, and others).

Hi: Dilated subepidermal venules without acanthosis. Immunohistochemical positivity for GB3 (intracytoplasmic ceramid deposits in endothelia, nerves, smooth muscles); PAS-stained formalin-fixed – but not paraffin-embedded – cryo-sections show intracytoplasmic granules.

Variant: Acral Pseudolymphomatous Angiokeratoma of Children (APACHE)

This rare entity belongs to pseudolymphomatous reactions.

Cl: Solitary or multiple slightly hyperkeratotic red papules on the hands of children.

Hi: In the upper dermis there are nodular lymphocytic infiltrates in association with dilated small vessels.

References

Fabry, H. (2002) Angiokeratoma corporis diffusum – Fabry disease: historical review from the original description to the introduction of enzyme replacement therapy. *Acta Paediatr* **91**(439) (Suppl): 3–5.

Fimiani, M., Mazzatenta, C., Rubegni, P., and Andreassi, L. (1997) Idiopathic angiokeratoma corporis diffusum. *Clin Exp Dermatol* **22**(4): 205–6.

Gerbig, A.W., Wiesmann, U., Gaeng, D., and Hunziker, T. (1995) [Angiokeratoma corporis diffusum without associated metabolic disorder] *Hautarzt* **46**(11): 785–8.

Jansen, W., Lentner, A., and Genzel, I. (1994) Capillary changes in angiokeratoma corporis diffusum Fabry. *J Dermatol Sci* **7**(1): 68–70.

Kanda, A., Tsuyama, S., Murata, F., Kodama, K., Hirabayashi, Y., and Kanzaki, T. (2002) Immunoelectron microscopic analysis of lysosomal deposits in alpha-N-acetylgalactosaminidase deficiency with angiokeratoma corporis diffusum. *J Dermatol Sci* **29**(1): 42–8.

Kanzaki, T., Yokota, M., Irie, F., Hirabayashi, Y., Wang, A.M., and Desnick, R.J. (1993) Angiokeratoma corporis diffusum with glycopeptiduria due to deficient lysosomal alpha-N-acetylgalactosaminidase activity. Clinical, morphologic, and biochemical studies. *Arch Dermatol* **129**(4): 460–5.

Laxmisha, C., Thappa, D.M., and Karthikeyan, K. (2003) Cutaneous variant of angiokeratoma corporis diffusum. *Dermatol Online J* **9**(1): 13.

Lu, Y.Y., Lu, C.C., Wu, C.S., and Wu, C.H. (2015) Familial angiokeratoma corporis diffusum without identified enzyme defect. *Indian J Dermatol Venereol Leprol* **81**(1): 46–9.

Suzuki, N., Konohana, I., Fukushige, T., and Kanzaki, T. (2004) Beta-mannosidosis with angiokeratoma corporis diffusum. *J Dermatol* **31**(11): 931–5.

Yokota, M., Koji, M., and Yotsumoto, S. (1995) Histopathologic and ultrastructural studies of angiokeratoma corporis diffusum in Kanzaki disease. *J Dermatol* **22**(1): 10–18.

Hyperplasias

Granuloma Pyogenicum (Lobular Capillary Hemangioma; Botryomykoma)

Exophytic vascular partially eroded lesion

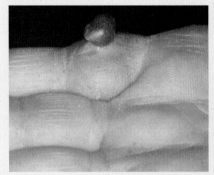
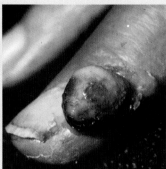

Nodular lesion with collarette of acanthotic and hyperkeratotic epidermis

Lobular arrangement of capillary tufts-separated by broad fibrous septa

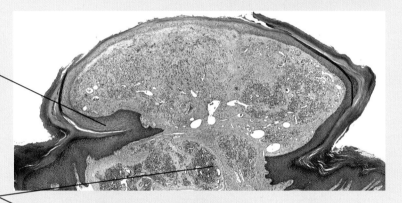
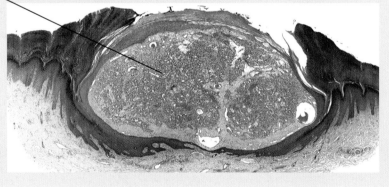

Granuloma Pyogenicum (Lobular Capillary Hemangioma; Botryomykoma)

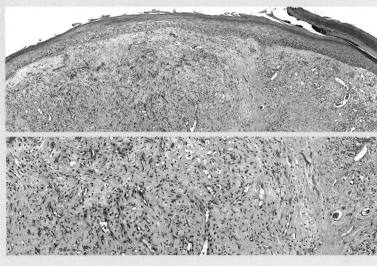

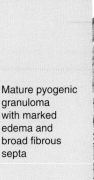

Mature pyogenic granuloma with marked edema and broad fibrous septa

Benign vascular tumor histologically showing a lobular structure accompanied by variable inflammatory infiltrate, without granulomatous features (the term refers to granulomatous tissue). These lesions are not neoplastic but rather reactive, following superficial injury.

Cl: Soft, friable, easily vulnerable and bleeding, peduncular exophytic nodular lesion. The small basis is surrounded by a collarette of normal surrounding skin. Fingers, palms, face, and scalp are preferential sites but it can develop on any other part of the body, including oral mucosa, possibly as a consequence of superficial trauma. The growth of the lesion can be boosted by hormonal (pregnancy) or other factors (tretinoin).

Hi:

- Dome-shaped lesion
- Epithelial collarette and epidermal lip formation on the borders
- Flat epidermis; superficial ulceration and crust formation possible
- Multilobular architecture with fibrous septae between vascular lobules
- Proliferation of capillaries (CD31, CD34): central feeding vessel
- Mitoses of endothelial cells without cellular atypia
- Variable inflammatory neutrophil-rich infiltrate and edema; fibrosis in elderly lesion

- Subcutaneous forms and extramedullary hematopoiesis in a pyogenic granuloma have been reported

DD: Granulation tissue; amelanotic malignant melanoma; capillary hemangioma; nodular Kaposi's sarcoma; angiosarcoma; acquired tufted angioma; epithelioid angiomatous nodule.

References

Blackwell, M.G., Itinteang, T., Chibnall, A.M., Davis, P.F., and Tan, S.T. (2016) Expression of embryonic stem cell markers in pyogenic granuloma. *J Cutan Pathol* **43**(12): 1096–101.

Brenn, T. and Fletcher, C.D. (2004) Cutaneous epithelioid angiomatous nodule: a distinct lesion in the morphologic spectrum of epithelioid vascular tumors. *Am J Dermatopathol* **26**(1): 14–21.

Fortna, R.R. and Junkins-Hopkins, J.M. (2007) A case of lobular capillary hemangioma (pyogenic granuloma), localized to the subcutaneous tissue, and a review of the literature. *Am J Dermatopathol* **29**(4): 408–11.

Fukunaga, M. (2000) Kaposi's sarcoma-like pyogenic granuloma. *Histopathology* **37**(2): 192–3.

McClain, C.M., Haws, A.L., Galfione, S.K., Rapini, R.P., and Hafeez Diwan, A. (2016) Pyogenic granuloma-like Kaposi's sarcoma. *J Cutan Pathol* **43**(6): 549–51.

Nakamura, T. (2000) Apoptosis and expression of Bax/Bcl-2 proteins in pyogenic granuloma: a comparative study with granulation tissue and capillary hemangioma. *J Cutan Pathol* **27**(8): 400–5.

Richey, J.D. and North, J.P. (2015) Extramedullary hematopoiesis in a pyogenic granuloma. *J Cutan Pathol* **42**(6): 375–8.

Rowlands, C.G., Rapson, D., and Morell, T. (2000) Extramedullary hematopoiesis in a pyogenic granuloma. *Am J Dermatopathol* **22**(5): 434–8.

Urquhart, J.L., Uzieblo, A., and Kohler, S. (2006) Detection of HHV-8 in pyogenic granuloma-like Kaposi sarcoma. *Am J Dermatopathol* **28**(4): 317–21.

Vega Harring, S.M., Niyaz, M., Okada, S., and Kudo, M. (2004) Extramedullary hematopoiesis in a pyogenic granuloma: a case report and review. *J Cutan Pathol* **31**(8): 555–7.

Differential Diagnosis: Pyogenic Granuloma-Like Granulation Tissue

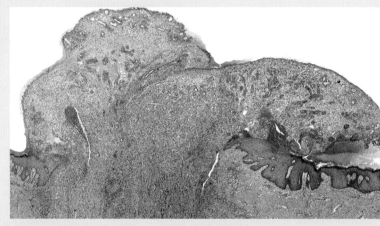

Protruding granulation tissue lacking the characteristic septa and capillary tufts of pyogenic granuloma

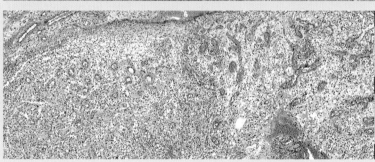

Cl: Excessive, oozing proliferation of granulation tissue, occurring in wound healing and chronic ulcerations. Spontaneous regression.

Hi: Loose suppurative granulation tissue, many capillaries, mixed inflammatory infiltrate with variable number of neutrophils.

Bacillary Angiomatosis

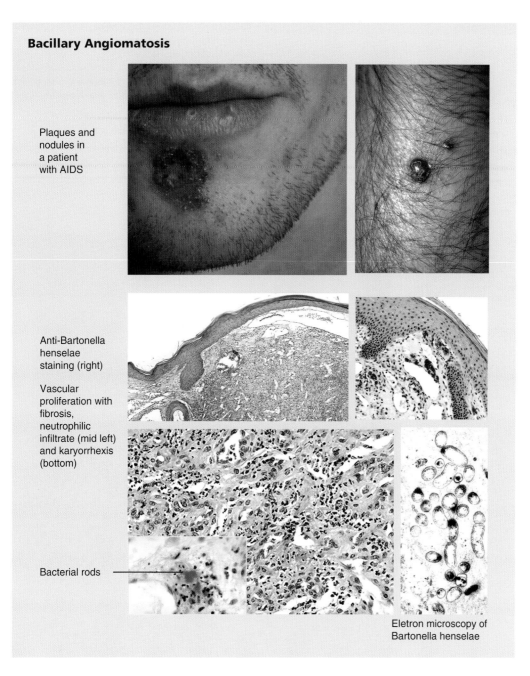

Plaques and nodules in a patient with AIDS

Anti-Bartonella henselae staining (right)

Vascular proliferation with fibrosis, neutrophilic infiltrate (mid left) and karyorrhexis (bottom)

Bacterial rods

Eletron microscopy of Bartonella henselae

Gram negative bacteria (*Bartonella henselae* or *Bartonella quintana*; formerly Rochalimaea) are the causative agents in immunodeficient individuals (AIDS).

Cl: Pyogenic granuloma-like, mostly multiple red hemorrhagic nodules or plaques.

Hi:
- Vascular proliferation resembling pyogenic granuloma or granulation tissue
- Blood vessels with large, activated epithelioid endothelia, high mitotic activity
- Conspicuous lack of fibrous septa between capillary lobules
- Edematous stroma
- Neutrophil-rich inflammatory infiltrate with karyorrhexis
- Causative bacteria can be demonstrated by Warthin–Starry stain or immunostains

DD: Pyogenic granuloma (lobular capillary hemangioma); epithelioid hemangioma (angiolymphoid hyperplasia with eosinophilia); Kaposi's sarcoma; verruga Peruana.

References

Amsbaugh, S., Huiras, E., Wang, N.S., Wever, A., and Warren, S. (2006) Bacillary angiomatosis associated with pseudoepitheliomatous hyperplasia. *Am J Dermatopathol* **28**(1): 32–5.

Perez-Piteira, J., Ariza, A., Mate, J.L., Ojanguren, I., and Navas-Palacios, J.J. (1995) Bacillary angiomatosis: a gross mimicker of malignancy. *Histopathology* **26**(5): 476–8.

Tsang, W.Y., Chan, J.K., and Wong, C.S. (1992) Giemsa stain for histological diagnosis of bacillary angiomatosis. *Histopathology* **21**(3): 299.

Zarraga, M., Rosen, L., and Herschthal, D. (2011) Bacillary angiomatosis in an immunocompetent child: a case report and review of the literature. *Am J Dermatopathol* **33**(5): 513–15.

Verruga Peruana

Multiple nodules on the legs

Vascular proliferation and inflammatory infiltrate in an edematous, inflammatory stroma (upper right and mid)

Bartonella bacilliformis. Grocott stain

Cl: Dermal papules and nodules, pedunculated, eroded or verrucous, resembling bacillary angiomatosis; due to infection by *Bartonella bacilliformis* in the Andes Mountains of South America, transmitted by sandflies.

Hi: Corresponds to bacillary angiomatosis, albeit with exclusively intracytoplasmic bacteria (Rocha–Lima bodies).

DD: See bacillary angiomatosis.

Reference

Arias-Stella, J., Lieberman, P.H., Erlandson, R.A., and Arias-Stella, J. Jr (1986) Histology, immunohistochemistry, and ultrastructure of the verruga in Carrion's disease. *Am J Surg Pathol* **10**(9): 595–610.

Intravascular Papillary Endothelial Hyperplasia (Masson)

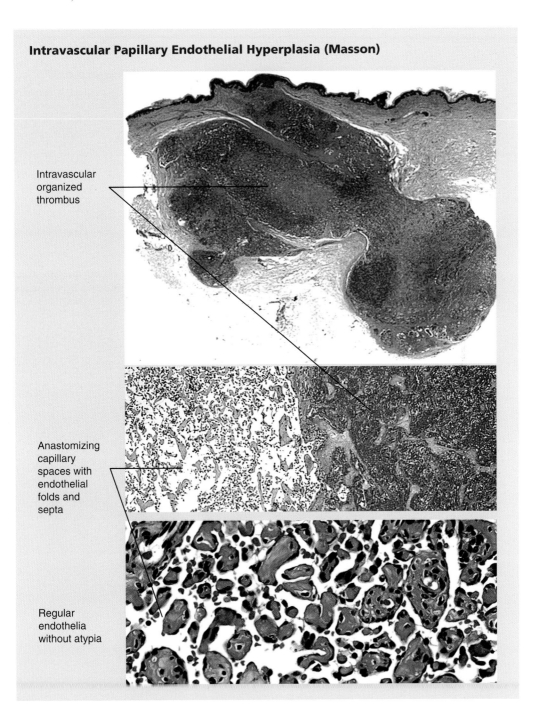

Intravascular organized thrombus

Anastomizing capillary spaces with endothelial folds and septa

Regular endothelia without atypia

Cl: This distinct reaction pattern was described by Masson 1923 as a vegetant intravascular angiosarcoma-like proliferation in thrombi of hemorrhoidal veins. It appears as subcutaneous violaceous nodular swelling preferentially on head, neck, and extremities but also in other localisations. Not necessarily associated with a pre-existing vascular lesion but can occur in a thrombosed blood vessel or within a vascular tumor or malformation.

Hi:

- Intravascular papillary endothelial proliferations in a thrombus undergoing organization and hyalinization
- Always within a pre-existing vessel (mostly veins); in exceptional cases "spilling over" into the adjacent dermis
- Anastomosing and labyrinthian vascular spaces, lined with flattened endothelial cells (endothelial septa and folds)
- Hyalinized papillary blebs and fibrous cores coated by endothelial cells
- Advanced stages with accompanying alpha smooth muscle actin-positive outer pericytic layers
- Myofibroblasts in the stroma
- Lack of cellular atypia

DD: Angiosarcoma; glomeruloid hemangioma; endovascular papillary angioendothelioma (Dabska tumor).

References

Albrecht, S., and Kahn, H.J. (1990) Immunohistochemistry of intravascular papillary endothelial hyperplasia. *J Cutan Pathol* **17**(1): 16–21.

Erol, O., Ozcakar, L., Uygur, F., Kecik, A., and Ozkaya, O. (2007) Intravascular papillary endothelial hyperplasia in the finger: not a premier diagnosis. *J Cutan Pathol* **34**(10): 806–7.

Korkolis, D.P., Papaevangelou, M., Koulaxouzidis, G., Zirganos, N., Psichogiou, H., and Vassilopoulos, P.P. (2005) Intravascular papillary endothelial hyperplasia (Masson's hemangioma) presenting as a soft-tissue sarcoma. *Anticancer Res* **25**(2B): 1409–12.

Kuo, T., Sayers, C.P., and Rosai, J. (1976).Masson's "vegetant intravascular hemangioendothelioma:" a lesion often mistaken for angiosarcoma: study of seventeen cases located in the skin and soft tissues. *Cancer* **38**(3): 1227–36.

Masson, M. (1923) Hemangioendotheliome vegetant intra-vasculaire. *Bull Soc Anat Paris* **93**: 517–23.

Paslin, D.A. (1981) Localized primary cutaneous intravascular papillary endothelial hyperplasia. *J Am Acad Dermatol* **4**(3): 316–18.

Salyer, W.R. and Salyer, D.C. (1975) Intravascular angiomatosis: development and distinction from angiosarcoma. *Cancer* **36**(3): 995–1001.

Acroangiodermatitis Mali (Pseudo-Kaposi's Sarcoma)

Red-violaceous plaques

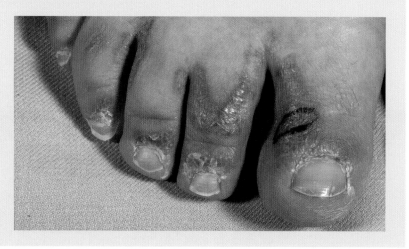

Acroangiodermatitis Mali (Pseudo-Kaposi's Sarcoma)

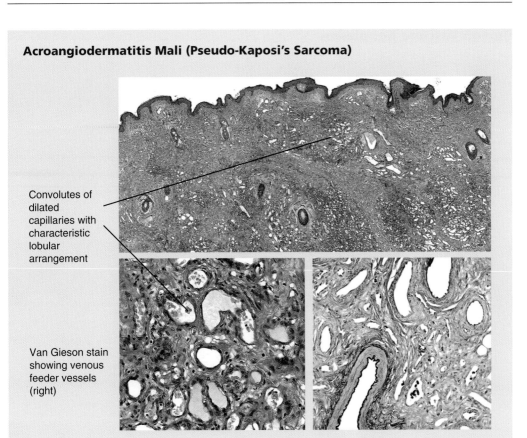

Convolutes of dilated capillaries with characteristic lobular arrangement

Van Gieson stain showing venous feeder vessels (right)

Cl: Blue-red or violaceous lichenoid macules and plaques in chronic venous insufficiency and venous stasis of the lower extremities, ankles, and toes. Similar lesions are seen in arteriovenous malformation or hemodialysis shunt.

Hi:

- Epidermal hyperplasia, occasionally verrucous hyperkeratosis
- Edema and subsequent fibrosis in the upper and mid dermis
- Proliferating capillaries convoluted and dilated in a markedly lobular arrangement
- Plump endothelial cells
- No cellular atypia; no mitoses
- Extravasation of erythrocytes
- Deposits of hemosiderin in siderophages
- Chronic inflammation

DD: Kaposi's sarcoma; pyogenic granuloma.

References

Dogan, S., Boztepe, G., and Karaduman, A. (2007) Pseudo-Kaposi sarcoma: a challenging vascular phenomenon. *Dermatol Online J* **13**(3): 22.

Lugovic, L., Pusic, J., Situm, M., et al. (2007) Acroangiodermatitis (pseudo-Kaposi sarcoma): three case reports. *Acta Dermatovenerol Croat* **15**(3): 152–7.

Mali, J.W., Kuiper, J.P., and Hamers, A.A. (1965) Acroangiodermatitis of the foot. *Arch Dermatol* **92**(5): 515–18.

Murakami, Y., Nagae, S., and Hori, Y. (1991) Factor XIIIa expression in pseudo-Kaposi sarcoma. *J Dermatol* **18**(11): 661–6.

Sbano, P., Miracco, C., Risulo, M., and Fimiani, M. (2005) Acroangiodermatitis (pseudo-Kaposi sarcoma) associated with verrucous hyperplasia induced by suction-socket lower limb prosthesis. *J Cutan Pathol* **32**(6): 429–32.

Singh, S.K. and Manchanda, K. (2014) Acroangiodermatitis (Pseudo-Kaposi sarcoma). *Indian Dermatol Online J* **5**(3): 323–5.

Benign Vascular Neoplasms

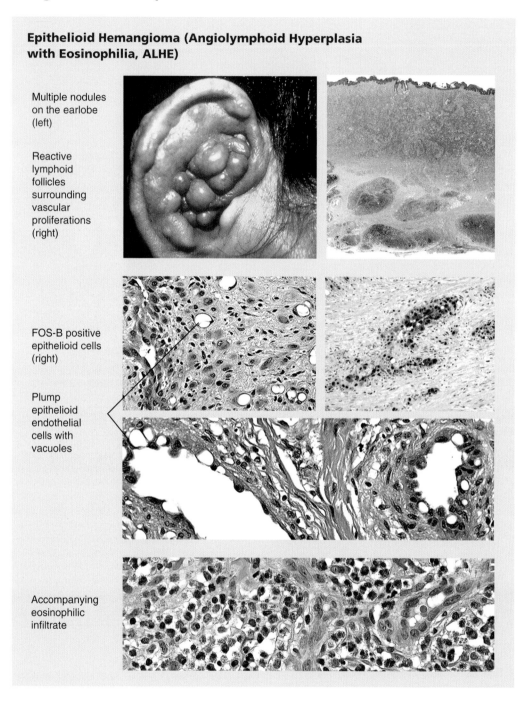

Epithelioid Hemangioma (Angiolymphoid Hyperplasia with Eosinophilia, ALHE)

Multiple nodules on the earlobe (left)

Reactive lymphoid follicles surrounding vascular proliferations (right)

FOS-B positive epithelioid cells (right)

Plump epithelioid endothelial cells with vacuoles

Accompanying eosinophilic infiltrate

Various forms of epithelioid vascular tumors have to be differentiated: (1) epithelioid hemangioma (angiolymphoid hyperplasia with eosinophilia), which is benign and is not related to HHV-8 infection; (2) epithelioid hemangioendothelioma, which is low grade malignant; and (3) epithelioid

angiosarcoma, which represents high-grade malignancy.

It is still a matter of debate whether ALHE is a reactive vascular proliferation or a primary benign vascular tumor. Recently, ALHE has been subsumed under the umbrella term *epithelioid hemangioma* that includes various morphological variants of benign hemangioma with epithelioid endothelial cells. Erroneously, the term *Kimura's disease* is sometimes used synonymously with angiolymphoid hyperplasia with eosinophilia. However, these diseases are nosologically and histologically totally unrelated.

Cl: Multiple grouped asymptomatic red nodules with a smooth surface, typically on the head and on the external earlobe.

Hi: Benign epithelioid hemangioma comprises superficial and deep variants of ALHE and classic solitary or multicentric solid epithelioid hemangioma. The common denominator is an epithelioid endothelial cell, sometimes with intracytoplasmic vacuoles ("blister cell") and immunohistochemical positivity for FOS-B.

- *Deep type of ALHE*: thick-walled venular vessels with prominent epithelioid endothelia. At the outer margin, there are eosinophil-rich lymphoid follicles
- *Superficial type of ALHE*: small protuberant papules with venular vessels in the upper and mid dermis. Epithelioid endothelia. Eosinophil-rich inflammatory infiltrate
- *Solid type of ALHE*: aggregated vessels with collapsed lumina. Predominance of epithelioid endothelia, sometimes in long rows or strands, simulating epithelioid hemangioendothelioma
- Large epithelioid endothelial cells without pleomorphism
- "Blister cells": endothelial cells with intracytoplasmic vacuoles
- Immunophenotype: FOS-B positive endothelia, rarely co-expressing cytokeratins

DD: Pyogenic granuloma; Kimura's disease; epithelioid hemangioendothelioma; epithelioid angiosarcoma; cutaneous epithelioid angiomatous nodule.

References

Bhattacharjee, P., Hui, P., and McNiff, J. (2004) Human herpesvirus-8 is not associated with angiolymphoid hyperplasia with eosinophilia. *J Cutan Pathol* **31**(9): 612–15.

Brenn, T. and Fletcher, C.D. (2004) Cutaneous epithelioid angiomatous nodule: a distinct lesion in the morphologic spectrum of epithelioid vascular tumors. *Am J Dermatopathol* **26**(1): 14–21.

Chun, S.I. and Ji, H.G. (1992) Kimura's disease and angiolymphoid hyperplasia with eosinophilia: clinical and histopathologic differences. *J Am Acad Dermatol* **27**(6 Pt 1): 954–8.

Fernandez-Flores, A. and Cassarino, D.S. (2017) Three unusual histopathological presentations of angiolymphoid hyperplasia with eosinophilia. *J Cutan Pathol* **44**(3): 300–6.

Googe, P.B., Harris, N.L., and Mihm, M.C. Jr (1987) Kimura's disease and angiolymphoid hyperplasia with eosinophilia: two distinct histopathological entities. *J Cutan Pathol* **14**(5): 263–71.

Helander, S.D., Peters, M.S., Kuo, T.T., and Su, W.P. (1995) Kimura's disease and angiolymphoid hyperplasia with eosinophilia: new observations from immunohistochemical studies of lymphocyte markers, endothelial antigens, and granulocyte proteins. *J Cutan Pathol* **22**(4): 319–26.

Kempf, W., Haeffner, A.C., Zepter, K., et al. (2002) Angiolymphoid hyperplasia with eosinophilia: evidence for a T-cell lymphoproliferative origin. *Hum Pathol* **33**(10): 1023–9.

Koubaa, W., Verdier, M., Perez, M., and Wechsler, J. (2008) Intra-arterial angiolymphoid hyperplasia with eosinophilia. *J Cutan Pathol* **35**(5): 495–8.

Kung, I.T., Gibson, J.B., and Bannatyne, P.M. (1984) Kimura's disease: a clinico-pathological study of 21 cases and its distinction from angiolymphoid hyperplasia with eosinophilia. *Pathology* **16**(1): 39–44.

Macarenco, R. S., do Canto, A.L., and Gonzalez, S. (2006) Angiolymphoid hyperplasia with eosinophilia showing prominent granulomatous and fibrotic reaction: a morphological and immunohistochemical study. *Am J Dermatopathol* **28**(6): 514–17.

Manton, R.N., Itinteang, T., de Jong, S., Brasch, H.D., and Tan, S.T. (2016) Angiolymphoid hyperplasia with eosinophilia developing within a port wine stain. *J Cutan Pathol* **43**(1): 53–6.

Miteva, M., Galimberti, M. L., Ricotti, C., Breza, T., Kirsner, R., and Romanelli, P. (2009) D2-40 highlights lymphatic vessel proliferation of angiolymphoid hyperplasia with eosinophilia. *J Cutan Pathol* **36**(12): 1316–22.

Olsen, T.G. and Helwig, E.B. (1985) Angiolymphoid hyperplasia with eosinophilia. A clinicopathologic study of 116 patients. *J Am Acad Dermatol* **12**(5 Pt 1) 781–96.

Rosai, J. (1982) Angiolymphoid hyperplasia with eosinophilia of the skin. Its nosological position in the spectrum of histiocytoid hemangioma. *Am J Dermatopathol* **4**(2): 175–84.

Sakamoto, F., Hashimoto, T., Takenouchi, T., Ito, M., and Nitto, H. (1998) Angiolymphoid hyperplasia with eosinophilia presenting multinucleated cells in histology: an ultrastructural study. *J Cutan Pathol* **25**(6): 322–6.

Tsang, W.Y. and Chan, J.K. (1993) The family of epithelioid vascular tumors. *Histol Histopathol* **8**(1): 187–212.

Urabe, A., Tsuneyoshi, M., and Enjoji, M. (1987) Epithelioid hemangioma versus Kimura's disease. A comparative clinicopathologic study. *Am J Surg Pathol* **11**(10): 758–66.

ENDOTHELIAL DIFFERENTIATION

Endothelial Differentiation

Infantile Capillary and Congenital Hemangioma

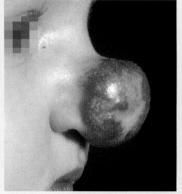
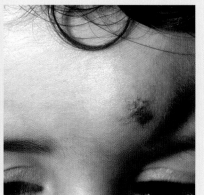

Superficial (left) and deep (right) hemangiomas

Cl: Common benign vascular tumor present at birth or acquired within the first weeks of life in 1% of newborns. Infantile and congenital hemangioma present as red or bluish erythemas, patches, and nodules of variable size, with marked predominance of the small-nodular type. Rapid enlargement before spontaneous regression within 4–8 years. Regression is indicated by replacement of the red color (blood vessels) by whitish fibrosis. Capillary hemangiomas are red and more superficial. Cavernous hemangiomas tend to be more bluish due to the deeper localisation of wider vascular spaces.

Infantile Capillary and Congenital Hemangioma

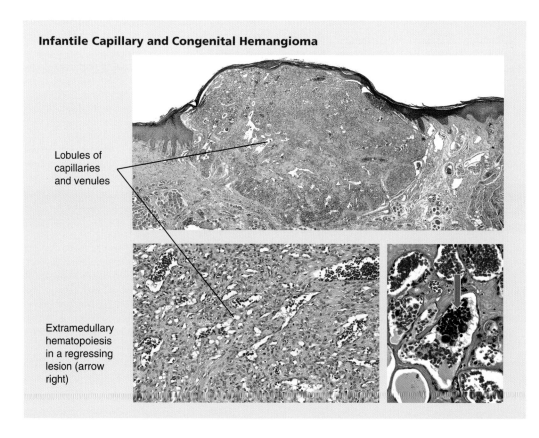

Lobules of capillaries and venules

Extramedullary hematopoiesis in a regressing lesion (arrow right)

ENDOTHELIAL DIFFERENTIATION

Hi: Lobular lesion with circumscribed borders, albeit with frequent multicentricity. While early lesions may be very cellular with densely packed capillary vessels and few patent lumina, late lesions may be hypocellular with isolated capillary lobules and massive fibrosis (signs of regression). No cellular atypia, regular capillary vessel walls. Differentiation between infantile hemangioma (GLUT1-positive endothelia) and congenital hemangioma (GLUT1-negative endothelia) is paramount, mostly for clinical reasons. Congenital hemangioma is further subdivided into NICH (non-involuting) and RICH (rapidly involuting) variants.

DD: Angiosarcoma; kaposiform hemangioendothelioma; tufted hemangioma.

References

Calonje, E., Mentzel, T., and Fletcher, C.D. (1995). Pseudomalignant perineurial invasion in cellular ('infantile') capillary haemangiomas. *Histopathology* **26**(2): 159–64.

Coffin, C.M. and Dehner, L.P. (1993) Vascular tumors in children and adolescents: a clinicopathologic study of 228 tumors in 222 patients. *Pathol Annu* **28**(Pt 1): 97–120.

Smoller, B.R. and Apfelberg, D.B. (1993) Infantile (juvenile) capillary hemangioma: a tumor of heterogeneous cellular elements. *J Cutan Pathol* **20**(4): 330–6.

Cherry Angioma (Senile Hemangioma)

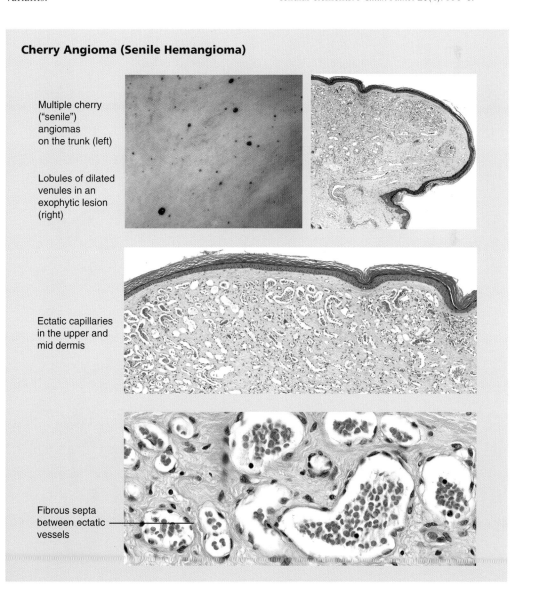

Multiple cherry ("senile") angiomas on the trunk (left)

Lobules of dilated venules in an exophytic lesion (right)

Ectatic capillaries in the upper and mid dermis

Fibrous septa between ectatic vessels

ENDOTHELIAL DIFFERENTIATION

Cl: Common finding appearing in midlife and increasing in number with age, often multiple. Trunk but also any other localisation. Tiny, multiple disseminated deep-red skin papules or macules.

Hi: Exophytic lesions consisting of small lobules of thin-walled endothelial vessels and vascular channels, separated by fibrous septa. Overlying epidermis may be flattened.

DD: Angioma serpiginosum; pyogenic granuloma.

References

Karadag, A.S. and Parish, L.C. (2016) Campbell de Morgan spot, better known as a cherry angioma. *Skinmed* **14**(5): 331–3.

Mukherjee, S., Salphale, P., and Singh, V. (2014) Late onset angioma serpiginosum of the breast with co-existing cherry angioma. *Indian Dermatol Online J* **5**(3): 316–19.

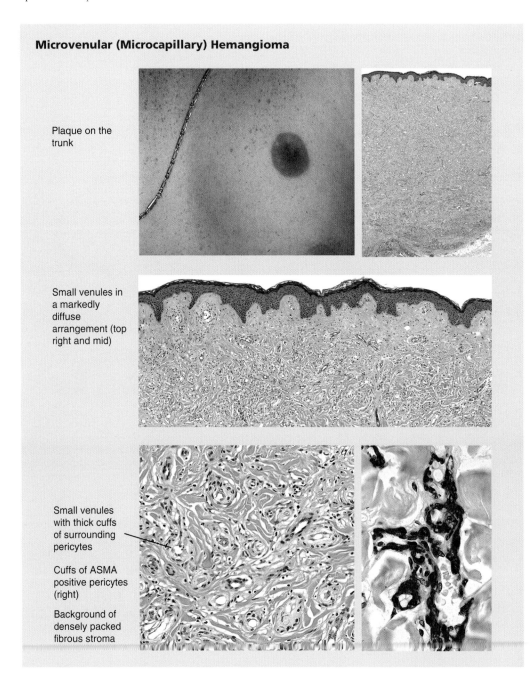

Microvenular (Microcapillary) Hemangioma

Plaque on the trunk

Small venules in a markedly diffuse arrangement (top right and mid)

Small venules with thick cuffs of surrounding pericytes

Cuffs of ASMA positive pericytes (right)

Background of densely packed fibrous stroma

ENDOTHELIAL DIFFERENTIATION

Cl: Mostly solitary, small, slowly enlarging purple or red-brown nodule or plaque lesion in young to middle-aged adults.

Hi:

- Diffuse, non-lobulated proliferation of multiple small blood vessels with thickened outer vessel walls
- Moderately fibrotic stroma
- Inconspicuous layer of alpha smooth muscle actin-positive pericytes (hallmark of venular differentiation) around these vessels (differentiation from angiosarcoma and Kaposi's sarcoma)
- No pleomorphism or mitoses
- Endothelia are negative for HHV8 and MYC

DD: Capillary hemangioma; tufted hemangioma; Kaposi's sarcoma; sclerosing hemangioma (dermatofibroma).

References

Aloi, F., Tomasini, C., and Pippione, M. (1993) Microvenular hemangioma. *Am J Dermatopathol* **15**(6): 534–8.

Bantel, E., Grosshans, E., and Oertone, J. (1989) Zur Kenntnis mikropapillärer Angiome. Beobachtungen bei schwangeren bzw unter hormoneller Antikonzeption stehender Frauen. *Z Hautkr* **64**: 1071–4.

Fernandez-Flores, A. (2008) Lack of expression of podoplanin by microvenular hemangioma. *Pathol Res Pract* **204**(11): 817–21.

Fukunaga, M. and Ushigome, S. (1998) Microvenular hemangioma. *Pathol Int* **48**(3): 237–9.

Hunt, S.J., Santa Cruz, D.J., and Barr, R.J. (1991) Microvenular hemangioma. *J Cutan Pathol* **18**(4): 235–40.

Kim, Y.C., Park, H.J., and Cinn, Y.W. (2003) Microvenular hemangioma. *Dermatology* **206**(2): 161–4.

Napekoski, K.M., Fernandez, A.P., and Billings, S.D. (2014) Microvenular hemangioma: a clinicopathologic review of 13 cases. *J Cutan Pathol* **41**(11): 816–22.

Stefanaki, C., Stefanaki, K., Floros, K., Rontogiani, D., and Georgala, S. (2005) Microvenular hemangioma: a rare vascular lesion. *J Dermatol* **32**(5): 402–4.

Trindade, F., Kutzner, H., Requena, L., Tellechea, O., and Colmenero, I. (2012) Microvenular hemangioma – an immunohistochemical study of 9 cases. *Am J Dermatopathol* **34**(8): 810–12.

Tufted Angioma

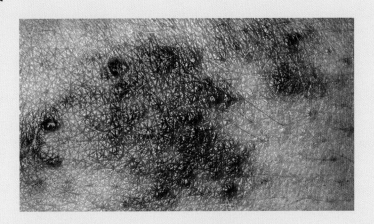

Erythema with "tufts" of protruding vascular proliferations

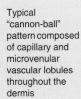

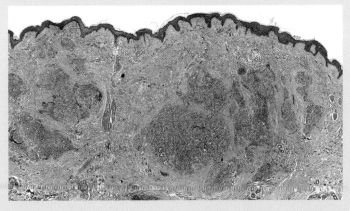

Typical "cannon-ball" pattern composed of capillary and microvenular vascular lobules throughout the dermis

ENDOTHELIAL DIFFERENTIATION

Tufted Angioma

Venular half-moon–like spaces at the periphery of capillary lobules (left and right)

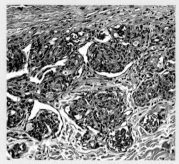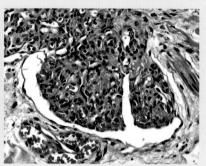

Tufted hemangioma (TH) and kaposiform hemangioendothelioma (KH) are closely related vascular tumors; kaposiform hemangioendothelioma is considered to be the deep variant of tufted hemangioma. Both tumors may be associated with Kasabach–Merritt syndrome.

CI: Rare tumor present at birth or developing in the first years of life, presenting as flat red-brown bruise-like slowly growing macules, patches or papular lesions of variable size, preferentially in the head, neck or upper trunk areas. Spontaneous regression may occur.

Hi:

- Multicentric roundish sharply circumscribed nodules of capillaries
- Dissemination of small capillary lobules throughout the dermis ("cannonball pattern")
- All levels of the dermis involved, extending into the subcutis
- Slit-like dilated blood vessels in half-moon arrangement at outer periphery of capillary lobules
- Regular capillary vessels
- No inflammatory infiltrate
- No cellular atypia
- Focal thromboses may occur (hallmark of Kasabach–Merritt syndrome)
- No deposits of hemosiderin

Immunohistochemistry: CD31-positive endothelia and alpha smooth muscle actin-positive pericytes. Importantly, both TH and KH express foci of strong positivity for podoplanin (marker of endothelia with lymphatic differentiation).

DD: Granuloma pyogenicum; infantile capillary hemangioma; glomeruloid hemangioma.

References

Arai, E., Kuramochi, A., Tsuchida, T., et al. (2006) Usefulness of D2-40 immunohistochemistry for differentiation between kaposiform hemangioendothelioma and tufted angioma. *J Cutan Pathol* **33**(7): 492–7.

Hebeda, C.L., Scheffer, E., and Starink, T.M. (1993) Tufted angioma of late onset. *Histopathology* **23**(2): 191–3.

Lam, W.Y., Mac-Moune Lai, F., Look, C.N., Choi, P.C., and Allen, P.W. (1994) Tufted angioma with complete regression. *J Cutan Pathol* **21**(5): 461–6.

Mentzel, T., Wollina, U., Castelli, E., and Kutzner, H. (1996) [Tufted hemangioma. Clinicopathologic and immunohistologic analysis of 5 cases of a distinct entity within the spectrum of capillary hemangioma] *Hautarzt* **47**(5): 369–75.

Padilla, R.S., Orkin, M., and Rosai, J. (1987) Acquired "tufted" angioma (progressive capillary hemangioma). A distinctive clinicopathologic entity related to lobular capillary hemangioma. *Am J Dermatopathol* **9**(4): 292–300.

Sadeghpour, M., Antaya, R.J., Lazova, R., and Ko, C.J. (2012) Dilated lymphatic vessels in tufted angioma: a potential source of diagnostic confusion. *Am J Dermatopathol* **34**(4): 400–3.

Wang, L., Liu, L., Wang, G., and Gao, T. (2013) Congenital disseminated tufted angioma. *J Cutan Pathol* **40**(4): 405–8.

ENDOTHELIAL DIFFERENTIATION

Kaposiform Hemangioendothelioma

Nodular infiltrate in the dermis and the subcutis (left); podoplanin positive (right)

Inset: large hemangioma on the hip of a child

Lethal outcome has been reported in 50% of patients due to the aggressive and invasive growth, and massive thrombocytopenia and consumption coagulopathy in the context of Kasabach–Merritt syndrome.

Cl: Rare vascular neoplasm in children and occasionally in adults. Considered to be the deep variant of tufted hemangioma. The deep soft tissue, especially the retroperitoneum, is involved and particularly the skin in 75% of patients. In the skin, ill-defined violaceous masses, reaching into the deep tissue levels, and purpuric lesions are found. Frequent association with Kasabach–Merritt syndrome. The tumor may be multifocal but does not metastasize.

Kaposiform Hemangioendothelioma

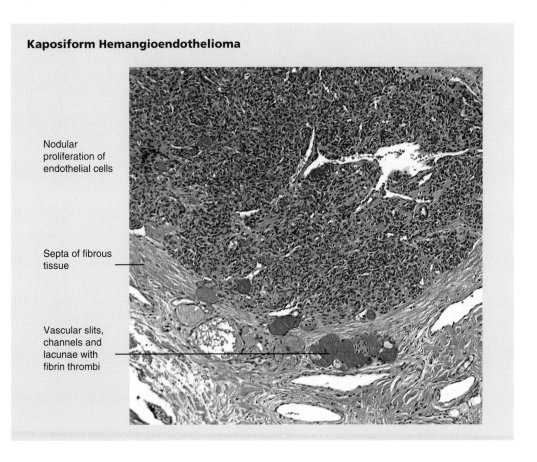

Nodular proliferation of endothelial cells

Septa of fibrous tissue

Vascular slits, channels and lacunae with fibrin thrombi

ENDOTHELIAL DIFFERENTIATION

Hi:
- Involvement of the dermis and subcutis
- Capillary lobules and sheets with peripheral half moon-shaped spaces
- Vascular cannonball pattern and sheets of densely aggregated capillaries and spindled myofibroblasts

- No cytological atypia
- Multifocal fibrin thrombi within vascular lumina, as indicators of Kasabach–Merritt syndrome

Immunohistochemistry: Multifocal positivity for podoplanin, similar to tufted hemangioma.

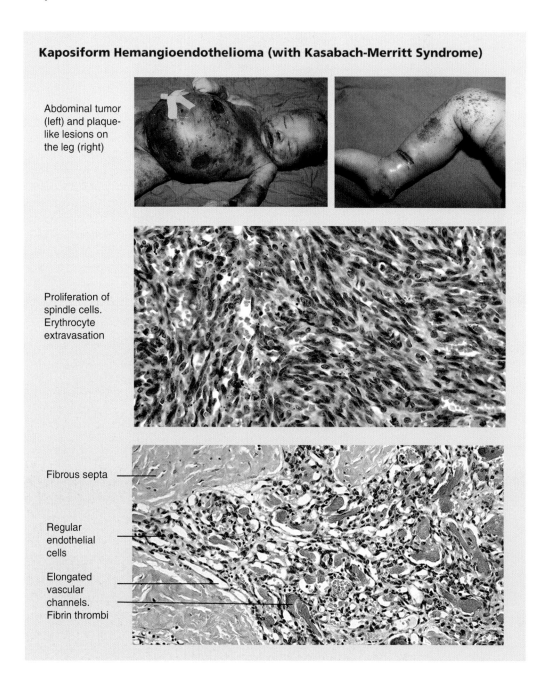

Kaposiform Hemangioendothelioma (with Kasabach-Merritt Syndrome)

Abdominal tumor (left) and plaque-like lesions on the leg (right)

Proliferation of spindle cells. Erythrocyte extravasation

Fibrous septa

Regular endothelial cells

Elongated vascular channels. Fibrin thrombi

ENDOTHELIAL DIFFERENTIATION

DD: Kaposi's sarcoma; capillary hemangioma; spindle cell hemangioma; tufted angioma.

References

Arai, E., Kuramochi, A., Tsuchida, T., et al. (2006) Usefulness of D2-40 immunohistochemistry for differentiation between kaposiform hemangioendothelioma and tufted angioma. *J Cutan Pathol* **33**(7): 492–7.

Gianotti, R., Gelmetti, C., and Alessi, E. (1999) Congenital cutaneous multifocal kaposiform hemangioendothelioma. *Am J Dermatopathol* **21**(6): 557–61.

Mentzel, T., Mazzoleni, G., Dei Tos, A.P., and Fletcher, C.D. (1997) Kaposiform hemangioendothelioma in adults. Clinicopathologic and immunohistochemical analysis of three cases. *Am J Clin Pathol* **108**(4): 450–5.

Vin-Christian, K., McCalmont, T.H., and Frieden, I.J. (1997) Kaposiform hemangioendothelioma. An aggressive, locally invasive vascular tumor that can mimic hemangioma of infancy. *Arch Dermatol* **133**(12): 1573–8.

Zukerberg, L.R., Nickoloff, B.J., and Weiss, S.W. (1993) Kaposiform hemangioendothelioma of infancy and childhood. An aggressive neoplasm associated with Kasabach-Merritt syndrome and lymphangiomatosis. *Am J Surg Pathol* **17**(4): 321–8.

Glomeruloid Hemangioma in POEMS Syndrome

Multiple red papules on the trunk (left)

Ectatic vascular spaces, surrounding intraluminal conglomerates of capillaries, resembling renal glomeruli (right top and mid)

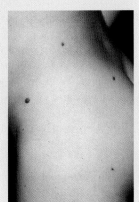
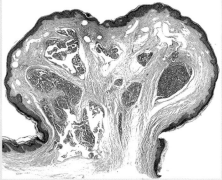

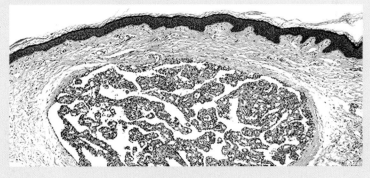

Intravascular "glomeruli" (mid and bottom left)

CD 31-staining (right)

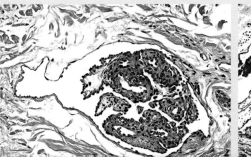
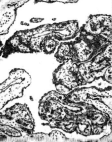

ENDOTHELIAL DIFFERENTIATION

Cl: This type of angioma, which histologically simulates renal glomeruli, presents as single or multiple red papules and is associated with POEMS (**p**olyneuropathy, **o**rganomegaly, **e**ndocrine disorders, **M** protein, and **s**kin changes) syndrome. Prevalence in Japanese ethnics.

Hi:

- Ectatic vascular spaces, surrounding intraluminal conglomerates of "free-floating" capillaries, resembling renal glomeruli
- Mostly flat, occasionally plump endothelial cells
- Presence of eosinophilic globules in some cases
- PAS-positive inclusions in some endothelial cells (immunoglobulins)
- Sinusoidal spaces

DD: Acquired tufted angioma; intravascular pyogenic granuloma; intravascular proliferation in cryoglobulinemia; reactive angioendotheliomatosis; papillary intralymphatic angioendothelioma (Dabska tumor); nodular Kaposi's sarcoma.

References

Chan, J.K., Fletcher, C.D., Hicklin, G.A., and Rosai, J. (1990) Glomeruloid hemangioma. A distinctive cutaneous lesion of multicentric Castleman's disease associated with POEMS syndrome. *Am J Surg Pathol, Pathol* **14**(11): 1036–46.

Chung, W.K., Lee, D.W., Yang, J.H., Lee, M.W., Choi, J.H., and Moon, K.C. (2009) Glomeruloid hemangioma as a very early presenting sign of POEMS syndrome. *J Cutan Pathol* **36**(10): 1126–8.

Gupta, J., Kandhari, R., Ramesh, V., and Singh, A. (2013) Glomeruloid hemangioma in normal individuals. *Indian J Dermatol* **58**(2): 160.

Hernandez Aragues, I., Pulido Perez, A., Ciudad Blanco, C., Parra Blanco, V., and Suarez Fernandez, R. (2017) Glomeruloid hemangioma and POEMS syndrome. *Actas Dermosifiliogr* **108**(2): e15–19.

Kishimoto, S., Takenaka, H., Shibagaki, R., Noda, Y., Yamamoto, M., and Yasuno, H. (2000) Glomeruloid hemangioma in POEMS syndrome shows two different immunophenotypic endothelial cells. *J Cutan Pathol* **27**(2): 87–92.

Lee, H., Meier, F.A., Ma, C.K., Ormsby, A.H., and Lee, M.W. (2008) Eosinophilic globules in 3 cases of glomeruloid hemangioma of the head and neck: a characteristic offering more evidence for thanatosomes with or without POEMS. *Am J Dermatopathol* **30**(6): 539–44.

Lee, J.Y., Choi, J.K., Ha, J.W., Park, S.E., Kim, C.W., and Kim, S.S. (2017) Glomeruloid hemangioma as a marker for the early diagnosis of POEMS syndrome. *Ann Dermatol* **29**(2): 249–51.

Tsai, C.Y., Lai, C.H., Chan, H L., and Kuo, T. (2001) Glomeruloid hemangioma – a specific cutaneous marker of POEMS syndrome. *Int J Dermatol* **40**(6): 403–6.

Yuri, T., Yamazaki, F., Takasu, K., Shikata, N., and Tsubura, A. (2008) Glomeruloid hemangioma. *Pathol Int* **58**(6): 390–5.

Pericytic Differentiation

Solitary fibrous tumor is a nodular lesion with the clinical aspect of a dermatofibroma, cyst or adnexal tumor. There are multiple sites, including the mucosa. *Myopericytoma* and *infantile myofibromatosis* are plaque-like tumors, often with a hemangioma-like or dermatofibroma-like morphology. In infants, regression may occur. Poorly vascularized and myofibroblast-rich variants are called *myofibroma*.

References

Brown, J.A. and Morgan, M.B. (2008) Pedunculated hemangiopericytoma-like tumor: peculiar fibroepithelial polyp or fibrous histiocytoma variant. *J Cutan Pathol* **35**(8): 748–51.

Fletcher, C.D.M. (1994) Haemangiopericytoma – a dying breed? Reappraisal of an "entity" and its variants: a hypothesis. *Curr Diagn Pathol* **1**: 19–23.

Goodlad, J.R. and Fletcher, C.D. (1991) Solitary fibrous tumour arising at unusual sites: analysis of a series. *Histopathology* **19**(6): 515–22.

Hasegawa, T., Hirose, T., Seki, K., Yang, P., and Sano, T. (1996) Solitary fibrous tumor of the soft tissue. An immunohistochemical and ultrastructural study. *Am J Clin Pathol* **106**(3): 325–31.

High, W.A. and Golitz, L.E. (2006) Epithelioid cell histiocytoma with hemangiopericytoma-like features. *Am J Dermatopathol* **28**(4): 369–71.

Mentzel, T., Calonje, E., Nascimento, A.G., and Fletcher, C.D. (1994) Infantile hemangiopericytoma versus infantile myofibromatosis. Study of a series suggesting a continuous spectrum of infantile myofibroblastic lesions. *Am J Surg Pathol* **18**(9): 922–30.

Nappi, O., Ritter, J.H., Pettinato, G., and Wick, M.R. (1995) Hemangiopericytoma: histopathological pattern or clinicopathologic entity? *Semin Diagn Pathol* **12**(3): 221–32.

PERICYTIC DIFFERENTIATION

Imitator: Solitary Fibrous Tumor of the Skin (SFT)

Solitary fibrous tumor is an imitator of pericytic differentiation.

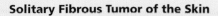

Solitary Fibrous Tumor of the Skin

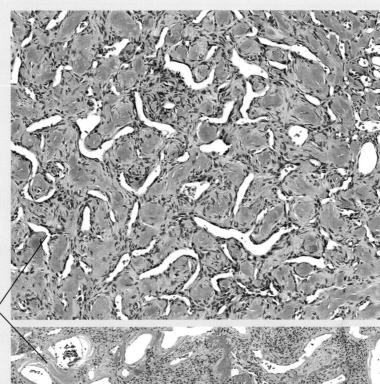

Staghorn-like vessels with broad sclerotic rims

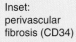

Inset: perivascular fibrosis (CD34)

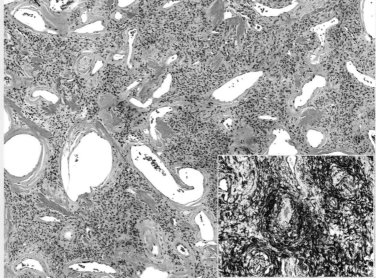

PERICYTIC DIFFERENTIATION

Cl: The most common localisation is the pleura but extrapleural localisations such as the mucosa and the head and neck area of the skin have been reported. These tumors formerly were subsumed under the umbrella term *hemangiopericytoma*.

Hi:

- Broad spectrum of histo- and cytomorphological presentation ("patternless pattern")
- Hypo- and hypercellular areas
- Prominent hemangiopericytoma-like pattern: antler-like branching of vascular spaces
- Perivascular eosinophilic sclerotic rims

Immunohistochemistry: STAT6 and CD34.

DD: Hemangiopericytoma; myopericytoma; dermatofibroma; dermatofibrosarcoma protuberans.

References

Creytens, D., Ferdinande, L., and Van Dorpe, J. (2016) Histopathologically malignant solitary fibrous tumor of the skin: a report of an unusual case. *J Cutan Pathol* **43**(7): 629–31.

Gengler, C. and Guillou, L. (2006) Solitary fibrous tumour and haemangiopericytoma: evolution of a concept. *Histopathology* **48**(1): 63–74.

Ide, F. and Kusama, K. (2002) Solitary fibrous tumor is rich in factor XIIIa + dendrocytes. *Am J Dermatopathol* **24**(5): 449–50.

Lee, J.Y., Park, S.E., Shin, S.J., Kim, C.W., Kim, S.S., and Kim, K.H. (2015) Solitary fibrous tumor with myxoid stromal change. *Am J Dermatopathol* **37**(7): 570–3.

Sigel, J.E. and Goldblum, J.R. (2001) Solitary fibrous tumor of the skin. *Am J Dermatopathol* **23**(3): 275–8.

Smith, K.J. and Skelton, H.G. (2001) Solitary fibrous tumor. *Am J Dermatopathol* **23**(1): 81–2.

Soldano, A.C. and Meehan, S.A. (2008) Cutaneous solitary fibrous tumor: a report of 2 cases and review of the literature. *Am J Dermatopathol* **30**(1): 54–8.

Vivero, M., Doyle, L.A., Fletcher, C.D., Mertens, F., and Hornick, J.L. (2014) GRIA2 is a novel diagnostic marker for solitary fibrous tumour identified through gene expression profiling. *Histopathology* **65**(1): 71–80.

Wood, L., Fountaine, T.J., Rosamilia, L., Helm, K.F., and Clarke, L.E. (2010) Cutaneous CD34+ spindle cell neoplasms: histopathologic features distinguish spindle cell lipoma, solitary fibrous tumor, and dermatofibrosarcoma protuberans. *Am J Dermatopathol* **32**(8): 764–8.

Myopericytoma (Infantile Myofibromatosis; Perivascular Myoma (incl. Myofibroma))

Perivascular tumors, evolving from pericytes and myogenic cells of the external vessel wall. Infantile myofibroma, adult myofibroma, and infantile myofibromatosis are closely related morphological variants of the same entity.

Myopericytoma

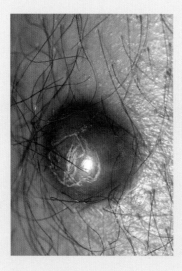
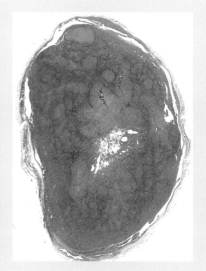

Nodular tumor on the trunk (left), sharply demarcated but not encapsulated (right)

PERICYTIC DIFFERENTIATION

Myopericytoma

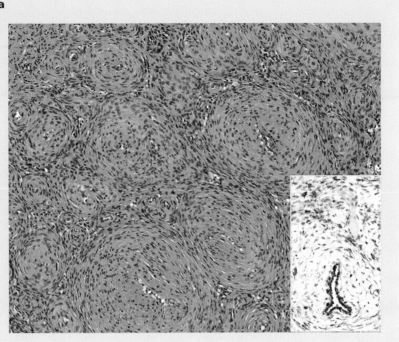

Bizarre blood vessels surrounded by plump spindled myoid tumor cells

CD34-positive endothelia and interspersed fibroblasts (inset)

Cl: Solitary or multiple firm cutaneous or subcutaneous nodules or plaques.

Myofibroma

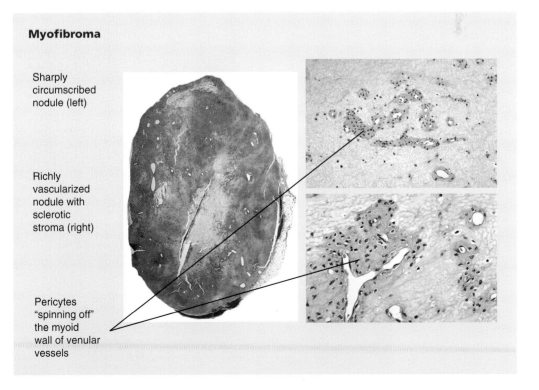

Sharply circumscribed nodule (left)

Richly vascularized nodule with sclerotic stroma (right)

Pericytes "spinning off" the myoid wall of venular vessels

PERICYTIC DIFFERENTIATION

Hi:
- Solitary or multicentric nodular tumors
- Richly vascularized sheets of small pericytic cells (positive for alpha smooth muscle actin)
- Intermingled deeply basophilic hypocellular nodules with pseudochondroid stroma and spindled myofibroblasts
- Adjacent staghorn-like, thin-walled vessels

- Characteristic "spinning off" of small fascicles of pericytes from the outer vessel walls
- In infantile myofibromatosis, "inversed zonation" versus adult and solitary myopericytoma, with peripheral vessels and internal basophilic nodules in the former
- In adult and solitary myofibroma, predominance of desmin-negative myofibroblasts

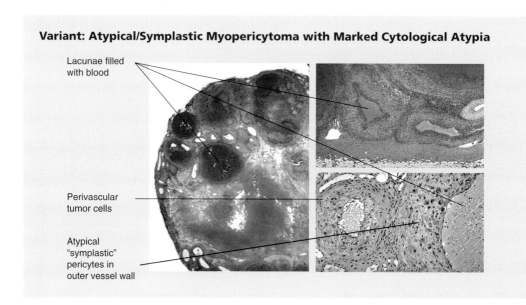

Variant: Atypical/Symplastic Myopericytoma with Marked Cytological Atypia

Lacunae filled with blood

Perivascular tumor cells

Atypical "symplastic" pericytes in outer vessel wall

DD: Hemangiopericytoma; glomus tumor; angioleiomyoma.

Reference

Requena, L., Kutzner, H., Hugel, H., Rutten, A., and Furio, V. (1996) Cutaneous adult myofibroma: a vascular neoplasm. *J Cutan Pathol* **23**(5): 445–57.

Glomoid and Myoid Differentiation

Glomus Tumor

Bluish subcutaneous nodule on the forehead (left) and subungual (right)

GLOMOID AND MYOID DIFFERENTIATION

Glomus Tumor

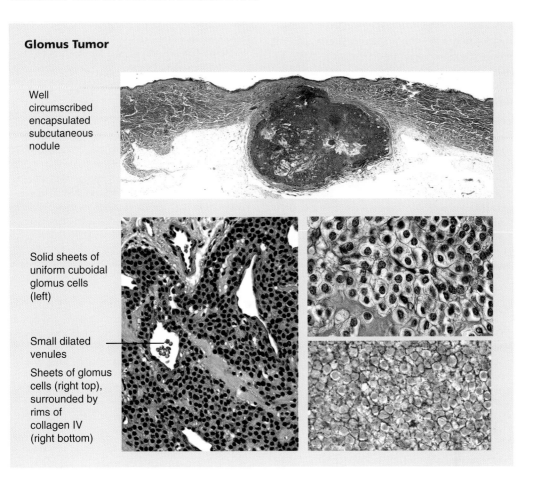

Well circumscribed encapsulated subcutaneous nodule

Solid sheets of uniform cuboidal glomus cells (left)

Small dilated venules

Sheets of glomus cells (right top), surrounded by rims of collagen IV (right bottom)

Glomus tumor is a genuine tumor composed exclusively of glomus cells, while glomuvenular malformation (obsolete term *glomangioma*) is a venous malformation with adjacent glomus cells in the outer vessel walls. The terms *glomus tumor* and *glomangioma* refer to the neuromyoarterial shunt ("glomera cutanea"), found preferentially in the reticular dermis of the nailbeds, toes, fingers, and other distinct anatomical sites. They regulate the blood flow in arteriovenous anastomoses and are composed of glomus cells, myoid spindle cells, and blood vessels. Genetic underpinnings of proliferations with glomus cells may be found in mutations of the glomulin gene.

Cl: Solitary or multiple small bluish subcutaneous pressure-sensitive or spontaneously painful nodule, preferentially in a subungual localisation. Multiple lesions may present as larger congenital plaques. Malignant variants (glomangiosarcoma or malignant glomus tumor) are rare.

Hi:
- Normal epidermis
- Monomorphous round or cuboidal glomus cells (alpha smooth muscle actin positive) surrounded by collagen IV-positive outer collagenous rims
- No pleomorphism or mitoses
- Variants:
  - Large vascular spaces, incompletely lined by glomus cells in the outer vascular layer (glomuvenular malformation)
  - Solid sheets of cuboidal glomus cells (solid glomus tumor); myxoid variants are CD34 positive
  - Predominance of spindle-shaped smooth muscle cells in conjunction with banal glomus cells (glomangiomyoma)

GLOMOID AND MYOID DIFFERENTIATION

DD: Blue rubber bleb nevus syndrome; painful vascular or soft tissue tumors; mastocytoma; adnexal tumors (eccrine acrospiroma; nodular hidradenoma); melanocytic nevus; Merkel cell carcinoma.

References

Acebo, E., Val-Bernal, J.F., and Arce, F. (1997) Giant intravenous glomus tumor. *J Cutan Pathol* **24**(6): 384–9.

Bozdogan, N., Dilek, G.B., Benzer, E., Karadeniz, M., and Bozdogan, O. (2017) Transducing-like enhancer of split 1: a potential immunohistochemical marker for glomus tumor. *Am J Dermatopathol* **39**(7): 524–7.

Calonje, E. and Fletcher, C.D. (1995) Cutaneous intraneural glomus tumor. *Am J Dermatopathol* **17**(4): 395–8.

Chakrapani, A., Warrick, A., Nelson, D., Beadling, C., and Corless, C.L. (2012) BRAF and KRAS mutations in sporadic glomus tumors. *Am J Dermatopathol* **34**(5): 533–5.

Chong, Y., Eom, M., Min, H.J., Kim, S., Chung, Y.K., and Lee, K.G. (2009) Symplastic glomus tumor: a case report. *Am J Dermatopathol* **31**(1): 71–3.

Damavandy, A.A., Anatelli, F., and Skelsey, M.K. (2016) Malignant glomus tumor arising in a long standing precursor lesion. *Am J Dermatopathol* **38**(5): 384–7.

Dervan, P.A., Tobbia, I.N., Casey, M., O'Loughlin, J., and O'Brien, M. (1989) Glomus tumours: an immunohistochemical profile of 11 cases. *Histopathology* **14**(5): 483–91.

Haupt, H.M., Stern, J.B., and Berlin, S.J. (1992) Immunohistochemistry in the differential diagnosis of nodular hidradenoma and glomus tumor. *Am J Dermatopathol* **14**(4): 310–14.

Herbst, W.M., Nakayama, K., and Hornstein, O.P. (1991) Glomus tumours of the skin: an immunohistochemical investigation of the expression of marker proteins. *Br J Dermatol* **124**(2): 172–6.

Kamarashev, J., French, L.E., Dummer, R., and Kerl, K. (2009) Symplastic glomus tumor – a rare but distinct benign histological variant with analogy to other 'ancient' benign skin neoplasms. *J Cutan Pathol* **36**(10): 1099–102.

Khoury, T., Balos, L., McGrath, B., Wong, M.K., Cheney, R.T., and Tan, D. (2005) Malignant glomus tumor: a case report and review of literature, focusing on its clinicopathologic features and immunohistochemical profile. *Am J Dermatopathol* **27**(5): 428–31.

Landthaler, M., Braun-Falco, O., Eckert, F., Stolz, W., Dorn, M., and Wolff, H.H. (1990) Congenital multiple plaquelike glomus tumors. *Arch Dermatol* **126**(9): 1203–7.

Mentzel, T., Hugel, H., and Kutzner, H. (2002) CD34-positive glomus tumor: clinicopathologic and immunohistochemical analysis of six cases with myxoid stromal changes. *J Cutan Pathol* **29**(7): 421–5.

Requena, L., Galvan, C., Sanchez Yus, E., Sangueza, O., Kutzner, H., and Furio, V. (1998) Solitary plaque-like telangiectatic glomangioma. *Br J Dermatol* **139**(5): 902–5.

Vigovich, F.A., Hurt, M.A., and Santa Cruz, D.J. (2010) Sclerotic glomus tumor. *Am J Dermatopathol* **32**(1): 76–8.

Angioleiomyoma (Angiomyoma; Vascular Leiomyoma)

Solitary painful nodule on the toe (left)

Well circumscribed solid myoid nodule extending into the subcutis (right)

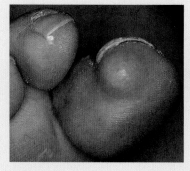
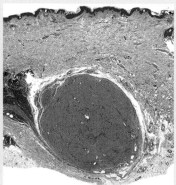

Cl: Benign solitary blue-red firm cutaneous nodules, preferentially located on the legs and feet of adult women. Painful, spontaneously or upon pressure. Recently, angioleiomyoma has been subsumed under the heading of the myoid perivascular tumors, including glomus tumor, and myopericytoma/myofibroma.

Angioleiomyoma (Angiomyoma; Vascular Leiomyoma)

Thick-walled aggregated venous vessels with compressed lumina

Compressed lumina of veins

Desmin-positivity of myoid cells of vessel wall

Hi:
- Well-circumscribed solid nodule in the cutis or subcutis
- Composed of confluent thick-walled veins with collapsed lumina
- Myoid spindle cells positive for desmin

DD: Leiomyosarcoma; pilar leiomyoma; myopericytoma; pleomorphic angioleiomyoma; hyalinized angioleiomyoma; adult myofibroma; angiolipoleiomyoma.

References

Baugh, W., Quigley, M.M., and Barrett, T.L. (2000) Palisaded angioleiomyoma. *J Cutan Pathol* **27**(10): 526–8.

Fox, S.B., Heryet, A., and Khong, T.Y. (1990) Angioleiomyomas: an immunohistological study. *Histopathology* **16**(5): 495–6.

Gomez-Bernal, S., Rodriguez-Pazos, L., Concheiro, J., Ginarte, M., and Toribio, J. (2010) Calcified acral angioleiomyoma. *J Cutan Pathol* **37**(6): 710–11.

Hachisuga, T., Hashimoto, H., and Enjoji, M. (1984) Angioleiomyoma. A clinicopathologic reappraisal of 562 cases. *Cancer* **54**(1): 126–30.

Kawagishi, N., Kashiwagi, T., Ibe, M., et al. (2000) Pleomorphic angioleiomyoma. *Am J Dermatopathol* **22**(3): 268–71.

Kutzner, H., Hügel, H., Rütten, A., and Braun, M. (1993) Erworbenes gutartiges Myofibrom der Haut (Adultes Myofibrom). *Hautarzt* **4**: 561–8.

Liu, J.Y., Liao, S.L., and Zheng, J. (2007) Cutaneous epithelioid angioleiomyoma with clear-cell change. *Am J Dermatopathol* **29**(2): 190–3.

Marco, V.S., Bosch, S.B., and Almeida, L.V. (2017) Acral angioleiomyoma with tumoral calcinosis: a complication of the insertional Achilles tendinopathy. *J Cutan Pathol* May 11. doi: 10.1111/cup.12956 [epub ahead of print].

Martinez, J.A., Quecedo, E., Fortea, J.M., Oliver, V., and Aliaga, A. (1996) Pleomorphic angioleiomyoma. *Am J Dermatopathol* **18**(4): 409–12.

Rütten, A. (1993) Das kutane Angiolipoleiomyom. *Z Hautkr* **68**: 165–7.

Varela-Duran, J., Oliva, H., and Rosai, J. (1979) Vascular leiomyosarcoma: the malignant counterpart of vascular leiomyoma. *Cancer* **44**(5): 1684–91.

Recently Described Benign Vascular Tumors

Symplastic Hemangioma

Protuberant hemangioma with thrombosed vascular spaces

Atypical cells with bizarre hyperchromatic nuclei in the myoid cell wall of medium-sized veins, showing normal endothelia; inset: CD 34

Cl: Protuberant banal hemangioma.

Hi: Hemangioma with highly characteristic "ancient changes" within stroma and myoid cell wall, but not among the endothelia.

- Small hemangioma with dilated venules and medium-sized dermal veins
- Some of them thrombosed or with eosinophilic rims

- Regular endothelia without atypia and without mitoses; low proliferative activity
- Bizarre hyperchromatic stroma cells within the adjacent stroma
- No mitoses

DD: Angiosarcoma.

References

Goh, S.G., Dayrit, J.F., and Calonje, E. (2006) Symplastic hemangioma: report of two cases. *J Cutan Pathol* **33**(11): 735–40.

Kutzner, H., Winzer, M., and Mentzel, T. (2000) [Symplastic hemangioma] *Hautarzt* **51**(5): 327–31.

Papillary Hemangioma

Bluish soft papules on the neck (left)

Sheets and tufts of aggregated capillaries (right)

Glomeruloid vascular spaces and capillary lobules

Inset: protuberant roundish endothelia, CD68 positive

Cl: Multiple papular solitary small hemangiomas.

Hi:

- Solid sheets and tufts of aggregated capillaries
- Small capillary lobules "free-floating" within glomeruloid vascular spaces
- Protuberant roundish endothelia with intracytoplasmic PAS-positive deposits
- PAS-positive endothelia express histiocytic markers CD68, CD163, and NKIC3

DD: Glomeruloid hemangioma; Kaposi's sarcoma; tufted hemangioma.

References

Ide, F., Mishima, K., and Saito, I. (2009) Papillary hemangioma on the face. *J Cutan Pathol* **36**(5): 601–2.

Rammeh, S., Fazaa, B., Ajouli, W., Labbene, I., Kharfi, M., and Zermani, R. (2014) Papillary haemangioma: a case report of multiple facial location. *Pathologica* **106**(2): 67–9.

Suurmeijer, A.J. and Fletcher, C.D. (2007) Papillary haemangioma. A distinctive cutaneous haemangioma of the head and neck area containing eosinophilic hyaline globules. *Histopathology* **51**(5): 638–48.

Vascular Neoplasms of Intermediate Malignant Potential

This group of tumors mainly comprises the hemangioendotheliomas, i.e. Kaposi's sarcoma, papillary intralymphatic angioendothelioma, retiform hemangioendothelioma, pseudomyogenic (epithelioid sarcoma-like) hemangioendothelioma, and epithelioid hemangioendothelioma). Remarkably, recent reclassification subsumes epithelioid hemangioendothelioma under the classic angiosarcomas. Common clinical denominators of the hemangioendotheliomas are aggressive growth with common recurrences, rare metastases in local lymph nodes, but no lethal outcome.

The hemangioendotheliomas co-express endothelial markers (ERG, CD31) and podoplanin. There are important immunohistochemical hallmark markers: epithelioid hemangioendothelioma (CAMTA-1 or TFE-3) and epithelioid sarcoma-like hemangioendothelioma (FOS-B and AE1/AE3).

Kaposi's Sarcoma (KS)

Kaposi's sarcoma is a multisystem vascular neoplasm of low-grade malignancy, which is considered as a "vascular lesion of indeterminate or borderline status" by some authors. Its origin (blood or lymphatic vessels or pluripotential stem cells) and its definite reactive or neoplastic character are still issues of debate. From a clinical and etiological point of view, KS has to be differentiated into several categories: (1) classic KS; (2) endemic in sub-saharan Africans (adults and children); (3) iatrogenic immunodeficiency in transplant recipients due to immunosuppressive therapies or chronic renal failure; (4) epidemic HIV/AIDS-related KS, induced by human herpesvirus 8 (HHV 8) infection. The histological features are basically the same.

In the new WHO classification of skin tumors (2018), KS will be renamed as "HHV-8 associated vascular tumor."

Kaposi's Sarcoma (Macular Stage)

Livid maculae on both plantae

Kaposi's Sarcoma (Macular Stage)

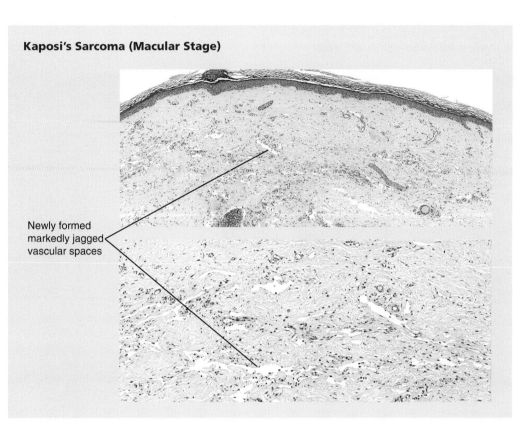

Newly formed markedly jagged vascular spaces

Cl: In classic KS, there is a high prevalence of males, who are 15 times more often affected than females; most patients are Jews or Mediterranean Europeans.

The disease starts with blue-red or brown macules and lymphedema at the lower extremities, which slowly spread and after some months or even years transform into infiltrated plaques and nodules, which finally result in ulcerated, bleeding, and crusted tumorous lesions. Mucosal involvement is rare. Patients may die from involvement of liver or the gastrointestinal tract.

In KS associated with immunodeficiency (HIV/ AIDS; immunosuppressive therapy; chronic renal failure), small red or blue-red firm papules and elongated nodules appear preferentially on the trunk along the skin lines and as blue patches in the mucosal areas.

Hi:
- Macular stage: the histological picture may be inconspicuous and almost normal
  - Stratum papillare uninvolved
  - Increased cellularity within the upper dermis
  - Irregular microvessels between collagen fibers lined by endothelium
  - Newly formed vessels protrude into vascular lumen or surround adnexal structures (promontory sign)
  - Focal accumulation of erythrocytes
  - Newly formed vascular spaces with HHV8- and podoplanin-positive endothelia

Kaposi's Sarcoma (Plaque Stage)

Blue-red plaques on the legs and feet

Vascular slits in conjunction with regular vessels (top right and mid)

Thin-walled vascular spaces surrounding pre-existing vessels ("promontory sign")

- Plaque stage:
  - Involvement of entire reticular dermis
  - Angulated irregular thin-walled small vascular lumina and slits adjacent to pre-existing vessels, adnexal structures, and between strands of collagen (promontory sign)
  - Dense proliferation of spindle cells (CD31+; CD34+; podoplanin+; HHV8+) arranged as fascicles
  - Mitotic activity
  - Hemorrhage with intra- and extravascular erythrocytes and hemosiderin and coin-like arrangement of erythrocytes

- Eosinophilic hyalin globules (PAS) (phago-
  cytized red blood cells) in fusiform cells
- Fibrosis

- Inflammatory infiltrate containing plasma
  cells (pseudogranulomatous inflammatory
  pattern)

Kaposi's Sarcoma (Tumor Stage)

Multiple tumors of Kaposi sarcoma on the leg. Moulages (right)

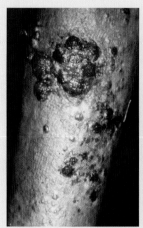 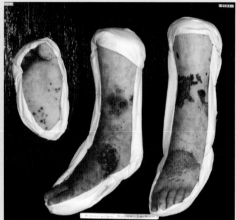

Cellular richly vascularized tumor

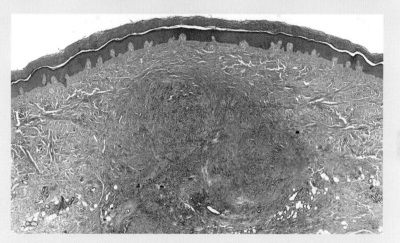

Dense proliferation of spindle cells. Thin vascular spaces filled with erythrocytes

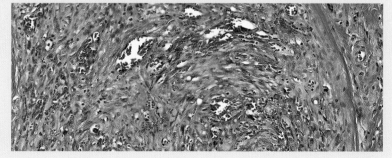

Kaposi's Sarcoma (Tumor Stage)

Dense proliferation of spindle cells. Thin vascular spaces filled with erythrocytes

Eosinophilic phagocytosed erythrocytes ("hyaline globi")

Characteristic hemosiderin deposits (Prussian blue)

- Nodular/tumorous stage:
  - Exaggeration of the histological changes seen in plaque stage
  - Small vascular slits
  - Nodules of densely proliferating fusiform cells
  - Mitotic activity but no pleomorphism
  - Hyalin globules
  - Erythrophagocytosis

Kaposi's Sarcoma (AIDS Associated)

Typical brown-red papular and nodular lesions on the trunk in AIDS-related epidemic Kaposi sarcoma

Nodular proliferation of round and spindle cells showing little pleomorphism

Thin-walled lymphatic spaces surrounding cellular infiltrate

Kaposi's Sarcoma (Lymphangioma-Like Pattern)

Bizarre lymphatic spaces in the upper and mid dermis closely reminiscent of progressive lymphangioma

Jagged vascular spaces amidst a dense collagenous stroma (left)

"Promontory sign" (right)

DD: Scar tissue; kaposiform hemangioendothelioma; hemangiosarcoma; dermatofibroma; acroangiodermatitis (pseudo-Kaposi); benign lymphangioendothelioma; leiomyoma; granuloma pyogenicum; bacillary angiomatosis; other spindle cell tumors; melanoma.

References

Castelli, E. and Wollina, U. (2000) Histopathologic features of progression in Mediterranean and immunodeficiency-related Kaposi sarcoma. *Am J Dermatopathol* **22**(1): 89–91.

Chadburn, A., Hyjek, E.M., Tam, W., et al. (2008) Immunophenotypic analysis of the Kaposi sarcoma herpesvirus (KSHV; HHV-8)-infected B cells in HIV+ multicentric Castleman disease (MCD). *Histopathology* **53**(5): 513–24.

Chan, J. (1997) Vascular tumours with a prominent spindle cell component. *Curr Diagn Pathol* **4**: 76–90.

Chor, P.J. and Santa Cruz, D.J. (1992) Kaposi's sarcoma. A clinicopathologic review and differential diagnosis. *J Cutan Pathol* **19**(1): 6–20.

Cossu, S., Satta, R., Cottoni, F., and Massarelli, G. (1997) Lymphangioma-like variant of Kaposi's sarcoma: clinicopathologic study of seven cases with review of the literature. *Am J Dermatopathol* **19**(1): 16–22.

Cota, C., Lora, V., Facchetti, F., and Cerroni, L. (2014) Localized post-radiation Kaposi sarcoma in a renal transplant immunosuppressed patient. *Am J Dermatopathol* **36**(3): 270–3.

Cottoni, F., Satta, R., and Montesu, M.A. (2000) "Early" in Kaposi sarcoma: signifier and signified. *Am J Dermatopathol* **22**(3): 294–5.

Gottlieb, G. and Ackerman, A. (1989) Kaposi's Sarcoma. A Text and Atlas. Philadelphia: Lea and Febiger.

Kao, G.F., Johnson, F.B., and Sulica, V.I. (1990) The nature of hyaline (eosinophilic) globules and vascular slits of Kaposi's sarcoma. *Am J Dermatopathol* **12**(3): 256–67.

O'Donnell, P.J., Pantanowitz, L., and Grayson, W. (2010) Unique histologic variants of cutaneous Kaposi sarcoma. *Am J Dermatopathol* **32**(3): 244–50.

Ramirez, J.A., Laskin, W.B., and Guitart, J. (2005) Lymphangioma-like Kaposi sarcoma. *J Cutan Pathol* **32**(4): 286–92.

Sbano, P., Miracco, C., Risulo, M., and Fimiani, M. (2005) Acroangiodermatitis (pseudo Kaposi sarcoma) associated with verrucous hyperplasia induced by suction-socket lower limb prosthesis. *J Cutan Pathol* **32**(6): 429–32.

Sutton, A.M., Tarbox, M., and Burkemper, N.M. (2014) Cavernous hemangioma-like Kaposi sarcoma: a unique histopathologic variant. *Am J Dermatopathol* **36**(5): 440–42.

Tappero, J.W., Conant, M.A., Wolfe, S.F., and Berger, T.G. (1993) Kaposi's sarcoma. Epidemiology, pathogenesis, histology, clinical spectrum, staging criteria and therapy. *J Am Acad Dermatol* **28**(3): 371–95.

Urquhart, J.L., Uzieblo, A., and Kohler, S. (2006) Detection of HHV-8 in pyogenic granuloma-like Kaposi sarcoma. *Am J Dermatopathol* **28**(4): 317–21.

Yang, S.H. and LeBoit, P.E. (2014) Angiomatous kaposi sarcoma: a variant that mimics hemangiomas. *Am J Dermatopathol* **36**(3): 229–37.

Retiform Hemangioendothelioma

Plaques and nodules on the hand

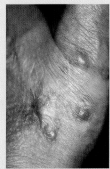
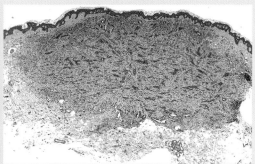

Retiform pattern of thin-walled vessels with protuberant hobnail endothelia (top right and mid)

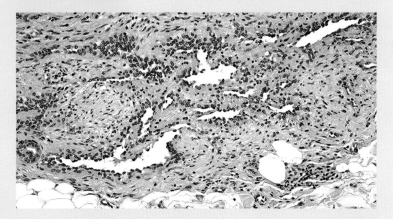

Solid strands of hobnail endothelia (left)

Hobnail endothelia (right)

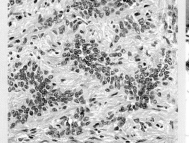
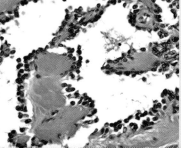

Cl: Slowly growing, poorly demarcated plaque or nodule, occasionally hyperkeratotic, preferentially located on the extremities. Recurrences are common, metastases uncommon.

Hi:

- Circumscribed nodule in the reticular dermis and subcutis without sharp borders
- Labyrinth-like retiform vascular pattern
- Vertically oriented, branching and arborizing thin-walled vessels, forming bizarre vascular spaces
- Solid strands of proliferating endothelial cells
- Prominent ("lymphocyte-like") endothelial cells protruding into vascular spaces (hobnail endothelia) (CD31+, CD34+, podoplanin+, HHV8 negative)
- Intravascular papillary projections
- Broad collagen bundles with hyalinization between vascular spaces
- Patchy lymphocytic infiltrate

DD: Papillary intralymphatic angioendothelioma; hobnail hemangioma; progressive lymphangioma; targetoid hemosiderotic hemangioma; radiation-induced angiosarcoma.

References

Arriola, A.G., Taylor, L.., Asemota, E., et al. (2017) Atypical retiform hemangioendothelioma arising in a patient with Milroy disease: a case report and review of the literature. *J Cutan Pathol* **44**(1): 98–103.

Calonje, E., Fletcher, C.D., Wilson-Jones, E., and Rosai, J. (1994) Retiform hemangioendothelioma. A distinctive form of low-grade angiosarcoma delineated in a series of 15 cases. *Am J Surg Pathol* **18**(2): 115–25.

Duke, D., Dvorak, A., Harris, T.J., and Cohen, L.M. (1996) Multiple retiform hemangioendotheliomas. A low-grade angiosarcoma. *Am J Dermatopathol* **18**(6): 606–10.

Emberger, M., Laimer, M., Steiner, H., and Zelger, B. (2009) Retiform hemangioendothelioma: presentation of a case expressing D2-40. *J Cutan Pathol* **36**(9): 987–90.

Mentzel, T., Stengel, B., and Katenkamp, D. (1997) [Retiform hemangioendothelioma. Clinico-pathologic case report and discussion of the group of low malignancy vascular tumors] *Pathologe* **18**(5): 390–4.

Parsons, A., Sheehan, D.J., and Sangueza, O.P. (2008) Retiform hemangioendotheliomas usually do not express D2-40 and VEGFR-3. *Am J Dermatopathol* **30**(1): 31–3.

Tan, D., Kraybill, W., Cheney, R.T., and Khoury, T. (2005) Retiform hemangioendothelioma: a case report and review of the literature. *J Cutan Pathol* **32**(9): 634–7.

Tsang, W. (1995) Retiform hemangioendothelioma: a new member of the group of hemangioendotheliomas. *Adv Anatom Pathol* **1**: 33–8.

Zheng, L.Q., Han, X.C., Huang, Y., and Fan, J.Y. (2014) Cutaneous retiform hemangioendothelioma on the right foot with an unusual clinicopathological feature. *Am J Dermatopathol* **36**(9): 757–9.

Composite Hemangioendothelioma

Cl: Rare solitary tumor on hands and feet of adults; other localisations have been reported.

Hi:

- Situated mainly within the deep dermis and the subcutaneous fat tissue
- Combination of various histological types of vascular tumors (benign, intermediate, and malignant) in the same lesion

References

Liau, J.Y., Lee, F.Y., Chiu, C.S., Chen, J.S., and Hsiao, T.L. (2013) Composite hemangioendothelioma presenting as a scalp nodule with alopecia. *J Am Acad Dermatol* **69**(2): e98–9.

Mahmoudizad, R., Samrao, A., Bentow, J.J., Peng, S.K., and Bhatia, N. (2014) Composite hemangioendothelioma: an unusual presentation of a rare vascular tumor. *Am J Clin Pathol* **141**(5): 732–6.

McNab, P.M., Quigley, B.C., Glass, L.F., and Jukic, D.M. (2013) Composite hemangioendothelioma and its classification as a low-grade malignancy. *Am J Dermatopathol* **35**(4): 517–22.

Nayler, S.J., Rubin, B.P., Calonje, E., Chan, J.K., and Fletcher, C.D. (2000) Composite hemangioendothelioma: a complex, low-grade vascular lesion mimicking angiosarcoma. *Am J Surg Pathol* **24**(3): 352–61.

Requena, L., Luis Diaz, J., Manzarbeitia, F., Carrillo, R., Fernandez-Herrera, J., and Kutzner, H. (2008) Cutaneous composite hemangioendothelioma with satellitosis and lymph node metastases. *J Cutan Pathol* **35**(2): 225–30.

Stojsic, Z., Brasanac, D., Stojanovic, M., and Boricic, M. (2014) Cutaneous composite hemangioendothelioma: case report and review of published reports. *Ann Saudi Med* **34**(2): 182–8.

Tejera-Vaquerizo, A., Herrera-Ceballos, E., Bosch-Garcia, R., Fernandez-Orland, A., and Matilla, A. (2008) Composite cutaneous hemangioendothelioma on the back. *Am J Dermatopathol* **30**(3): 262–4.

Papillary Intralymphatic Angioendothelioma (PILA) (Malignant Endovascular Papillary Angioendothelioma (Dabska Tumor); Endovascular Papillary Hemangioendothelioma)

Malignant endovascular papillary angioendothelioma (Dabska tumor) is an exceedingly rare vascular proliferation of borderline malignancy. Histologically and probably also nosologically, it is identical with papillary intralymphatic angioendothelioma.

Malignant Endovascular Papillary Angioendothelioma (Dabska Tumor)

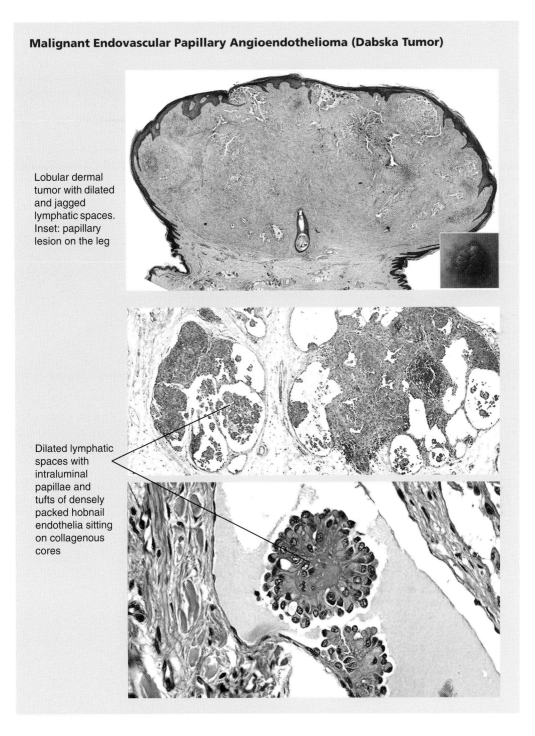

Lobular dermal tumor with dilated and jagged lymphatic spaces. Inset: papillary lesion on the leg

Dilated lymphatic spaces with intraluminal papillae and tufts of densely packed hobnail endothelia sitting on collagenous cores

Cl: Locally aggressive growing dermal tumor occurring in children and adults. No metastases.

Hi:
- Compact sheets and dilated vascular spaces, expressing lymphatic endothelial markers (podoplanin)
- Monomorphous epithelioid or "large lymphocyte-like" hobnail endothelia
- Intraluminal papillary projections with collagenous cores and aggregated hobnail endothelia on the surface ("Dabskoid tufts")

DD: Lymphangioma circumscriptum; retiform hemangioendothelioma.

References

Fanburg-Smith, J.C., Michal, M., Partanen, T.A., Alitalo, K., and Miettinen, M. (1999) Papillary intralymphatic angioendothelioma (PILA): a report of twelve cases of a distinctive vascular tumor with phenotypic features of lymphatic vessels. *Am J Surg Pathol* **23**(9): 1004–10.

Kugler, A., Koelblinger, P., Zelger, B., Ahlgrimm-Siess, V., and Laimer, M. (2016) Papillary intralymphatic angioendothelioma (PILA), also referred to as Dabska tumour, in an 83-year-old woman. *J Eur Acad Dermatol Venereol* **30**(10): e59–e61.

Radiation-Induced Atypical Vascular Lesion (AVL) (Benign Lymphangiomatous Papule (BLAP))

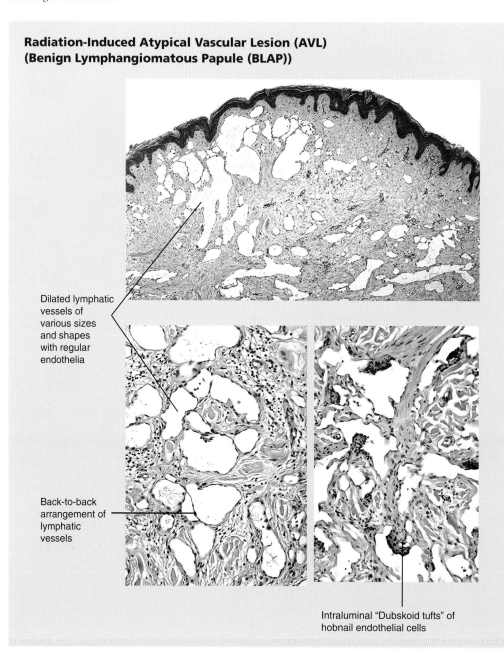

Dilated lymphatic vessels of various sizes and shapes with regular endothelia

Back-to-back arrangement of lymphatic vessels

Intraluminal "Dubskoid tufts" of hobnail endothelial cells

Atypical vascular lesions (AVL) after radiotherapy (syn: benign lymphangiomatous papules (BLAP)) present with an almost identical clinicopathological setting. Their role as precursor lesion of angiosarcoma is still a matter of debate. Histopathological differentiation from incipient angiosarcoma may be cumbersome without cytogenetic (FISH) and immunohistochemical methods. Remarkably, AVL/BLAP are clearly negative for MYC expression and MYC amplification; there is no significant proliferative activity (Ki67 < 5%).

Cl: Small red papular or plaque-like vascular lesions, mostly in women after radiation therapy for breast or ovarian cancer.

Hi:

- Lacuna-like wide and slit-like thin-walled vascular spaces in the dermis
- Increased number of small thin-walled vessels with slightly hyperchromatic endothelia
- Small endothelia with little pleomorphism
- Endothelia express the lymphatic marker podoplanin
- Projections with plump hobnail endothelia into the vascular lumina

DD: Lymphangiomatosis; incipient angiosarcoma.

References

Diaz-Cascajo, C., Borghi, S., Weyers, W., Retzlaff, H., Requena, L., and Metze, D. (1999) Benign lymphangiomatous papules of the skin following radiotherapy: a report of five new cases and review of the literature. *Histopathology* **35**(4): 319–27.

Fineberg, S. and Rosen, P.P. (1994) Cutaneous angiosarcoma and atypical vascular lesions of the skin and breast after radiation therapy for breast carcinoma. *Am J Clin Pathol* **102**(6): 757–63.

Vascular Neoplasms with High Malignant Potential

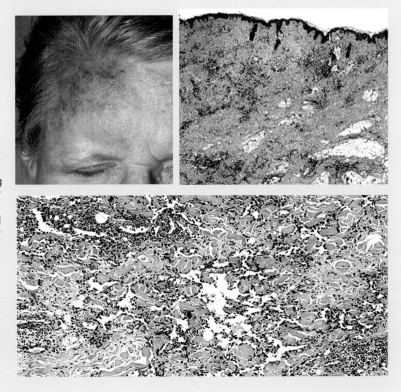

Cutaneous Angiosarcoma

Bruise-like lesion on the forhead (left)

Bizarre arborising slits and vascular spaces with markedly atypical endothelial tumor cells (top right and bottom)

Cutaneous Angiosarcoma

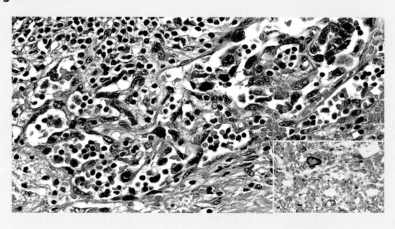

Pleomorphic and hyperchromatic atypical endothelial tumor cells lining atypical vascular spaces

Inset: CD31

The skin is the most common organ affected by this highly malignant tumor of blood or lymphatic vessels, which also can develop in various visceral organs and bone and which has a very poor prognosis.

Cl: Angiosarcoma of the skin can appear in various clinical settings, usually with ill-defined borders.

- Spontaneously on the head of elderly people. Angiosarcomas present as macular or plaque-like red or violaceous bruise-like slowly growing lesions, often imitating inflammatory facial dermatoses (e.g. "unilateral" rosacea or erysipelas). Later, infiltrated plaques, nodules, tumors and ulceration occur
- Secondary to chronic lymphedema of the limbs (Stewart–Treves), and following mastectomy
- Dermal tumors, following ionizing irradiation or after trauma and ulceration

Hi:

- Epidermis normal or atrophic
- Infiltrative growth pattern
- Atypical endothelial tumor cells with marked pleomorphism
- Many mitoses
- Intraluminal multilayering ("piling up") of atypical endothelia
- Tumor cells positive for endothelial markers ERG and CD31, often co-expressing podoplanin and myc

- Multiple histological variants. The most common are:
  - ○ Angiomatous: irregular bizarre vascular channels, with jagged spaces, slits, and lacunae throughout the dermis, dissecting collagen bundles
  - ○ Spindle cell variant
  - ○ Granular cell and foamy cell variant
  - ○ Anaplastic variant with atypical pleomorphic endothelial cells
- Erythrocytes intra- and extravascular ("bloody dermis")

Immunohistochemistry: Remarkably, cytokeratins may be focally expressed.

DD: Kaposi's sarcoma; epithelioid angiosarcoma; epithelioid hemangioendothelioma; hemangiopericytoma; pseudoangiosarcomatous carcinoma; acantholytic squamous cell carcinoma; Indian file metastasis of adenocarcinoma or malignant melanoma; pyogenic granuloma; dermatofibroma.

References

Aust, M.R., Olsen, K.D., Lewis, J.E., et al. (1997) Angiosarcomas of the head and neck: clinical and pathologic characteristics. *Ann Otol Rhinol Laryngol* **106**(11): 943–51.

Cooper, P. (1987). Angiosarcomas of the skin. *Semin Diagnost Pathol* **4**: 2–17.

Daniels, B.H., Ko, J.S., Rowe, J.J., Downs-Kelly, E., and Billings, S.D. (2017) Radiation-associated angiosarcoma in the setting of breast cancer mimicking radiation dermatitis: a diagnostic pitfall. *J Cutan Pathol* **44**(5): 456–61.

Hara, H. (2012) Endoglin (CD105) and claudin-5 expression in cutaneous angiosarcoma. *Am J Dermatopathol* **34**(7): 779–82.

Jarell, A. and McCalmont, T.H. (2012) Granular cell angiosarcoma. *J Cutan Pathol* **39**(5): 475–8.

Kiyohara, T., Kumakiri, M., Kobayashi, H., et al. (2002) Spindle cell angiosarcoma following irradiation therapy for cervical carcinoma. *J Cutan Pathol* **29**(2): 96–100.

Lazova, R., McNiff, J.M., Glusac, E.J., and Godic, A. (2009). Promontory sign – present in patch and plaque stage of angiosarcoma! *Am J Dermatopathol* **31**(2): 132–6.

Llamas-Velasco, M., Kutzner, H., and Requena, L. (2016) Cutaneous angiosarcoma mimicking xanthoma: a challenging histopathologic diagnosis with important consequences. *J Cutan Pathol* **43**(9): 792–7.

Macias-Garcia, L., Lara-Bohorquez, C., Jorquera-Barquero, E., and Rios-Martin, J.J. (2017) Recurrent cutaneous angiosarcoma of the scalp with aberrant expression of S100: a case report. *Am J Dermatopathol* Apr 25. doi: 10.1097/DAD [epub ahead of print].

Naresh, K.N., Francis, N., Sarwar, N., and Bower, M. (2007) Expression of human herpesvirus 8 (HHV-8), latent nuclear antigen 1 (LANA1) in angiosarcoma in acquired immunodeficiency syndrome (AIDS) – a report of two cases. *Histopathology* **51**(6): 861–4.

North, J.P. and McCalmont, T.H. (2011) Angiosarcoma with tingible body macrophages. *J Cutan Pathol* **38**(9): 683; discussion 684–6.

Orchard, G.E., Zelger, B., Jones, E.W., and Jones, R.R. (1996) An immunocytochemical assessment of 19 cases of cutaneous angiosarcoma. *Histopathology* **28**(3): 235–40.

Paolino, G., Lora, V., Cota, C., Panetta, C., Muscardin, L.M., and Donati, P. (2016) Early angiosarcoma of the scalp: a clinicopathological pitfall. *Am J Dermatopathol* **38**(9): 690–4.

Requena, L., Santonja, C., Stutz, N., et al. (2007) Pseudolymphomatous cutaneous angiosarcoma: a rare variant of cutaneous angiosarcoma readily mistaken for cutaneous lymphoma. *Am J Dermatopathol* **29**(4): 342–50.

Salviato, T., Bacchi, C.E., Luzar, B., and Falconieri, G. (2013) Signet ring cell angiosarcoma: a hitherto unreported pitfall in the diagnosis of epithelioid cutaneous malignancies. *Am J Dermatopathol* **35**(6): 671–5.

Shon, W., Jenkins, S.M., Ross, D.T., et al. (2011) Angiosarcoma: a study of 98 cases with immunohistochemical evaluation of TLE3, a recently described marker of potential taxane responsiveness. *J Cutan Pathol* **38**(12): 961–6.

Svajdler, M., Benicky, M., Frohlichova, L., Benes, T., Hojstricova, Z., and Kazakov, D.V. (2014) Foamy cell angiosarcoma is a diagnostic pitfall: a case report of an angiosarcoma mimicking xanthoma. *Am J Dermatopathol* **36**(8): 669–72.

Tatsas, A.D., Keedy, V.L., Florell, S.R., et al. (2010) Foamy cell angiosarcoma: a rare and deceptively bland variant of cutaneous angiosarcoma. *J Cutan Pathol* **37**(8): 901–6.

Wood, A., Mentzel, T., van Gorp, J., et al. (2015) The spectrum of rare morphological variants of cutaneous epithelioid angiosarcoma. *Histopathology* **66**(6): 856–63.

Radiation-Induced (Postradiation) Angiosarcoma

Foci of dermal infiltrates

Mostly spindle-shaped atypical cells and slit-like spaces with intraluminal and extraluminal red blood cells (left)

CD31 (upper right) and ASMA-positivity (bottom right)

Cl: Solitary or multiple papular blue-black skin lesions.

Hi:

- Epidermis not affected
- Solid epithelioid or solid spindle cell foci in the dermis
- Slit-like spaces, containing intraluminal or extravasated erythrocytes
- Importantly, endothelia co-express podoplanin and myc, with concomitant high (>10%) proliferative activity (Ki67)
- *MYC* gene amplification (FISH)

References

Fineberg, S. and Rosen, P.P. (1994) Cutaneous angiosarcoma and atypical vascular lesions of the skin and breast after radiation therapy for breast carcinoma. *Am J Clin Pathol* **102**(6): 757–63.

Gao, Z. and Chen, S. (2006) Postradiation angiosarcoma of the skin featuring capillary lobules. *Am J Dermatopathol* **28**(4): 376.

Epithelioid Hemangioendothelioma

Due to its aggressive course, epithelioid hemangioendothelioma has been subsumed under the angiosarcomas. Together with epithelioid angio-sarcoma, it represents the malignant end of the spectrum of epithelioid vascular tumors. They metastasize early and have a poor prognosis.

Epithelioid Hemangioendothelioma

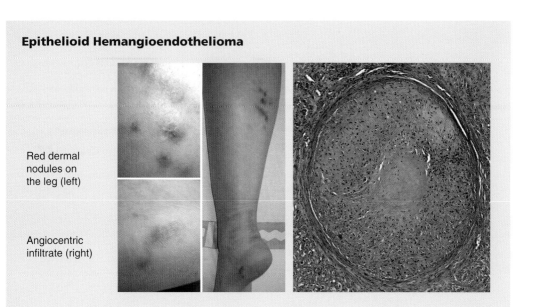

Red dermal nodules on the leg (left)

Angiocentric infiltrate (right)

Cl: Involvement of various organs and occasionally presenting in the skin, showing solitary or multiple cutaneous plaques or nodules, preferentially involving the extremities.

Epithelioid Hemangioendothelioma

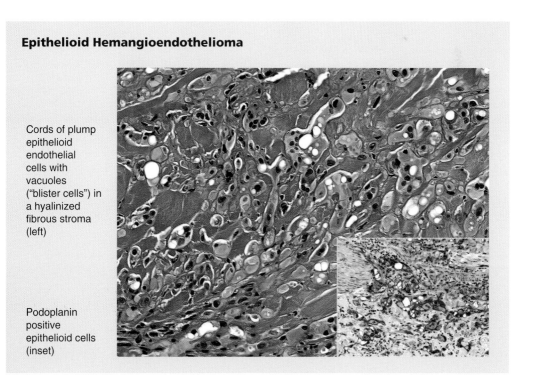

Cords of plump epithelioid endothelial cells with vacuoles ("blister cells") in a hyalinized fibrous stroma (left)

Podoplanin positive epithelioid cells (inset)

Hi:

- Angiocentric, multifocal neoplasm
- Nodules and sheets of large polygonal epithelioid cells with abundant eosinophilic cytoplasm and large nuclei with large nucleoli (CD31+, ERG+, vimentin+, epithelial membrane antigen (EMA) and cytokeratins variably expressed)
- Intracytoplasmic vacuoles ("blister cells")
- Few vascular spaces, sometimes with jagged contours
- Mitoses, pyknoses, necroses

Immunohistochemistry: Importantly, epithelioid angiosarcoma does not express hallmark markers of look-alike tumors with epithelioid endothelia: epithelioid hemangioma (FOS-B), epithelioid hemangioendothelioma (CAMTA-1 or TFE-3), epithelioid-sarcoma like hemangioendothelioma (FOS-B and AE1/AE3).

DD: Epithelioid hemangioma; metastasizing squamous cell carcinoma; metastasizing malignant melanoma; granulomatous or infectious lesions.

References

Brightman, L.A., Demierre, M.F., and Byers, H.R. (2006) Macrophage-rich epithelioid angiosarcoma mimicking malignant melanoma. *J Cutan Pathol* **33**(1): 38–42.

Eusebi, V., Carcangiu, M.L., Dina, R., and Rosai, J. (1990) Keratin-positive epithelioid angiosarcoma of thyroid. A report of four cases. *Am J Surg Pathol* **14**(8): 737–47.

Farina, M.C., Casado, V., Renedo, G., Estevez, L., Martin, L., and Requena, L. (2003) Epithelioid angiosarcoma of the breast involving the skin: a highly aggressive neoplasm readily mistaken for mammary carcinoma. *J Cutan Pathol* **30**(2): 152–6.

Fletcher, C.D., Beham, A., Bekir, S., Clarke, A.M., and Marley, N.J. (1991) Epithelioid angiosarcoma of deep soft tissue: a distinctive tumor readily mistaken for an epithelial neoplasm. *Am J Surg Pathol* **15**(10): 915–24.

Gray, M.H., Rosenberg, A.E., Dickersin, G.R., and Bhan, A.K. (1990) Cytokeratin expression in epithelioid vascular neoplasms. *Hum Pathol* **21**(2): 212–17.

Marrogi, A.J., Hunt, S.J., and Cruz, D.J. (1990) Cutaneous epithelioid angiosarcoma. *Am J Dermatopathol* **12**(4): 350–6.

McCluggage, W.G., Clarke, R., and Toner, P.G. (1995) Cutaneous epithelioid angiosarcoma exhibiting cytokeratin positivity. *Histopathology* **27**(3): 291–4.

Meis-Kindblom, J.M. and Kindblom, L.G. (1998) Angiosarcoma of soft tissue: a study of 80 cases. *Am J Surg Pathol* **22**(6): 683–97.

Mobini, N. (2009) Cutaneous epithelioid angiosarcoma: a neoplasm with potential pitfalls in diagnosis. *J Cutan Pathol* **36**(3): 362–9.

Perez-Atayde, A.R., Achenbach, H., and Lack, E.E. (1986) High-grade epithelioid angiosarcoma of the scalp. An immunohistochemical and ultrastructural study. *Am J Dermatopathol* **8**(5): 411–18.

Prescott, R.J., Banerjee, S.S., Eyden, B.P., and Haboubi, N.Y. (1994) Cutaneous epithelioid angiosarcoma: a clinicopathological study of four cases. *Histopathology* **25**(5): 421–9.

Salviato, T., Bacchi, C.E., Luzar, B., and Falconieri, G. (2013) Signet ring cell angiosarcoma: a hitherto unreported pitfall in the diagnosis of epithelioid cutaneous malignancies. *Am J Dermatopathol* **35**(6): 671–5.

Tsang, W.Y. and Chan, J.K. (1993) The family of epithelioid vascular tumors. *Histol Histopathol* **8**(1): 187–212.

Wood, A., Mentzel, T., van Gorp, J., et al. (2015) The spectrum of rare morphological variants of cutaneous epithelioid angiosarcoma. *Histopathology* **66**(6): 856–63.

Epithelioid Angiosarcoma

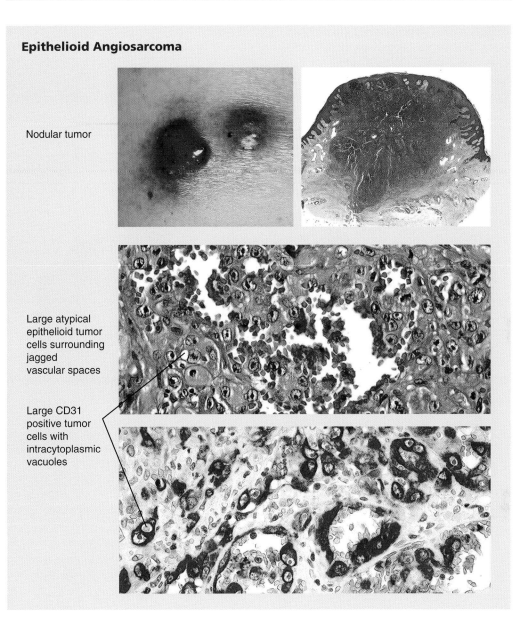

Nodular tumor

Large atypical epithelioid tumor cells surrounding jagged vascular spaces

Large CD31 positive tumor cells with intracytoplasmic vacuoles

Cl: Most aggressive vascular tumor, which metastasizes early and has a poor prognosis.

Hi:

- Epithelioid endothelial cells protruding into vascular spaces
- Significant cytological atypia and mitotic activity
- Intracytoplasmic vacuoles
- Dissection of collagen bundles by tumor cells

Immunocytochemistry: Pan-cytokeratin expression within endothelial cells is not uncommon and can lead to confusion in differential diagnosis with an acantholytic squamous cell carcinoma.

DD: Poorly differentiated carcinoma or melanoma.

References

Fetsch, J.F., Sesterhenn, I.A., Miettinen, M., and Davis, C.J. Jr (2004) Epithelioid hemangioma of the penis: a clinicopathologic and immunohistochemical analysis of 19 cases, with special reference to exuberant examples often confused with epithelioid hemangioendothelioma and epithelioid angiosarcoma. *Am J Surg Pathol* **28**(4): 523–33.

Marrogi, A.J., Hunt, S.J., and Cruz, D.J. (1990) Cutaneous epithelioid angiosarcoma. *Am J Dermatopathol* **12**(4): 350 6.

Differential Diagnosis: Acantholytic (Angiosarcoma-Like) Squamous Cell Carcinoma

See also acantholytic squamous cell carcinoma (epithelioma spinocellulare segregans Delacretaz Chapter 1)

Differential Diagnosis: Acantholytic (Angiosarcoma-Like) Squamous Cell Carcinoma

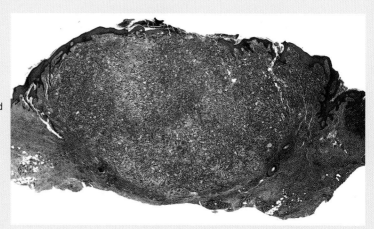

Circumscribed tumor, originating from the ulcerated epidermis, extending throughout the dermis

Cl: Exo- or endophytic tumor with criteria of squamous cell carcinoma.

Differential Diagnosis: Acantholytic (Angiosarcoma-Like) Squamous Cell Carcinoma

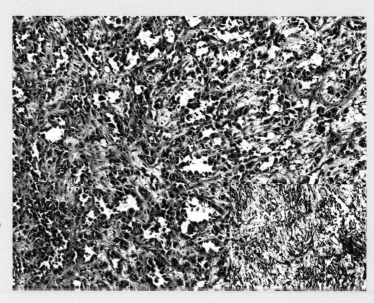

Acantholytic squamous cells, simulating angiomatous slits and lacunae

Inset: tumor cells express cytokeratin (CK4)

Hi:
- Squamous cell carcinoma with large atypical keratinocytes and a conspicuous dyscohesive tumor pattern ("neoplastic acantholysis")
- Simulation of angiomatous slits and lacunae

Immunophenotype: Expression of cytokeratins. Negative for endothelial markers.

DD: Epithelioid angiosarcoma; epithelioid hemangioendothelioma.

Glomangiosarcoma (Malignant Glomus Tumor)

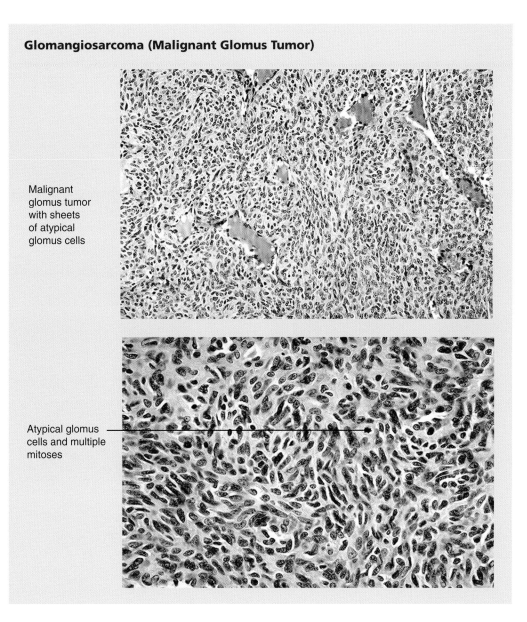

Malignant glomus tumor with sheets of atypical glomus cells

Atypical glomus cells and multiple mitoses

Cl: Rare malignant transformation of glomus tumor.

Hi: Areas of classic glomangioma gradually blending into zones with pleomorphic tumor cells and mitoses. Most glomangiosarcomas present as homogeneous highly pleomorphic tumors with a desmin-negative and alpha-SMA-positive immunophenotype. Many mitoses.

References

Aiba, M., Hirayama, A., and Kuramochi, S. (1988) Glomangiosarcoma in a glomus tumor. An immunohistochemical and ultrastructural study. *Cancer* **61**(7): 1467–71.

Brathwaite, C.D. and Poppiti, R. J. Jr (1996) Malignant glomus tumor. A case report of widespread metastases in a patient with multiple glomus body hamartomas. *Am J Surg Pathol* **20**(2): 233–8.

Cibull, T.L., Gleason, B.C., O'Malley, D.P., Billings, S.D., Wiersema, P., and Hiatt, K.M. (2008) Malignant cutaneous glomus tumor presenting as a rapidly growing leg mass in a pregnant woman. *J Cutan Pathol* **35**(8): 765–9.

D'Antonio, A., Addesso, M., Caleo, A., Altieri, R., and Boscaino, A. (2014) Glomus tumor of uncertain malignant potential on the forehead. *Cutis* **94**(3): E13–16.

Hiruta, N., Kameda, N., Tokudome, T., et al. (1997) Malignant glomus tumor: a case report and review of the literature. *Am J Surg Pathol* **21**(9): 1096–103.

Kayal, J.D., Hampton, R.W., Sheehan, D.J., and Washington, C.V. (2001) Malignant glomus tumor: a case report and review of the literature. *Dermatol Surg* **27**(9): 837–40.

Lancerotto, L., Salmaso, R., Sartore, L., and Bassetto, F. (2012) Malignant glomus tumor of the leg developed in the context of a superficial typical glomus tumor. *Int J Surg Pathol* **20**(4): 420–4.

Lopez-Rios, F., Rodriguez-Peralto, J.L., Castano, E., and Ballestin, C. (1997) Glomangiosarcoma of the lower limb: a case report with a literature review. *J Cutan Pathol* **24**(9): 571–4.

Oh, S.D., Stephenson, D., Schnall, S., Fassola, I., and Dinh, P. (2009) Malignant glomus tumor of the hand. *Appl Immunohistochem Mol Morphol* **17**(3): 264–9.

Terada, T., Fujimoto, J., Shirakashi, Y., Kamo, M., and Sugiura, M. (2011) Malignant glomus tumor of the palm: a case report. *J Cutan Pathol* **38**(4): 381–4.

Other Neoplasms with Significant Vascular Component

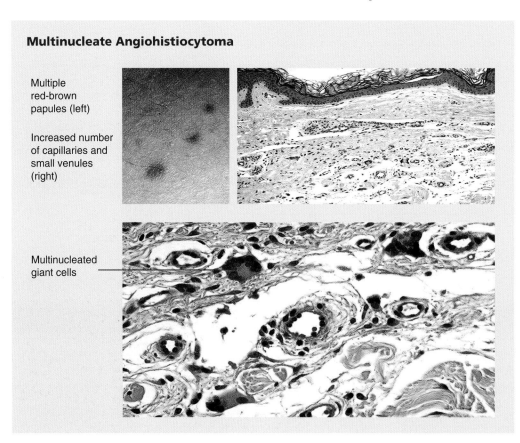

Multinucleate Angiohistiocytoma

Multiple red-brown papules (left)

Increased number of capillaries and small venules (right)

Multinucleated giant cells

Cl: Solitary or multiple brownish nodules and small plaques, preferentially on the dorsa of hands, feet, and on the knee. Facial lesions are not uncommon

Hi:
- At scanning magnification, close resemblance to richly vascularized dermatofibroma

Dense stroma

- Increased number of capillaries and venules
- Interspersed multinucleated giant cells

References

Annessi, G., Girolomoni, G., and Giannetti, A. (1992) Multinucleate cell angiohistiocytoma. *Am J Dermatopathol* **14**(4): 340–4.

Cesinaro, A.M., Roncati, L., and Maiorana, A. (2010) Estrogen receptor alpha overexpression in multinucleate cell angiohistiocytoma: new insights into the pathogenesis of a reactive process. *Am J Dermatopathol* **32**(7): 655–9.

Chang, S.N., Kim, H.S., Kim, S.C., and Yang, W.I. (1996) Generalized multinucleate cell angiohistiocytoma. *J Am Acad Dermatol* **35**(2 Pt 2): 320–2.

Puig, L., Fernandez-Figueras, M.T., Bielsa, I., Lloveras, B., and Alomar, A. (2002) Multinucleate cell angiohistiocytoma: a fibrohistiocytic proliferation with increased mast cell numbers and vascular hyperplasia. *J Cutan Pathol* **29**(4): 232–7.

Shapiro, P.E., Nova, M.P., Rosmarin, L.A., and Halperin, A.J. (1994) Multinucleate cell angiohistiocytoma: a distinct entity diagnosable by clinical and histologic features. *J Am Acad Dermatol* **30**(3): 417–22.

Wang, M., Abdul-Fattah, B., Wang, C., et al. (2017) Generalized multinucleate cell angiohistiocytoma: case report and literature review. *J Cutan Pathol* **44**(2): 125–34.

Wilk, M., Zelger, B.G., and Zelger, B. (2016) Generalized eruptive histiocytosis with features of multinucleate cell angiohistiocytoma. *Am J Dermatopathol* **38**(6): 470–2.

Angiofibroma (Adenoma Sebaceum Associated with Pringle–Bourneville Disease)

This particular variant of the angiofibromas represents the cutaneous manifestation of tuberous sclerosis (Pringle–Bourneville disease).

Angiofibroma

Multiple dense firm papules on the face and at the nasolabial fold (left). Moulage (right)

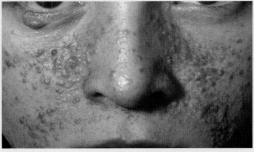
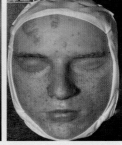

Fibrous nodule with dilated vessels

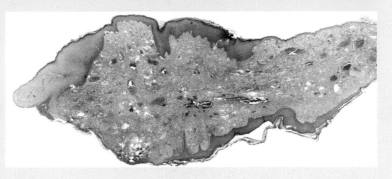

Cl: Preferentially the nasolabial fold and the cheeks, but also other facial and extrafacial localisations are involved. Multiple tiny pink or skin-colored papules; pink periungual tumors, typically on lower extremities; other organs involved: CNS, eyes, bones, inner organs (phacomatosis).

Angiofibroma

Dilated venules with fibrotic stroma

CD31 stain of regular endothelia

Hi:

- Increased swirly collagen fibers
- Increased number of thick-walled dilated blood vessels
- Stellate fibroblasts
- Atrophic sebaceous glands

DD: Trichoepitheliomas; cylindromas; rosacea; dermal nevi; angiofibroma of the nose (fibrous papule of the nose).

References

Creytens, D. (2016) Cellular angiofibroma with sarcomatous transformation showing pleomorphic liposarcoma-like and atypical lipomatous tumor-like features. *Am J Dermatopathol* **38**(9): 712–14.

Darling, T.N., Skarulis, M.C., Steinberg, S.M., Marx, S.J., Spiegel, A.M., and Turner, M. (1997) Multiple facial angiofibromas and collagenomas in patients with multiple endocrine neoplasia type 1. *Arch Dermatol* **133**(7): 853–7.

Dei Tos, A.P., Seregard, S., Calonje, E., Chan, J.K., and Fletcher, C.D. (1995) Giant cell angiofibroma. A distinctive orbital tumor in adults. *Am J Surg Pathol* **19**(11): 1286–93.

Ganesan, R., Hammond, C.J., and van der Walt, J.D. (1997) Giant cell angiofibroma of the orbit. *Histopathology* **30**(1): 93–6.

Maggiani, F., Debiec-Rychter, M., Vanbockrijck, M., and Sciot, R. (2007) Cellular angiofibroma: another mesenchymal tumour with 13q14 involvement, suggesting a link with spindle cell lipoma and (extra)-mammary myofibroblastoma. *Histopathology* **51**(3): 410–12.

Misago, N., Kimura, T., and Narisawa, Y. (2009) Fibrofolliculoma/trichodiscoma and fibrous papule (perifollicular fibroma/angiofibroma): a revaluation of the histopathological and immunohistochemical features. *J Cutan Pathol* **36**(9): 943–51.

Nucci, M.R., Granter, S.R., and Fletcher, C.D. (1997) Cellular angiofibroma: a benign neoplasm distinct from angiomyofibroblastoma and spindle cell lipoma. *Am J Surg Pathol* **21**(6): 636–44.

Rosen, L.B. and Suster, S. (1988) Fibrous papules. A light microscopic and immunohistochemical study. *Am J Dermatopathol* **10**(2): 109–15.

Silverman, J.S. and Tamsen, A. (1998) A cutaneous case of giant cell angiofibroma occurring with dermatofibrosarcoma protuberans and showing bimodal CD34+ fibroblastic and FXIIIa+histiocytic immunophenotype. *J Cutan Pathol* **25**(5): 265–70.

Yamada, Y., Yamamoto, H., Kohashi, K., et al. (2016) Histological spectrum of angiofibroma of soft tissue: histological and genetic analysis of 13 cases. *Histopathology* **69**(3): 459–69.

Angiolipoma

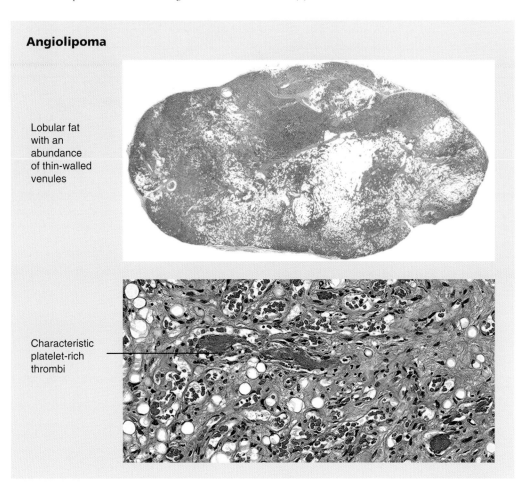

Lobular fat with an abundance of thin-walled venules

Characteristic platelet-rich thrombi

Richly vascularized lipoma. Recent findings suggest that angiolipoma is an acquired hemangioma variant with predilection of the lobular subcutaneous fat

Cl: Painful subcutaneous nodule. Often multiple and acquired.

Hi:

- Sharply demarcated subcutaneous nodule with thin pseudocapsule
- Diffuse proliferation of small venules and rare capillaries within the subcutaneous fat
- Cellular variant: vessels may coalesce to large intralobular sheets
- Hallmarks are eosinophilic CD61-positive platelet thrombi within some or all of the vessels

DD: Lipoma; hemangioma; angiomyolipoma; Kaposi's sarcoma.

References

Belcher, R.W., Czarnetzki, B.M., Carney, J.F., and Gardner, E. (1974) Multiple (subcutaneous) angiolipomas. Clinical, pathologic, and pharmacologic studies. *Arch Dermatol* **110**(4): 583–5.

Hunt, S.J., Santa Cruz, D.J., and Barr, R.J. (1990) Cellular angiolipoma. *Am J Surg Pathol* **14**(1): 75–81.

Kanik, A.B., Oh, C.H., and Bhawan, J. (1995) Cellular angiolipoma. *Am J Dermatopathol* **17**(3): 312–15.

Sheng, W., Lu, L., and Wang, J. (2013) Cellular angiolipoma: a clinicopathological and immunohistochemical study of 12 cases. *Am J Dermatopathol* **35**(2): 220–5.

Angiolipoleiomyoma (Angiomyolipoma)

Combination of fatty tissue, smooth muscle bundles, and thick-walled venules ("angiolipoleiomyoma")

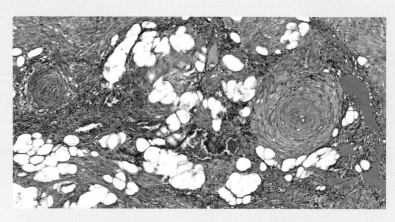

Cl: Benign tumor, most likely angioleiomyoma variant with accompanying (metaplastic) fat. Renal angiomyolipoma with strong expression of HMB-45 may be associated with Birt–Hogg–Dubé syndrome.

Hi: Sharply circumscribed combined proliferation of blood vessels, smooth muscle, and fat.

DD: Cellular angiolipoma.

References

Argenyi, Z.B., Piette, W.W., and Goeken, J.A. (1991) Cutaneous angiomyolipoma. A light-microscopic, immunohistochemical, and electron-microscopic study. *Am J Dermatopathol* **13**(5): 497–502.

Byrne, M., Mallipeddi, R., Pichert, G., and Whittaker, S. (2012) Birt–Hogg–Dube syndrome with a renal angiomyolipoma: further evidence of a relationship between Birt–Hogg–Dube syndrome and tuberous sclerosis complex. *Australas J Dermatol* **53**(2): 151–4.

Dow, E. and Winship, I. (2016) Renal angiomyolipoma in Birt–Hogg–Dube syndrome: a case study supporting overlap with tuberous sclerosis complex. *Am J Med Genet A* **170**(12): 3323–6.

Fitzpatrick, J.E., Mellette, J.R. Jr, Hwang, R.J., Golitz, L.E., Zaim, M.T., and Clemons, D. (1990) Cutaneous angiolipoleiomyoma. *J Am Acad Dermatol* **23**(6 Pt 1): 1093–8.

Mehregan, D.A., Mehregan, D.R., and Mehregan, A.H. (1992) Angiomyolipoma. *J Am Acad Dermatol* **27**(2 Pt 2): 331–3.

Pea, M., Bonetti, F., Zamboni, G., et al. (1991) Melanocyte-marker-HMB-45 is regularly expressed in angiomyolipoma of the kidney. *Pathology* **23**(3): 185–8.

Rütten, A. (1993) Das kutane Angiolipoleiomyom. *Z Hautkr* **68**: 165–7.

Yaldiz, M., Kilinc, N., and Ozdemir, E. (2004) Strong association of HMB-45 expression with renal angiomyolipoma. *Saudi Med J* **25**(8): 1020–3.

Angiomyxoma

Mucinous stroma and delicate vessels in the dermis

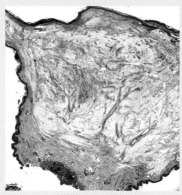
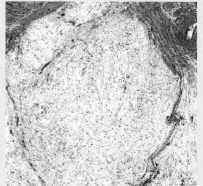

Angiomyxoma

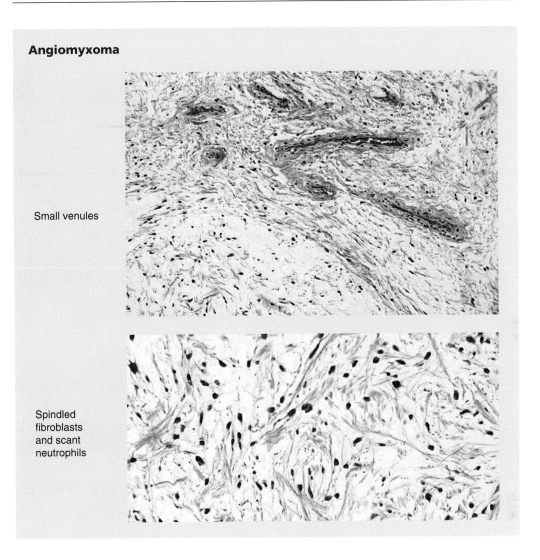

Small venules

Spindled
fibroblasts
and scant
neutrophils

Cl: Small nodule resembling a cyst.

Hi:

- Mucinous stroma in the dermis and subcutis with prominent vessels
- Spindled and stellate fibroblasts
- Mast cells and neutrophilic granulocytes ("sprinkle of neutrophils")

References

Granter, S.R., Nucci, M.R., and Fletcher, C.D. (1997) Aggressive angiomyxoma: reappraisal of its relationship to angiomyofibroblastoma in a series of 16 cases. *Histopathology* **30**(1): 3–10.

Satter, E.K. (2009) Solitary superficial angiomyxoma: an infrequent but distinct soft tissue tumor. *J Cutan Pathol* **36**(Suppl 1): 56–9.

Zamecnik, M., Skalova, A., Michal, M., and Gomolcak, P. (2000).Aggressive angiomyxoma with multinucleated giant cells: a lesion mimicking liposarcoma. *Am J Dermatopathol* **22**(4): 368–71.

Intralymphatic Histiocytosis

Diffuse tumorous swelling of the cheek and eyebrows (left) due to nodular infiltrates in the dermis, edema and fibrosis (right)

Intralymphatic histiocytes; CD68 positive (right)

Inflammatory lymphocytic infiltrate

Lymph vessels; CD31 positive

Cl: Erythemas or flat erythematous plaques, sometimes with nodular surface. Often in association with underlying endoprosthesis (hip, knee).

Hi:
- Dilated thin-walled lymphatic vessels in all levels of the dermis
- Podoplanin-positive endothelia
- Dense aggregates of intraluminal histocytic cells (CD14+, CD68+, CD163+)
- Perivascular mixed infiltrate composed of lymphocytes, plasma cells, histiocytes, and granulocytes

- Importantly, endothelial marker CD31 may be misleading due to its cross-reactivity with histiocytes

DD: Intravascular lymphomatosis (intravascular T- or B-cell lymphoma, intravascular malignant histiocytosis); reactive angioendotheliomatosis.

Reference

Takiwaki, H., Adachi, A., Kohno, H., and Ogawa, Y. (2004) Intravascular or intralymphatic histiocytosis associated with rheumatoid arthritis: a report of 4 cases. *J Am Acad Dermatol* **50**(4): 585–90

Kimura's Disease

Subcutaneous
swelling on the
forehead (left)

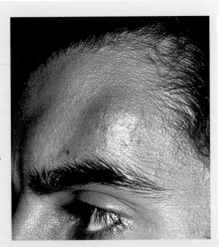

Lymphoid follicles
in the dermis and
subcutis (right)

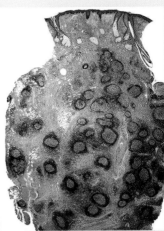

Lymph follicles
with germinal
center formation.
Thick-walled
vessels with
enlarged
endothelia (left)

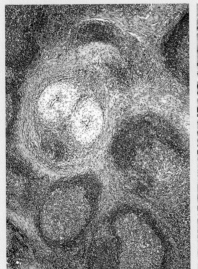

Lymphocytic
infiltrate rich with
eosinophils
(right)

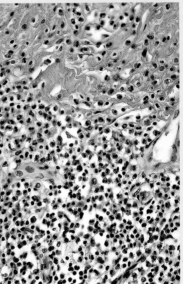

Courtesy of L Requena, Madrid

Kimura's disease occurs as an immune-reactive lymphocytic condition in Asian individuals. The skin is rarely involved. It is not a vascular tumor and does not belong to the family of epithelioid vascular tumors.

Cl: Subcutaneous swelling, preferentially in the parotid and submandibular regions of young adult males, associated with marked lymphadenopathy, blood eosinophilia, and increased serum levels of immunoglobulin (IgE).

Hi:
- Dense lymphocytic infiltrate with admixture of eosinophils
- Dilated blood vessels
- Prominent lymphoid follicles with germinal center formation

- Tissue eosinophilia
- No epithelioid endothelial cells
- Septal fibrosis

DD: Epithelioid hemangioma; cutaneous B-cell lymphomas (marginal zone and follicle center lymphoma); pseudolymphoma; bacillary angiomatosis; epithelioid angiosarcoma.

References

Dargent, J.L., Vannuffel, P., Saint-Remy, J.M., Fisogni, S., and Facchetti, F. (2009) Plasmacytoid dendritic cells in Kimura disease. *Am J Dermatopathol* **31**(8): 854–6.

Helander, S.D., Peters, M.S., Kuo, T.T., and Su, W.P. (1995) Kimura's disease and angiolymphoid hyperplasia with eosinophilia: new observations from immunohistochemical studies of lymphocyte markers, endothelial antigens, and granulocyte proteins. *J Cutan Pathol* **22**(4): 319–26.

Jang, K.A., Ahn, S.J., Choi, J.H., et al. (2001) Polymerase chain reaction (PCR) for human herpesvirus 8 and heteroduplex PCR for clonality assessment in angiolymphoid hyperplasia with eosinophilia and Kimura's disease. *J Cutan Pathol* **28**(7): 363–7.

Watanabe, C., Koga, M., Honda, Y., and Oh, I.T. (2002) Juvenile temporal arteritis is a manifestation of Kimura disease. *Am J Dermatopathol* **24**(1): 43–9.

Wong, K.T. and Shamsol, S. (1999) Quantitative study of mast cells in Kimura's disease. *J Cutan Pathol* **26**(1): 13–16.

CHAPTER 7

Fat

Atlas of Dermatopathology: Tumors, Nevi, and Cysts, First Edition. Günter Burg, Heinz Kutzner,
Werner Kempf, Josef Feit, and Bruce R. Smoller.
© 2019 John Wiley & Sons Ltd. Published 2019 by John Wiley & Sons Ltd.

Nevus (Hamartoma)

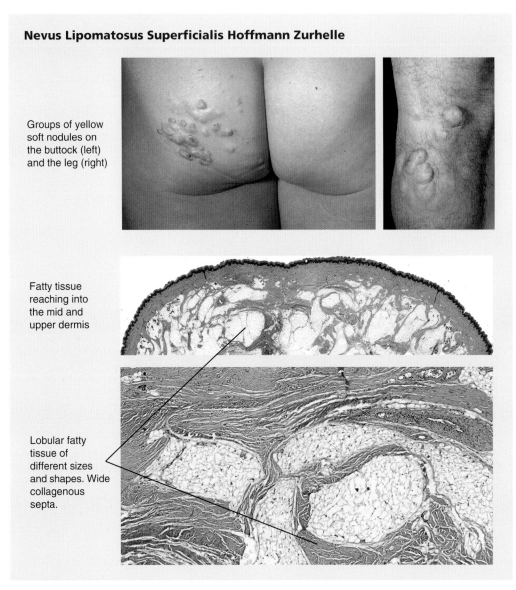

Nevus Lipomatosus Superficialis Hoffmann Zurhelle

Groups of yellow soft nodules on the buttock (left) and the leg (right)

Fatty tissue reaching into the mid and upper dermis

Lobular fatty tissue of different sizes and shapes. Wide collagenous septa.

Cl: Soft yellowish papules and nodules, single or in groups or in linear arrangement, on the buttocks and thighs but also in other areas, frequently unilateral. The surface may be wrinkled or cobblestone-like. Lesions are present at birth or appear during infancy.

Hi:
- Thinned dermis
- Multiple lobules of normal fat in the mid- and deep dermis, usually sparing the papillary dermis
- Fibrotic septa

DD: Focal dermal hypoplasia; myxoma; clinically, neurofibroma, melanocytic nevi.

References

Chopra, R., Al Marzooq, Y.M., Siddiqui, F.A., Aldawsari, S., and Al Ameer, A. (2015) Nevus lipomatosus cutaneous superficialis with focal lipocytic pagetoid epidermal spread and secondary calcinosis cutis: a case report. *Am J Dermatopathol* **37**(4): 326–8.

BENIGN NEOPLASMS

Goyal, M., Wankhade, V.H., Mukhi, J.I., and Singh, R.P. (2016) Nevus lipomatosus cutaneous superficialis – a rare hamartoma: report of two cases. *J Clin Diagn Res* **10**(10): WD01–WD02.

Gutierrez-Gonzalez, E., Montero, I., Sanchez-Aguilar, D., Ginarte, M., and Toribio, J. (2014) Adult-onset verrucous nevus lipomatosus cutaneous superficialis. *Int J Dermatol* **53**(1): e69–71.

Ioannidou, D.J., Stefanidou, M.P., Panayiotides, J.G., and Tosca, A.D. (2001) Nevus lipomatosus cutaneous superficialis (Hoffmann–Zurhelle) with localized scleroderma like appearance. *Int J Dermatol* **40**(1): 54–7.

Kim, E.J., Jo, S.J., and Cho, K.H. (2014) A case of mucinous nevus clinically mimicking nevus lipomatosus superficialis. *Ann Dermatol* **26**(4): 549–50.

Pujani, M., Choudhury, M., Garg, T., and Madan, N.K. (2014) Nevus lipomatosus superficialis: A rare cutaneous hamartoma. *Indian Dermatol Online J* **5**(1): 109–10.

Sendhil Kumaran, M., Narang, T., Dogra, S., Saikia, U.N., and Kanwar, A.J. (2013) Nevus lipomatosus superficialis unseen or unrecognized: a report of eight cases. *J Cutan Med Surg* **17**(5): 335–9.

Takashima, H., Toyoda, M., Ikeda, Y., Kagoura, M., and Morohashi, M. (2003) Nevus lipomatosus cutaneous superficialis with perifollicular fibrosis. *Eur J Dermatol* **13**(6): 584–6.

Neoplasms of Fat Tissue

Benign Neoplasms

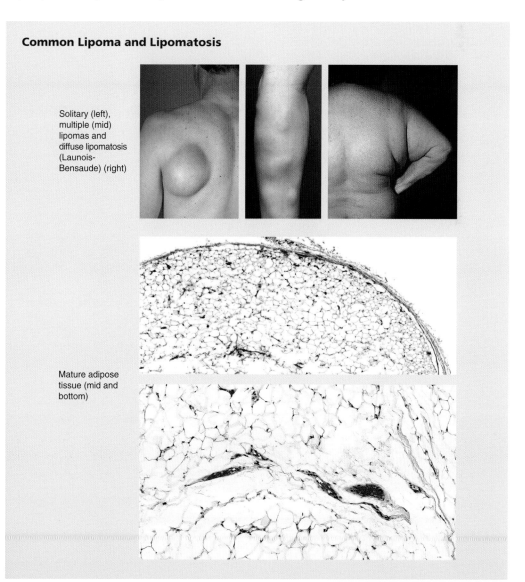

Common Lipoma and Lipomatosis

Solitary (left), multiple (mid) lipomas and diffuse lipomatosis (Launois-Bensaude) (right)

Mature adipose tissue (mid and bottom)

BENIGN NEOPLASMS

Cl: Poorly defined subcutaneous soft nodules or tumors, single, multiple or diffuse (Launois–Bensaude syndrome). Rarely painful, except when impinging on nerves.

Hi:

- Large lobules of mature adipose tissue
- Regular adipocytes
- No lipoblasts
- Rarely large macrophages ("pseudolipoblasts") – particularly in post-traumatic lesions

Immunohistochemistry: Negative for MDM2 and CDK2.

DD: Deep neurofibroma; cyst; any subcutaneous tumor.

References

French, C.A., Mentzel, T., Kutzner, H., and Fletcher, C.D. (2000) Intradermal spindle cell/pleomorphic lipoma: a distinct subset. *Am J Dermatopathol* **22**(6): 496–502.

Gonzalez, R.S., McClain, C.M., Chamberlain, B.K., Coffin, C.M., and Cates, J.M. (2013) Cyclin-dependent kinase inhibitor 2A (p16) distinguishes well-differentiated liposarcoma from lipoma. *Histopathology* **62**(7): 1109–11.

Laskin, W.B., Fetsch, J.F., Michal, M., and Miettinen, M. (2006) Sclerotic (fibroma-like) lipoma: a distinctive lipoma variant with a predilection for the distal extremities. *Am J Dermatopathol* **28**(4): 308–16.

Michal, M. and Zamecnik, M. (1998) Synovial metaplasia in lipoma. *Am J Dermatopathol* **20**(3): 285–9.

Silverman, J.S. and Tamsen, A. (1997) Fibrohistiocytic differentiation in subcutaneous fatty tumors. Study of spindle cell, pleomorphic, myxoid, and atypical lipoma and dedifferentiated liposarcoma cases composed in part of CD34+ fibroblasts and FXIIIa + histiocytes. *J Cutan Pathol* **24**(8): 484–93.

Templeton, S.F. and Solomon, A.R. Jr. (1996) Spindle cell lipoma is strongly CD34 positive. An immunohistochemical study. *J Cutan Pathol* **23**(6): 546–50.

Zelger, B.G., Zelger, B., Steiner, H., and Rutten, A. (1997) Sclerotic lipoma: lipomas simulating sclerotic fibroma. *Histopathology* **31**(2): 174–81.

Angiolipoma (see Vessels, Chapter 6)

Angiomyolipoma (see Vessels, Chapter 6)

Spindle Cell Lipoma

Sharply circumscribed spindle cell tumor with interspersed clusters of lipocytes

BENIGN NEOPLASMS

Spindle Cell Lipoma

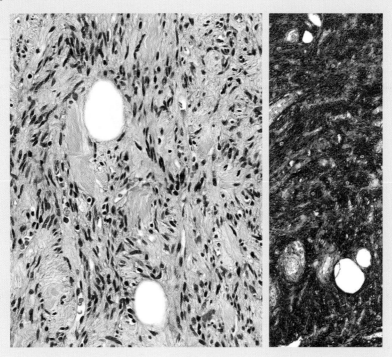

Solid proliferation of spindle cells entrapping lipocytes (left). CD34 positive spindle cells (right)

Cl: Benign subcutaneous well-circumscribed tumor; location preferentially in the neck, upper back or shoulders.

Hi:

- Solid nests and bundles of various proportion of CD34-positive spindle cells
- Entrapping of lobules of mature adipose tissue or fat vacuoles
- Wiry collagen between the adipocytes
- Basophilic mucinous stroma
- Spindled tumor cells show distinct loss of RB1

References

Duve, S., Muller-Hocker, J., and Worret, W.I. (1995).Spindle-cell lipoma of the skin. *Am J Dermatopathol* **17**(5): 529–33.

Forcucci, J.A., Sugianto, J.Z., Wolff, D.J., Maize, J.C. Sr, and Ralston, J.S. (2015) "Low-Fat" pseudoangiomatous spindle cell lipoma: a rare variant with loss of 13q14 region. *Am J Dermatopathol* **37**(12): 920–3.

Gurel, D., Kargi, A., and Lebe, B. (2010).Pedunculated cutaneous spindle cell/pleomorphic lipoma. *J Cutan Pathol* **37**(9): e57–9.

Hawley, I.C., Krausz, T., Evans, D.J., and Fletcher, C.D. (1994) Spindle cell lipoma – a pseudoangiomatous variant. *Histopathology* **24**(6): 565–9.

Kelley, C., Gleason, B., Fox, M., Thomas, A., Victor, T., and Cibull, T. (2011) Spindle cell lipoma with collagen rosettes. *J Cutan Pathol* **38**(9): 756–8.

Mandal, R.V., Duncan, L.M., Austen, W.G. Jr, and Nielsen, G.P. (2009) Infiltrating intramuscular spindle cell lipoma of the face. *J Cutan Pathol* **36**(Suppl 1): 70–3.

McInturff, M. and Graham, B. (2017) Spindle cell lipoma with prominent Verocay bodies: a potential diagnostic pitfall. *J Cutan Pathol* **44**(4): 317–19.

Sciot, R. and Bekaert, J. (2001) Spindle cell lipoma with extramedullary haematopoiesis. *Histopathology* **39**(2): 215–16.

Wood, L., Fountaine, T.J., Rosamilia, L., Helm, K.F., and Clarke, L.E. (2010) Cutaneous CD34+ spindle cell neoplasms: histopathologic features distinguish spindle cell lipoma, solitary fibrous tumor, and dermatofibrosarcoma protuberans. *Am J Dermatopathol* **32**(8): 764–8.

BENIGN NEOPLASMS

Pleomorphic Lipoma (see Pleomorphic Liposarcoma)

Pleomorphic lipoma may be interpreted as a morphological variant of spindle cell lipoma with hyperchromatic and floret-like tumor cells and loss of RB1. Mitotic activity is exceedingly low. There are no distinct pleomorphic lipoblasts as in pleomorphic liposarcoma.

Reference

Griffin, T.D., Goldstein, J., and Johnson, W.C. (1992).Pleomorphic lipoma. Case report and discussion of "atypical" lipomatous tumors. *J Cutan Pathol* **19**(4): 330–3.

Hibernoma

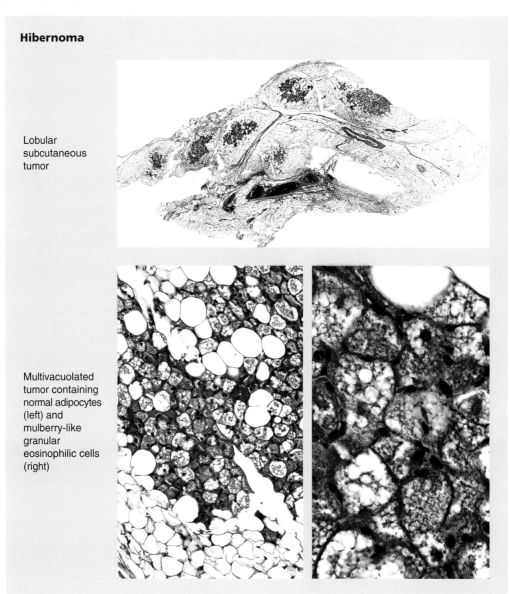

Lobular subcutaneous tumor

Multivacuolated tumor containing normal adipocytes (left) and mulberry-like granular eosinophilic cells (right)

Tumor of brown fat, which is especially abundant in newborns and decreases in adults. Its primary function is thermoregulation. Whereas white adipocytes contain a single lipid droplet, brown adipocytes contain numerous smaller droplets. The higher number of mitochondria, which contain iron, results in the brown appearance.

MALIGNANT NEOPLASMS

Cl: Subcutaneous well-circumscribed tumors, preferentially on the trunk of young adults.

Hi:
- Macroscopically yellow-brown cutting surface
- Lobular tumor
- Large mulberry-like cells with abundant eosinophilic granular cytoplasm
- Variants: lipoma-like, spindle cell or myxoid type

DD: Granular cell tumor; liposarcoma; rhabdomyoma.

References

Evers, L.H., Gebhard, M., Lange, T., Siemers, F., and Mailander, P. (2009) Hibernoma-case report and literature review. *Am J Dermatopathol* **31**(7): 685–6.

Furlong, M.A., Fanburg-Smith, J.C., and Miettinen, M. (2001) The morphologic spectrum of hibernoma: a clinicopathologic study of 170 cases. *Am J Surg Pathol* **25**(6): 809–14.

Novy, F.G. Jr and Wilson, J.W. (1956) Hibernomas, brown fat tumors. *AMA Arch Derm* **73**(2): 149–57.

Malignant Neoplasms
Cutaneous Liposarcoma

In the skin, the most common liposarcoma is atypical lipomatous tumor (ALT). This is a well-differentiated liposarcoma and shows identical histopathological features to well-differentiated liposarcoma of the retroperitoneum, albeit with a completely different biological course: ALT of the skin does recur, but is benign. However, there are genuine liposarcomas of the subcutis, including pleomorphic and chondroid variants.

Cutaneous Liposarcoma

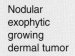

Nodular exophytic growing dermal tumor

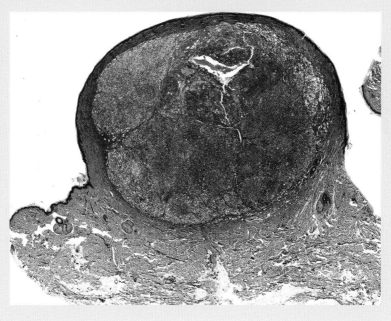

MALIGNANT NEOPLASMS

Cutaneous Liposarcoma

Multivacuolated
lipoblasts

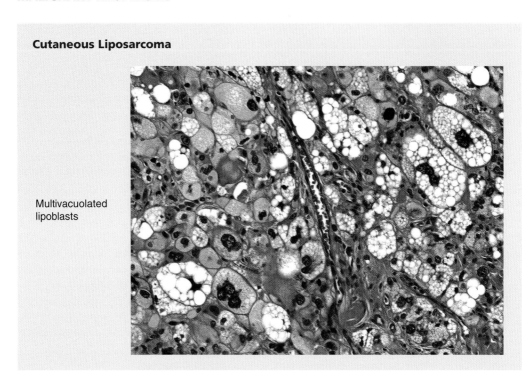

Cl: Deep subcutaneous tumor, morphology mostly similar to large banal lipoma.

Variants of Liposarcoma

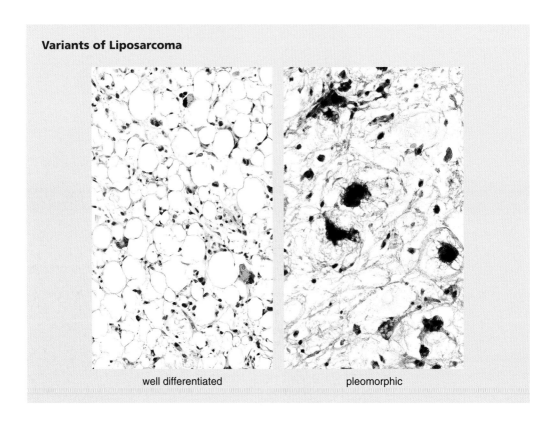

well differentiated   pleomorphic

MALIGNANT NEOPLASMS

Variants of Liposarcoma

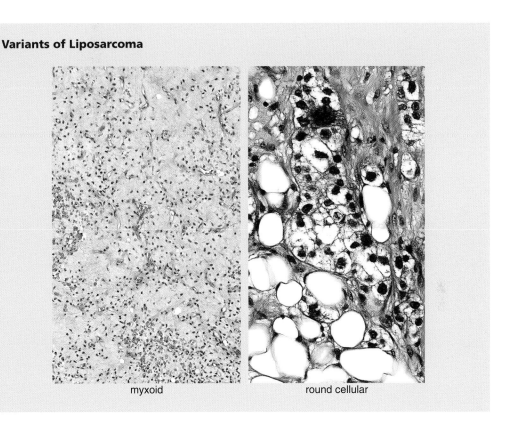

myxoid   round cellular

Hi: Under low power, these tumors appear as mature adipose tissue or as "normal" lipomas, albeit with interspersed lipoblasts ("busy fat"). Lipoblasts are the hallmark cell type, containing cytoplasmatic vacuoles with lipid, which cause wedge-shaped morphology of the nucleus. The nuclear polymorphism is variable, from low (ALT) to strikingly atypical (pleomorphic liposarcoma). High-grade liposarcomas show unequivocal signs of malignancy (mitotic activity, polymorphism, infiltrative growth). Various cytological subtypes can be differentiated.

• Well differentiated (ALT)
• Pleomorphic
• Myxoid
• Round cellular
• Chondroid
• Spindle cellular
• Mixed

Cytogenetic hallmarks of ALT and conventional liposarcoma are amplifications (FISH) of the *MDM2* and the *CDK4* genes that correlate with hyperexpression of their proteins. There is co-expression of p16. Remarkably, pleomorphic liposarcoma does not show amplifications of *MDM2* and *CDK4*.

DD: Lipoma; other sarcomas; angiomyxoma.

References

Al-Zaid, T., Frieling, G., and Rosenthal, S. (2013) Dermal pleomorphic liposarcoma resembling pleomorphic fibroma: report of a case and review of the literature. *J Cutan Pathol* **40**(8): 734–9.

Buehler, D., Marburger, T.B., and Billings, S.D. (2014) Primary subcutaneous myxoid liposarcoma: a clinicopathologic review of three cases with molecular confirmation and discussion of the differential diagnosis. *J Cutan Pathol* **41**(12): 907–15.

Dei Tos, A.P., Mentzel, T., and Fletcher, C.D. (1998) Primary liposarcoma of the skin: a rare neoplasm with unusual high grade features. *Am J Dermatopathol* **20**(4): 332–8.

Gonzalez, R.S., McClain, C.M., Chamberlain, B.K., Coffin, C.M., and Cates, J.M. (2013) Cyclin-dependent kinase inhibitor 2A (p16) distinguishes well-differentiated liposarcoma from lipoma. *Histopathology* **62**(7). 1109–11.

MALIGNANT NEOPLASMS

Liau, J.Y., Lee, J.C., Wu, C.T., Kuo, K.T., Huang, H.Y., and Liang, C.W. (2013) Dedifferentiated liposarcoma with homologous lipoblastic differentiation: expanding the spectrum to include low-grade tumours. *Histopathology* **62**(5): 702–10.

Martelosso, A., Bitencourt, P., Lima, R.B., et al. (2017) Giant primary pleomorphic dermal liposarcoma. *J Cutan Pathol* **44**(8): 724–5.

Mentzel, T. and Fletcher, C.D. (1997) Dedifferentiated myxoid liposarcoma: a clinicopathological study suggesting a closer relationship between myxoid and well-differentiated liposarcoma. *Histopathology* **30**(5): 457–63.

Paredes, B.E. and Mentzel, T. (2011) Atypical lipomatous tumor/"well-differentiated liposarcoma" of the skin clinically presenting as a skin tag: clinicopathologic, immunohistochemical, and molecular analysis of 2 cases. *Am J Dermatopathol* **33**(6): 603–7.

Ramirez-Bellver, J.L., Lopez, J., Macias, E., et al. (2017) Primary dermal pleomorphic liposarcoma: utility of adipophilin and MDM2/CDK4 immunostainings. *J Cutan Pathol* **44**(3): 283–8.

Suster, S. and Morrison, C. (2008) Sclerosing poorly differentiated liposarcoma: clinicopathological, immunohistochemical and molecular analysis of a distinct morphological subtype of lipomatous tumour of soft tissue. *Histopathology* **52**(3): 283–93.

Val-Bernal, J.F., Gonzalez-Vela, M.C., and Cuevas, J. (2003) Primary purely intradermal pleomorphic liposarcoma. *J Cutan Pathol* **30**(8): 516–20.

CHAPTER 8
Muscle

Atlas of Dermatopathology: Tumors, Nevi, and Cysts, First Edition. Günter Burg, Heinz Kutzner,
Werner Kempf, Josef Feit, and Bruce R. Smoller.
© 2019 John Wiley & Sons Ltd. Published 2019 by John Wiley & Sons Ltd.

BENIGN NEOPLASMS

Benign Neoplasms

Leiomyomas are benign tumors arising from structures containing smooth muscles (arrector pili, tunica dartos of the scrotum, labia major, nipple, and blood vessels). The most common variant is pilar leiomyoma.

Piloleiomyoma (Pilar Leiomyoma)

Solitary (left) and multiple agminated leiomyomas (right)

Fascicles of spindle-shaped smooth muscle cells. Longitudinal (left) and cross (right) section

BENIGN NEOPLASMS

Piloleiomyoma

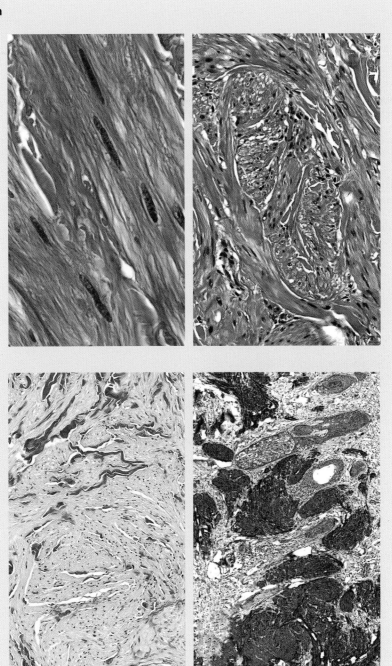

Fascicles of smooth muscle cells with typical cigar-shaped nuclei in longitudinal (left) and cross section (right)

van Gieson (left; yellow) and smooth muscle actin (ASMA) (right)

Fumarate hydratase deficiency (sporadic mutation or germline mutation) is a hallmark of a familial cancer syndrome. Atypical leiomyomas are considered to be borderline tumors or variants of low-grade cutaneous leiomyosarcoma, depending on grade and size of the tumor.

Cl: Solitary or multiple (zosteriform pattern), skin-colored or pink tender nodules.

Hi:
- Poorly circumscribed dermal tumor composed of fascicles of spindled smooth muscle cells
- Cells have blunt-ended cigar-shaped nuclei

BENIGN NEOPLASMS

- Variants may show giant cells, myxoid changes, and atypical nuclei (atypical leiomyoma, ancient leiomyoma)
- Immunohistochemical positivity for desmin. α-SMA often positive
- Diffuse positivity for fumarate hydratase
- Sporadic and syndromic variants are fumarate hydratase negative, reflecting underlying mutation or germline mutation of FH gene, resulting in early onset of uterine leiomyomas and hereditary leiomyomatosis and renal cell cancer syndrome

DD: Angioleiomyoma; myofibroma; neural tumors.

References

Dobashi, Y., Iwabuchi, K., Nakahata, J., Yanagimoto, K., and Kameya, T. (1999) Combined clear and granular cell leiomyoma of soft tissue: evidence of transformation to a histiocytic phenotype. *Histopathology* **34**(6): 526–31.

Idriss, M.H., Kazlouskaya, V., Malhotra, S., Andres, C., and Elston, D.M. (2013) Phosphohistone-H3 and Ki-67 immunostaining in cutaneous pilar leiomyoma and leiomyosarcoma (atypical intradermal smooth muscle neoplasm). *J Cutan Pathol* **40**(6): 557–63.

Lespi, P.J. and Smit, R. (1999) Verocay body-prominent cutaneous leiomyoma. *Am J Dermatopathol* **21**(1): 110–11.

Mesbah Ardakani, N., O'Brien, G., and Wood, B. (2016) Symplastic pilar leiomyoma: description of a rare entity. *Am J Dermatopathol* **38**(10): 787–9.

Raj, S., Calonje, E., Kraus, M., Kavanagh, G., Newman, P.L., and Fletcher, C.D. (1997) Cutaneous pilar leiomyoma: clinicopathologic analysis of 53 lesions in 45 patients. *Am J Dermatopathol* **19**(1): 2–9.

Usmani, N., Merchant, W., and Yung, A. (2008) A case of cutaneous symplastic leiomyoma – a rare variant of cutaneous pilar leiomyoma. *J Cutan Pathol* **35**(3): 329–31.

Angioleiomyoma (see Vessels, Chapter 6)

Rhabdomyoma, Adult Type

Nodules of rhabdoid cells in the dermis (left)

Rhabdoid cells (right top), ASMA positive (right bottom)

Infantile and adult types have to be differentiated. Rhabdomyomas of adult skin are rare benign tumors of striated skeletal muscle. More common are rhabdomyomatous hamartomas of extracutaneous organs (heart) in association with tuberous sclerosis in children.

Cl: In adults, mostly solitary dermal and subcutaneous lesions preferentially affect the head and neck area.

Hi: The histological picture shows foci of skeletal muscle tissue in the dermis. There are age-dependent variations: in the adult type, fascicles

MALIGNANT NEOPLASMS

of mature striated myofibers and polygonal, densely packed cells with abundant granular eosinophilic cytoplasm and eccentric nuclei are seen. The fetal type shows immature spindle-shaped skeletal muscle cells in a myxoid background. Mitotic activities or cellular atypias are lacking in all types.

DD: Rhabdomyosarcoma; granular cell tumor.

References

Bastian, B.C. and Brocker, E.B. (1998) Adult rhabdomyoma of the lip. *Am J Dermatopathol* **20**(1): 61–4.

Mengoli, M.C., Jukna, A., and Cesinaro, A.M. (2016) Rhabdomyoma of the lip: a case report with review of the literature. *Am J Dermatopathol* **38**(2): 154–7.

Sangueza, O., Sangueza, P., Jordan, J., and White, C.R. Jr (1990) Rhabdomyoma of the tongue. *Am J Dermatopathol* **12**(5): 492–5.

Verdolini, R., Goteri, G., Brancorsini, D., et al. (2000) Adult rhabdomyoma: report of two cases of rhabdomyoma of the lip and of the eyelid. *Am J Dermatopathol* **22**(3): 264–7.

Malignant Neoplasms

Rhabdomyosarcoma

Proliferation of atypical skeletal muscle tissue (left), myf4-positive (right)

This malignant neoplasm of childhood rarely arises primarily in the skin. Histologically, various subtypes have been reported, including spindle or epithelioid cell variants. Immunohistochemistry shows reactivity for muscle actin, desmin, and myf4.

References

Feasel, P.C., Marburger, T.B., and Billings, S.D. (2014) Primary cutaneous epithelioid rhabdomyosarcoma: a rare, recently described entity with review of the literature. *J Cutan Pathol* **41**(7): 588–91.

Li, J.J., Forstner, D., and Henderson, C. (2015) Cutaneous pleomorphic rhabdomyosarcoma occurring on sun-damaged skin: a case report. *Am J Dermatopathol* **37**(8): 653–7.

Marburger, T.B., Gardner, J.M., Prieto, V.G., and Billings, S.D. (2012) Primary cutaneous rhabdomyosarcoma: a clinicopathologic review of 11 cases. *J Cutan Pathol* **39**(11): 987–95.

MALIGNANT NEOPLASMS

Superficial Leiomyosarcoma

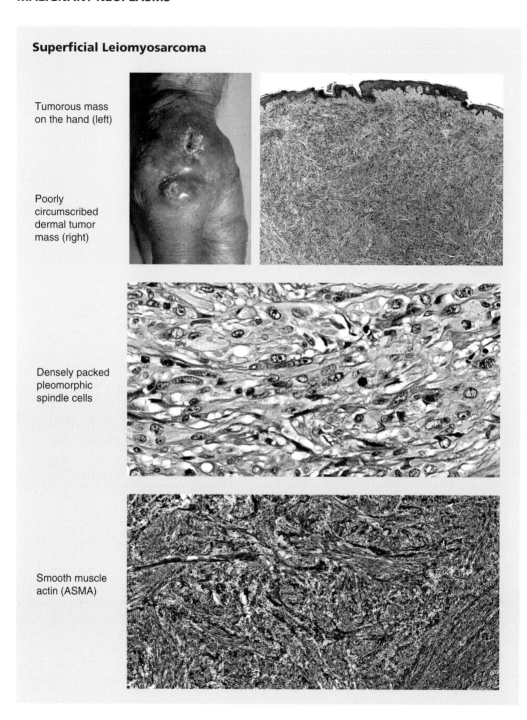

Tumorous mass on the hand (left)

Poorly circumscribed dermal tumor mass (right)

Densely packed pleomorphic spindle cells

Smooth muscle actin (ASMA)

CI: Dermal or subcutaneous pink nodules or tumors preferentially on the extremities of adults, arising from hair or blood vessel muscles. Recent findings suggest that superficial dermal leiomyosarcoma is a low-grade sarcoma showing morphological overlap with atypical leiomyoma. Nosologically, there is a clear-cut difference between low-grade superficial dermal leiomyosarcoma and leiomyosarcoma of soft tissue.

MALIGNANT NEOPLASMS

Hi:

- Poorly circumscribed tumor; tumor silhouette resembling leiomyoma
- Invasive growth pattern
- Fascicles of densely packed spindle cells, with abundant eosinophilic clear cytoplasm
- Pleomorphic, blunt-ended nuclei, sometimes vesicular with prominent nucleoli
- High mitotic activity
- Tumor cells positive for alpha-SMA and desmin. Focal cytokeratin positivity in larger anaplastic tumors
- Cutaneous metastasis of soft tissue leiomyosarcoma may present with identical morphology

Immunohistochemistry: Tumor cells positive for alpha-SMA and desmin. Focal cytokeratin positivity in larger anaplastic tumors.

DD: Dermatofibrosarcoma protuberans; leiomyoma; fibrous histiocytoma; malignant melanoma; granular cell tumor.

References

Alessi, E. and Sala, F. (1992) Leiomyosarcoma in ectopic areola. *Am J Dermatopathol* **14**(2): 165–9.

Berzal-Cantalejo, F., Sabater-Marco, V., Perez-Valles, A., and Martorell-Cebollada, M. (2006) Desmoplastic cutaneous leiomyosarcoma: case report and review of the literature. *J Cutan Pathol* **33**(Suppl 2): 29–31.

Diaz-Cascajo, C., Borghi, S., and Weyers, W. (2000) Desmoplastic leiomyosarcoma of the skin. *Am J Dermatopathol* **22**(3): 251–5.

Fauth, C.T., Bruecks, A.K., Temple, W., Arlette, J.P., and DiFrancesco, L.M. (2010) Superficial leiomyosarcoma: a clinicopathologic review and update. *J Cutan Pathol* **37**(2): 269–76.

Fons, M.E., Bachhuber, T., and Plaza, J.A. (2011) Cutaneous leiomyosarcoma originating in a symplastic pilar leiomyoma: a rare occurrence and potential diagnostic pitfall. *J Cutan Pathol* **38**(1): 49–53.

Idriss, M.H., Kazlouskaya, V., Malhotra, S., Andres, C., and Elston, D.M. (2013) Phosphohistone-H3 and Ki-67 immunostaining in cutaneous pilar leiomyoma and leiomyosarcoma (atypical intradermal smooth muscle neoplasm). *J Cutan, Pathol* **40**(6): 557–63.

Karroum, J.E., Zappi, E.G., and Cockerell, C.J. (1995) Sclerotic primary cutaneous leiomyosarcoma. *Am J Dermatopathol* **17**(3): 292–6.

Kempson, R.L., Fletcher, C.D.M., Evans, H.L., et al. (2001) Tumors of the Soft Tissues: Atlas of Tumor Pathology. Bethesda: AFIP.

Massi, D., Franchi, A., Alos, L., et al. (2010) Primary cutaneous leiomyosarcoma: clinicopathological analysis of 36 cases. *Histopathology* **56**(2): 251–62.

Montgomery, E., Goldblum, J.R., and Fisher, C. (2002) Leiomyosarcoma of the head and neck: a clinicopathological study. *Histopathology* **40**(6): 518–25.

CHAPTER 9

Nerves

Atlas of Dermatopathology: Tumors, Nevi, and Cysts, First Edition. Günter Burg, Heinz Kutzner,
Werner Kempf, Josef Feit, and Bruce R. Smoller.
© 2019 John Wiley & Sons Ltd. Published 2019 by John Wiley & Sons Ltd.

Benign Neoplasms

Neurofibroma and schwannoma are the most common neoplasms of the nerve sheath. They are composed of several components, mostly Schwann cells and endoneurial and perineurial fibroblasts. Axons may be present, albeit in rather low quantities.

Neurofibroma and Recklinghausen's Disease (Phakomatosis)

Kypho-scoliosis (left). Large neurofibroma of the planta (right)

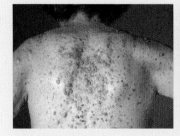
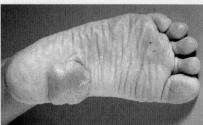

Multiple neurofibromas in Recklinghausen's disease

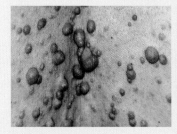
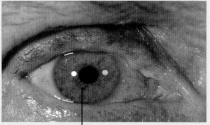

Brown Lisch nodules (iris hamartomas)

Dermal tumor, sparing the papillary dermis and showing capsule-like condensation of perineural tissue at the outer margin

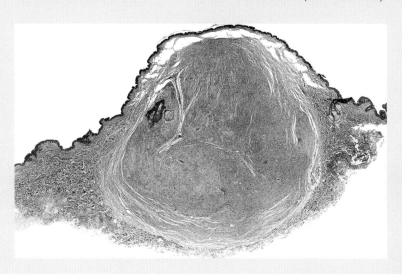

Neurofibroma and Recklinghausen's Disease (Phakomatosis)

Distinct wavy
nuclei of
Schwann cells
and interspersed
fibroblasts
in obliquely (left)
and longitudinally
(right) cut
fascicles

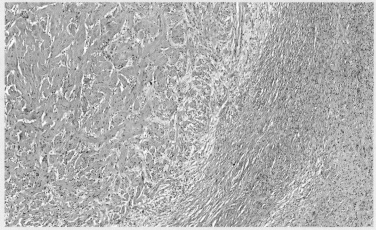

S100 + Schwann
cells in
neurofibroma
(left)

Alcian blue
staining of
myxoid stroma
(right)

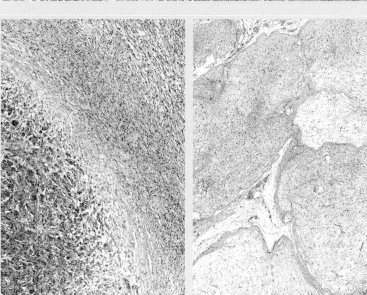

Plexiform Neurofibroma

Large dermal
tumor mass
(inset),
composed of
fascicles and
bundles of
spindle-shaped
nerve cells

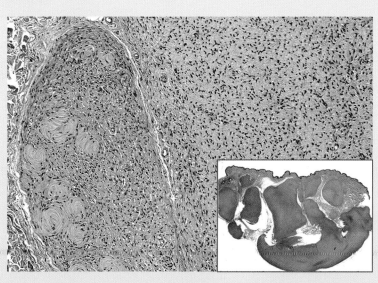

Plexiform Neurofibroma

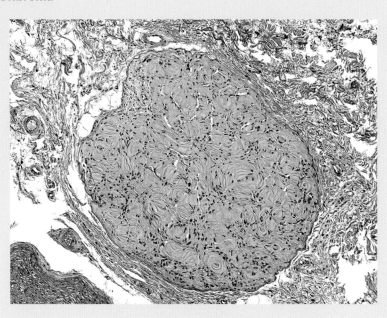

Whorly plexiform growth pattern of spindle cells and fibrous stroma reaction

Neurofibromas are proliferations of Schwann cells, endoneurial and perineurial cells, few axons, and mast cells. Sporadic forms have to be differentiated from neurofibromas associated with Reckling-hausen's phacomatosis (NF 1 and NF 2), which is an inherited autosomal dominant disorder. NF 1 presents with skin, neurological, and orthopedic symptoms. The diagnosis can be made if two or more of the following diagnostic criteria are present.

- Six or more café-au-lait spots
- 1–2 neurofibromas or 1 plexiform neurofibroma
- Axillary or inguinal freckles
- Optic nerve glioma
- Lisch nodules (iris hamartomas)
- Bone deformity and kyphoscoliosis

Cl: Multiple, molluscoid, polypoid, sometimes pedunculated, soft, pink or skin-colored tumors, preferentially on the trunk. Some tumors can be pushed into the skin (herniation from the subcutis). Large plexiform neurofibromas may affect large body areas or involve an entire extremity.

Hi:

- Circumscribed dermal tumor, surrounded by perineurial outer fibrous sheath simulating encapsulation
- Fusiform spindle cells (Schwann cells) with distinct cytoplasmic membrane and wavy nuclei with tapered ends

- Eosinophilic pale, myxoid or fibrotic stroma
- No Verocay bodies
- No mitoses
- Stroma rich in mast cells
- Fine, scattered nerve fibers may be present
- Variants of neurofibroma include plexiform, diffuse, myxoid, sclerotic, granular cellular, epithelioid and "ancient" forms with bizarre giant cells

Immunohistochemistry: Diffuse positivity for S100 (Schwann cells) and CD34 (stroma and perineurial fibroblasts). Few neurofilament positive axons.

DD: Large skin tag (acrochordon); dermatofibroma; schwannoma; smooth muscle neoplasms; melanocytic nevus; hypertrophic scar.

References

Gomez-Mateo M.C., Compan-Quilis, A., and Monteagudo, C. (2015) Microcystic pseudoglandular plexiform cutaneous neurofibroma. *J Cutan Pathol* **42**(11): 884–8.

Gonzalez-Vela, M.C., Val-Bernal, J.F., Gonzalez-Lopez, M.A., Drake, M., and Fernandez-Llaca, J.H. (2006) Pure sclerotic neurofibroma: a neurofibroma mimicking sclerotic fibroma. *J Cutan Pathol* **33**(1): 47–50.

Husain, S. and Silvers, D.N. (2013) Fingerprint CD34 immunopositivity to distinguish neurofibroma from an early/paucicellular desmoplastic melanoma can be misleading. *J Cutan Pathol* **10**(11): 905–7.

Jokinen, C.H. and Argenyi, Z.B. (2010) Atypical neurofibroma of the skin and subcutaneous tissue: clinicopathologic analysis of 11 cases. *J Cutan Pathol* **37**(1): 35–42.

Megahed, M. (1994) Histopathological variants of neurofibroma. A study of 114 lesions. *Am J Dermatopathol* **16**(5): 486–95.

Nakashima, K., Yamada, N., Yoshida, Y., and Yamamoto, O. (2008) Solitary sclerotic neurofibroma of the skin. *Am J Dermatopathol* **30**(3): 278–80.

Puri, P.K., Tyler, W.B., and Ferringer, T.C. (2009) Neurofibroma with clear cell change. *Am J Dermatopathol* **31**(5): 453–6.

Satter, E. (2009) Floret-like multinucleated giant cells in a neurofibroma outside the context of neurofibromatosis type 1. *Am J Dermatopathol* **31**(7): 724–5.

Shek, T.W. (2000) Sclerosing neurofibroma. *Histopathology* **36**(4): 377–8.

Swick, B.L. (2008) Floret-like multinucleated giant cells in a neurofibromatosis type 1-associated neurofibroma. *Am J Dermatopathol* **30**(6): 632–4.

Val-Bernal, J.F. and Gonzalez-Vela, M.C. (2005) Cutaneous lipomatous neurofibroma: characterization and frequency. *J Cutan Pathol* **32**(4): 274–9.

Yeh, I. and McCalmont, T.H. (2011) Distinguishing neurofibroma from desmoplastic melanoma: the value of the CD34 fingerprint. *J Cutan Pathol* **38**(8): 625–30.

Schwannoma (Neurilemmoma)

Well circumscribed nodular proliferations of Schwann cells

Palisading nuclei (Verocay bodies)

S100 (right)

"Ancient" Schwannoma

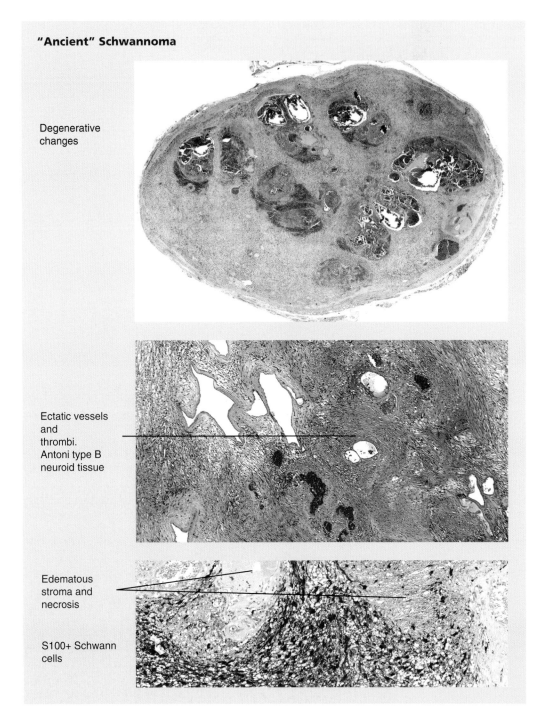

Degenerative changes

Ectatic vessels and thrombi. Antoni type B neuroid tissue

Edematous stroma and necrosis

S100+ Schwann cells

Schwannomas represent neural Schwann cell proliferations with embedded axons and perineurial fibroblasts. They are genuine nerve sheath tumors showing morphological overlap with genuine neuromas.

Cl: Mostly well-demarcated solitary tumors in adults, located in the deep dermis or subcutaneous tissue of the head and neck area or the extremities. Close attachment to peripheral nerves may be responsible for tenderness.

Hi:

- Well-demarcated nodular proliferation of S100-positive Schwann cells in the dermis or subcutaneous tissue
- CD34-positive perineurial outer sheath
- Adjacent nerves may be present
- Schwann cells show elongated nuclei with roundish poles and fine chromatin
- Tumor with a dual morphological pattern:
  - *Antoni A areas*. loosely textured fascicles with palisading nuclei aligned in parallel arrays and bordered on both sides by amphophilic masses (Verocay bodies)
  - *Antoni B areas*: fewer cellular areas, myxoid, edematous, without conspicuous aligning of nuclei
- Besides common schwannoma, there are several histological subtypes, including cellular, myxoid, plexiform psammomatous (associated with Carney's complex) and "ancient" schwannoma. The latter is composed of Antoni type B tissue and shows cellular atypia, degenerative changes, ectatic vessels with thrombi, stromal edema, and inflammatory infiltrate with many macrophages
- Vessels with thickened vessel walls and fibrosis may be present
- Neurofilament-positive axons in low numbers

DD: Encapsulated, palisaded neuroma; amputation neuroma; neurofibroma; dermatofibroma; angioleiomyoma.

References

Argenyi, Z.B., Balogh, K., and Abraham, A.A. (1993) Degenerative ("ancient") changes in benign cutaneous schwannoma. A light microscopic, histochemical and immunohistochemical study. *J Cutan Pathol* **20**(2): 148–53.

Deng, A., Petrali, J., Jaffe, D., Sina, B., and Gaspari, A. (2005) Benign cutaneous pseudoglandular schwannoma: a case report. *Am J Dermatopathol* **27**(5): 432–5.

Diaz-Cascajo, C. (2002).Epithelioid malignant schwannoma of the superficial soft tissues versus metastatic amelanotic melanoma. *J Cutan Pathol* **29**(6): 382–3.

Feany, M.B., Anthony, D.C., and Fletcher, C.D. (1998) Nerve sheath tumours with hybrid features of neurofibroma and schwannoma: a conceptual challenge. *Histopathology* **32**(5): 405–10.

Fisher, C., Chappell, M.E., and Weiss, S.W. (1995) Neuroblastoma-like epithelioid schwannoma. *Histopathology* **26**(2): 193–4.

Gao, Z., Palleschi, S.M., and Chen, S. (2007) Plexiform epithelioid schwannoma: a case report. *Am J Dermatopathol* **29**(1): 56–8.

Holliday, A.C., Mazloom, S.E., Coman, G.C., et al. (2017) Benign glandular schwannoma with ancient change. *Am J Dermatopathol* **39**(4): 300–3.

Lisle, A., Jokinen, C., and Argenyi, Z. (2011) Cutaneous pseudoglandular schwannoma: a case report of an unusual histopathologic variant. *Am J Dermatopathol* **33**(5): e63–5.

Luzar, B., Tanaka, M., Schneider, J., and Calonje, E. (2016) Cutaneous microcystic/reticular schwannoma: a poorly recognized entity. *J Cutan Pathol* **43**(2): 93–100.

Megahed, M. (1994) Plexiform schwannoma. *Am J Dermatopathol* **16**(3): 288–93.

Megahed, M. and Ruzicka, T. (1994) Cellular schwannoma. *Am J Dermatopathol* **16**(4): 418–21.

Nayler, S.J., Leiman, G., Omar, T., and Cooper, K. (1996) Malignant transformation in a schwannoma. *Histopathology* **29**(2): 189–92.

Orosz, Z. (1999) Cutaneous epithelioid schwannoma: an unusual benign neurogenic tumor. *J Cutan Pathol* **26**(4): 213–14.

Saad, A.G., Mutema, G.K., and Mutasim, D.F. (2005) Benign cutaneous epithelioid Schwannoma: case report and review of the literature. *Am J Dermatopathol* **27**(1): 45–7.

Shek, T.W. (2000) Sclerosing neurofibroma. *Histopathology* **36**(4): 377–8.

Sundarkrishnan, L., Bradish, J.R., Oliai, B.R., and Hosler, G.A. (2016) Cutaneous cellular pseudoglandular schwannoma: an unusual histopathologic variant. *Am J Dermatopathol* **38**(4): 315–18.

Yeh, I., Argenyi, Z., Vemula, S.S., Furmanczyk, P.S., Bouffard, D., and McCalmont, T.H. (2012) Plexiform melanocytic schwannoma: a mimic of melanoma. *J Cutan Pathol* **39**(5): 521–5.

Zamecnik, M. (2000) Hybrid neurofibroma/schwannoma versus schwannoma with Antoni B areas. *Histopathology* **36**(5): 473–4.

Zelger, B.G., Steiner, H., Kutzner, H., Rutten, A., and Zelger, B. (1997) Verocay body-prominent cutaneous schwannoma. *Am J Dermatopathol* **19**(3): 242–9.

Solitary Neuroma ("Palisaded Encapsulated Neuroma")

Non-capsulated
dermal nodule
with distinct
clefts

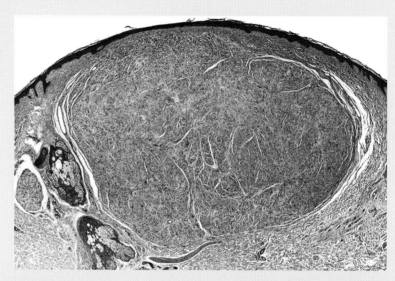

Interweaving
Schwann cell
fascicles
showing axons
and clefts

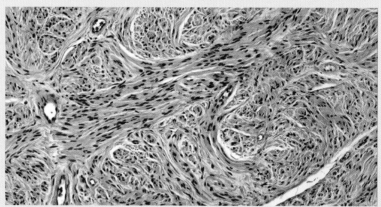

Neurofilament-
positive axons

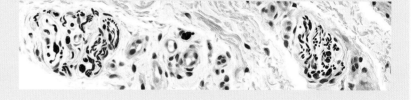

Cl: Small protuberant nodules with the clinical aspect of a papillomatous nevus. Predilection sites are the head and neck area. The tumor is a genuine dermal neuroma.

Hi:

- Sharp circumscription, but no encapsulation
- Densely packed interweaving nerve fascicles
- Prominent shrinkage clefts between nerve fascicles
- Neurofilament-positive axons throughout the tumor

References

Argenyi, Z.B. (1990) Immunohistochemical characterization of palisaded, encapsulated neuroma. *J Cutan Pathol* **17**(6): 329–35.

Argenyi, Z.B. and Penick, G.D. (1993) Vascular variant of palisaded encapsulated neuroma. *J Cutan Pathol* **20**(1): 92–3.

Argenyi, Z.B., Cooper, P.H., and Santa Cruz, D. (1993) Plexiform and other unusual variants of palisaded encapsulated neuroma. *J Cutan Pathol* **20**(1): 34–9.

Dakin, M.C., Leppard, B., and Theaker, J.M. (1992) The palisaded, encapsulated neuroma (solitary circumscribed neuroma). *Histopathology* **20**(5): 405–10.

Eckert, F. and Kutzner, H. (1995) Palisaded encapsulated neuroma (solitary circumscribed neuroma). *Am J Dermatopathol* **17**(3): 316.

Jokinen, C.H., Ragsdale, B.D., and Argenyi, Z.B. (2010) Expanding the clinicopathologic spectrum of palisaded encapsulated neuroma. *J Cutan Pathol* **37**(1): 43–8.

Kossard, S., Kumar, A., and Wilkinson, B. (1999) Neural spectrum: palisaded encapsulated neuroma and verocay body poor dermal schwannoma. *J Cutan Pathol* **26**(1): 31–6.

Megahed, M. (1994) Palisaded encapsulated neuroma (solitary circumscribed neuroma). A clinicopathologic and immunohistochemical study. *Am J Dermatopathol* **16**(2): 120–5.

Misago, N., Inoue, T., and Narisawa, Y. (2007) Unusual benign myxoid nerve sheath lesion: myxoid palisaded encapsulated neuroma (PEN) or nerve sheath myxoma with PEN/PEN-like features? *Am J Dermatopathol* **29**(2): 160–4.

Variant: Traumatic Neuroma

Cl: Traumatic neuromas are painful skin-colored, broad-based firm nodules following injury. They represent an incomplete repair process following nerve destruction and are related to rudimentary supernumerary digit, which develops at the lateral aspect of the hand.

Hi:

- Poorly circumscribed dermal tumor
- Confluent nerve fascicles with neurofilament-positive axons
- Fibrous stroma next to adjacent scar
- No Verocay bodies

DD: Supernumerary digit; schwannoma; neurofibroma; angioleiomyoma.

References

Ahn, S.K., Choi, E.H., Won, J.H., and Lee, SH. (1995). Idiopathic solitary neuroma of skin with unusual histologic changes. *J Cutan Pathol* **22**(6): 570–3.

Fung, M.A. (2012) Epithelial sheath neuroma: neoplasia or hyperplasia? *J Cutan Pathol* **39**(11): 1052–4.

Hirano-Ali, S.A., Bryant, E.A., and Warren, S.J. (2016) Epithelial sheath neuroma: evidence supporting a hyperplastic etiology and epidermal origin. *J Cutan Pathol* **43**(6): 531–4.

Jokinen, C.H., Ragsdale, B.D., and Argenyi, Z.B. (2010) Expanding the clinicopathologic spectrum of palisaded encapsulated neuroma. *J Cutan Pathol* **37**(1): 43–8.

Kossard, S., Kumar, A., and Wilkinson, B. (1999) Neural spectrum: palisaded encapsulated neuroma and verocay body poor dermal schwannoma. *J Cutan Pathol* **26**(1): 31–6.

Megahed, M. (1994) Palisaded encapsulated neuroma (solitary circumscribed neuroma). A clinicopathologic and immunohistochemical study. *Am J Dermatopathol* **16**(2): 120–5.

Requena, L. (2016) Epithelial sheath neuroma: hyperplasia or neoplasia? *J Cutan Pathol* **43**(11): 1088.

Tashiro, A., Imafuku, S., and Furue, M. (2008) Traumatic neuroma of the lower lip with intraepithelial nerve fibers. *J Cutan Pathol* **35**(3): 320–3.

Wang, J.Y., Nuovo, G., Kline, M., and Magro, C.M. (2017) Reexcision perineural invasion and epithelial sheath neuroma possibly on a spectrum of postinjury reactive hyperplasia mediated by IL-6. *Am J Dermatopathol* **39**(1): 49–52.

Granular Cell Tumor (Abrikossoff)

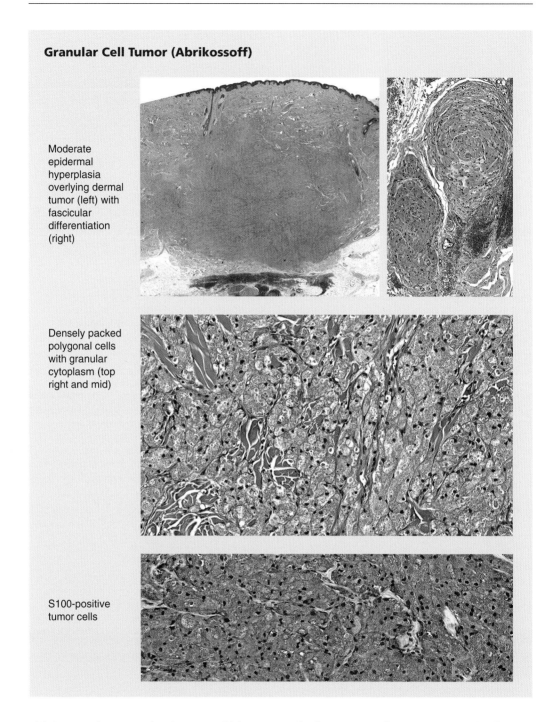

Moderate epidermal hyperplasia overlying dermal tumor (left) with fascicular differentiation (right)

Densely packed polygonal cells with granular cytoplasm (top right and mid)

S100-positive tumor cells

This is a genuine nerve sheath tumor which was originally considered to be derived from striated muscle cells ("granular cell myoblastoma"). Tumor cells show schwannian features with an abundance of lysosomes within the cytoplasm.

Cl: The tongue is the most common localisation for mostly solitary and sometimes multiple tumors, which also can appear on the skin and in extracutaneous organs. Malignant variants are rare.

Hi:
- Pseudocarcinomatous hyperplasia, sometimes with verrucous features
- Compact dermal tumor, extending into the subcutis
- Large, densely packed polygonal tumor cells with eosinophilic granular cytoplasm
- Uniformed small, round, centrally located nuclei
- No mitotic activity
- Cytoplasmic granules stain positive for PAS
- Schwannian tumor cells are positive for S100 protein; cross-reaction with CD68 may be misleading

DD: Malignant granular cell tumor; xanthoma; squamous cell carcinoma; basal cell carcinoma; leiomyoma; renal cell carcinoma; granular cell variants of other tumors.

References

Aldabagh, B., Azmi, F., Vadmal, M., Neider, S., and Usmani, A.S. (2009) Plexiform pattern in cutaneous granular cell tumors. *J Cutan Pathol* **36**(11): 1174–6.

Banerjee, S.S., Harris, M., Eyden, B.P., and Hamid, B.N. (1990) Granular cell variant of dermatofibrosarcoma protuberans. *Histopathology* **17**(4): 375–8.

Beer, T.W. (2010) Keloidal and granular cell change in a series of 171 atypical fibroxanthomas. *J Cutan Pathol* **37**(6): 712–13.

Caltabiano, R., Magro, G., Vecchio, G.M., and Lanzafame, S. (2010) Solitary cutaneous histiocytosis with granular cell changes: a morphological variant of reticulohistiocytoma? *J Cutan Pathol* **37**(2): 287–91.

Chaudhry, I.H. and Calonje, E. (2005) Dermal non-neural granular cell tumour (so-called primitive polypoid granular cell tumour): a distinctive entity further delineated in a clinicopathological study of 11 cases. *Histopathology* **47**(2): 179–85.

Claassen, S.L., Royer, M.C., and Rush, W.L. (2014) Granular cell basal cell carcinoma: report of a case and review of the literature. *Am J Dermatopathol* **36**(7): e121–4.

Fernandez-Flores, A., Cassarino, D.S., Riveiro-Falkenbach, E., Rodriguez-Peralto, J.L., Fernandez-Figueras, M.T., and Monteagudo, C. (2017) Cutaneous dermal non-neural granular cell tumor is a granular cell dermal root sheath fibroma. *J Cutan Pathol* **44**(6): 582–7.

Gokaslan, S.T., Terzakis, J.A., and Santagada, E.A. (1994).Malignant granular cell tumor. *J Cutan Pathol* **21**(3): 263–70.

Heerema, M.G. and Suurmeijer, A.J. (2012) Sox10 immunohistochemistry allows the pathologist to differentiate between prototypical granular cell tumors and other granular cell lesions. *Histopathology* **61**(5): 997–9.

Hitchcock, M.G., Hurt, M.A., and Santa Cruz, D.J. (1994) Cutaneous granular cell angiosarcoma. *J Cutan Pathol* **21**(3): 256–62.

Jarell, A. and McCalmont, T.H. (2012) Granular cell angiosarcoma. *J Cutan Pathol* **39**(5): 475–8.

Lee, J. (2007) Epithelioid cell histiocytoma with granular cells (another nonneural granular cell neoplasm). *Am J Dermatopathol* **29**(5): 475–6.

Mentzel, T., Wadden, C., and Fletcher, C.D. (1994) Granular cell change in smooth muscle tumours of skin and soft tissue. *Histopathology* **24**(3): 223–31.

Perez-Gonzalez, Y.C., Pagura, L., Llamas-Velasco, M., Cortes-Lambea, L., Kutzner, H., and Requena, L. (2015) Primary cutaneous malignant granular cell tumor: an immunohistochemical study and review of the literature. *Am J Dermatopathol* **37**(4): 334–40.

Rabkin, M.S. and Vukmer, T. (2012) Granular cell variant of epithelioid cell histiocytoma. *Am J Dermatopathol* **34**(7): 766–9.

Rios-Martin, J.J., Delgado, M.D., Moreno-Ramirez, D., Garcia-Escudero, A., and Gonzalez-Campora, R. (2007) Granular cell atypical fibroxanthoma: report of two cases. *Am J Dermatopathol* **29**(1): 84–7.

Rudisaile, S.N., Hurt, M.A., and Santa Cruz, D.J. (2005) Granular cell atypical fibroxanthoma. *J Cutan Pathol* **32**(4): 314–17.

Wright, N.A., Thomas, C.G., Calame, A., and Cockerell, C.J. (2010) Granular cell atypical fibroxanthoma: case report and review of the literature. *J Cutan Pathol* **37**(3): 380–5.

Yang, X.J., Takahashi, M., Schafernak, K.T., et al. (2007) Does 'granular cell' renal cell carcinoma exist? Molecular and histological reclassification. *Histopathology* **50**(5): 678–80.

Zedek, D.C., Murphy, B.A., Shea, C.R., Hitchcock, M.G., Reutter, J.C., and White, W.L. (2007) Cutaneous clear-cell granular cell tumors: the histologic description of an unusual variant. *J Cutan Pathol* **34**(5): 397–404.

Zelger, B.G., Steiner, H., Kutzner, H., Rutten, A., and Zelger, B. (1997) Granular cell dermatofibroma. *Histopathology* **31**(3): 258–62.

Dermal Nerve Sheath Myxoma (Myxoid Neurothekeoma)

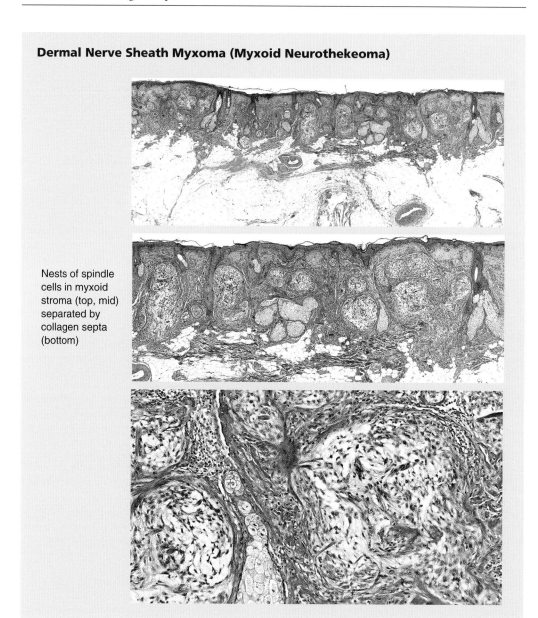

Nests of spindle cells in myxoid stroma (top, mid) separated by collagen septa (bottom)

The term *neurothekeoma* comprises a spectrum of histogenetically different benign neoplasms, ranging from hypocellular myxoid ("classic" neurothekeoma) to hypercellular lesions with immature cells in a collagenous stroma (cellular neurothekeoma). Recent findings suggest that myoid neurothekeoma and cellular neurothekeoma show no histogenetic relationship. The latter most likely is a variant of histiocytoma/dermatofibroma (with conspicuous immunohistochemical co-expression of NKIC3 and alpha-SMA).

Cl: Small, asymptomatic dome-shaped, firm, pink or red-brown papules and nodules, mostly on the head, neck or upper extremities of young women.

Hi:

- Multilobulated myxoid tumor in the dermis
- S100-positive stellate and spindled cells with hyperchromatic nuclei within a myxoid stroma
- Collagenous septa separating myxoid nests

References

Argenyi, Z.B., Kutzner, H., and Seaba, M.M. (1995) Ultrastructural spectrum of cutaneous nerve sheath myxoma/cellular neurothekeoma. *J Cutan Pathol* **22**(2): 137–45.

Barnhill, R.L. (1994) Nerve sheath myxoma (neurothekeoma). *J Cutan Pathol* **21**(1): 91–3.

Misago, N., Inoue, T., and Narisawa, Y. (2007) Unusual benign myxoid nerve sheath lesion: myxoid palisaded encapsulated neuroma (PEN) or nerve sheath myxoma with PEN/PEN-like features? *Am J Dermatopathol* **29**(2): 160–4.

Rudolph, P. and Schubert, C. (2002) Myxoid cellular neurothekeoma. *Am J Dermatopathol* **24**(1): 92–3.

Strumia, R., Lombardi, A.R., and Cavazzini, L. (2001) S-100 negative myxoid neurothekeoma. *Am J Dermatopathol* **23**(1): 82–3.

Variant: Cellular Neurothekeoma

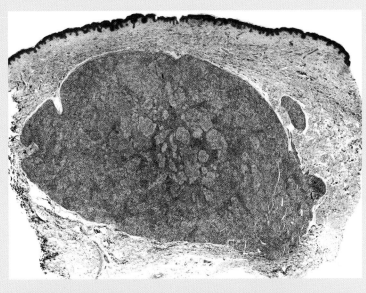

Nodular dermal tumor

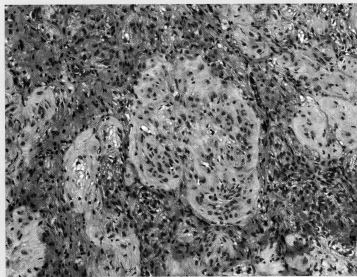

Nests of histiocytoid cells with slight epithelioid morphology in an eosinophilic stroma

Cellular neurothekeoma, which histologically imitates dermal Spitz nevus, is an important differential diagnosis.

Hi:

- Cellular nests of histiocytoid cells, imitating dermal Spitz nevus
- Collagenous septa
- Low mitotic activity

Immunohistochemical positivity for NKIC3, alpha-SMA, and CD68.

References

Argenyi, Z.B., LeBoit, P.E., Santa Cruz, D., Swanson, P.E., and Kutzner, H. (1993) Nerve sheath myxoma (neurothekeoma) of the skin: light microscopic and immunohistochemical reappraisal of the cellular variant. *J Cutan Pathol* **20**(4): 294–303.

Fox, M.D., Billings, S.D., Gleason, B.C., et al. (2012) Expression of MiTF may be helpful in differentiating cellular neurothekeoma from plexiform fibrohistiocytic tumor (histiocytoid predominant) in a partial biopsy specimen. *Am J Dermatopathol* **34**(2): 157–60.

Fried, I., Sitthinamsuwan, P., Muangsomboon, S., Kaddu, S., Cerroni, L., and McCalmont, T.H. (2014) SOX-10 and MiTF expression in cellular and 'mixed' neurothekeoma. *J Cutan Pathol* **41**(8): 640–5.

Lane, J.E., Mullins, S., and Davis, L.S. (2006) Clinical pathologic challenge. Cellular neurothekeoma. *Am J Dermatopathol* **28**(1): 65–6; answer and discussion 67–8.

Misago, N., Satoh, T., and Narisawa, Y. (2004) Cellular neurothekeoma with histiocytic differentiation. *J Cutan Pathol* **31**(8): 568–72.

Plaza, J.A., Torres-Cabala, C., Evans, H., Diwan, A.H., and Prieto, V.G. (2009) Immunohistochemical expression of S100A6 in cellular neurothekeoma: clinicopathologic and immunohistochemical analysis of 31 cases. *Am J Dermatopathol* **31**(5): 419–22.

Rudolph, P. and Schubert, C. (2002) Myxoid cellular neurothekeoma. *Am J Dermatopathol* **24**(1): 92–3.

Thakral, B., Gleason, B.C., Thomas, A.B., Billings, S.D., Victor, T.A., and Cibull, T.L. (2011) Cellular neurothekeoma with fascicular growth features mimicking cellular dermatofibroma. *Am J Dermatopathol* **33**(3): 281–4.

Pacinian Neurofibroma (Pacinoma)

Cl: The clinical setting is identical with genuine neurofibroma.

Hi: Hallmarks are tumor foci that exhibit Pacinian differentiation, imitating the morphological pattern of Pacinian bodies.

References

MacLennan, S.E., Melin-Aldana, H., and Yakuboff, K.P. (1999) Pacinian neurofibroma of the hand: a case report and literature review. *J Hand Surg Am* **24**(2): 413–16.

Nath, A.K., Timshina, D.K., Thappa, D.M., and Basu, D. (2011) Pacinian neurofibroma: a rare neurogenic tumor. *Indian J Dermatol Venereol Leprol* **77**(2): 204–5.

Malignant Neoplasms

Malignant Peripheral Nerve Sheath Tumor (Malignant Schwannoma)

Circumscribed dermal tumor

Malignant Peripheral Nerve Sheath Tumor (Malignant Schwannoma)

Undifferentiated spindle shaped tumor cells in a sparse myxoid stroma

Inset: characteristically unmethylated tumor cells (negative for H3K27me3; polyclonal antibody)

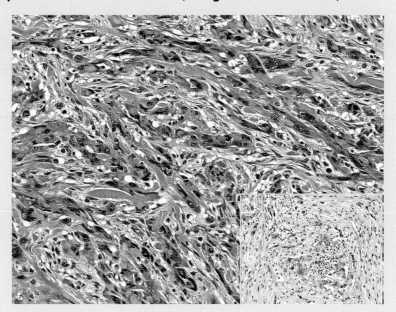

Cl: Large tumor masses involving the dermis and the adjacent upper subcutis.

Hi:

- Spindle-shaped atypical pleomorphic cells
- S100 positive
- Scarce myxoid stroma
- Tumor cells characteristically lack tri-methylation of lysine-residue in histone 3 complex (negative for H3K27me3; polyclonal antibody)

DD: Melanoma; fibrosarcoma.

References

Argenyi, Z.B., LeBoit, P.E., Santa Cruz, D., Swanson, P.E., and Kutzner, H. (1993) Nerve sheath myxoma (neurothekeoma) of the skin: light microscopic and immunohistochemical reappraisal of the cellular variant. *J Cutan Pathol* **20**(4): 294–303.

Barnhill, R.L. (1994) Nerve sheath myxoma (neurothekeoma). *J Cutan Pathol* **21**(1): 91–3.

Campanati, A., Brandozzi, G., Sisti, S., Bernardini, M.L., and Offidani, A.M. (2007) Atypical neurothekeoma: a new case and review of the literature. *J Cutan Pathol* **34**(5): 435–7.

Diaz-Cascajo, C. (2002). Epithelioid malignant schwannoma of the superficial soft tissues versus metastatic amelanotic melanoma. *J Cutan Pathol* **29**(6): 382–3.

Husain, S., Silvers, D.N., Halperin, A.J., and McNutt, N.S. (1994) Histologic spectrum of neurothekeoma and the value of immunoperoxidase staining for S-100 protein in distinguishing it from melanoma. *Am J Dermatopathol* **16**(5): 496–503.

Kikuchi, A., Akiyama, M., Han-Yaku, H., Shimizu, H., Naka, W., and Nishikawa, T. (1993) Solitary cutaneous malignant schwannoma. Immunohistochemical and ultrastructural studies. *Am J Dermatopathol* **15**(1): 15–19.

Nayler, S.J., Leiman, G., Omar, T., and Cooper, K. (1996) Malignant transformation in a schwannoma. *Histopathology* **29**(2): 189–92.

Shimizu, S., Teraki, Y., Ishiko, A., et al. (1993) Malignant epithelioid schwannoma of the skin showing partial HMB-45 positivity. *Am J Dermatopathol* **15**(4): 378–84.

Yamamoto, T. (2002) Epithelioid malignant schwannoma of the superficial soft tissues vs. metastatic amelanotic melanoma. *J Cutan Pathol* **29**(9): 569.

Yamamoto, T., Minami, R., and Ohbayashi, C. (2001) Subcutaneous malignant epithelioid schwannoma with cartilaginous differentiation. *J Cutan Pathol* **28**(9): 486–91.

Zelger, B.G., Steiner, H., Kutzner, H., Maier, H., and Zelger, B. (1998) Cellular 'neurothekeoma': an epithelioid variant of dermatofibroma? *Histopathology* **32**(5): 414–22.

Malignant Granular Cell Tumor

Cl: In most cases, this tumor variant is diagnosed retrospectively, after multiple metastases have occurred. **Hi**: Remarkably, it is exceedingly difficult to differentiate atypical granular cell tumor unequivocally from its malignant counterpart without the help of ancillary clinical information. Both tumors may show significant morphological overlap. Mitotic activity and pleomorphism may be low in the malignant variant, although mitoses and atypical nuclei as well as tumor size should be taken as signs of caution.

References

Gokaslan, S.T., Terzakis, J.A., and Santagada, E.A. (1994) Malignant granular cell tumor. *J Cutan Pathol* **21**(3): 263–70.

Mahoney, A., Garg, A., Wolpowitz, D., and Mahalingam, M. (2010) Atypical granular cell tumor-apropos of a case with indeterminate malignant potential. *Am J Dermatopathol* **32**(4): 370–3.

Perez-Gonzalez, Y.C., Pagura, L., Llamas-Velasco, M., Cortes-Lambea, L., Kutzner, H., and Requena, L. (2015) Primary cutaneous malignant granular cell tumor: an immunohistochemical study and review of the literature. *Am J Dermatopathol* **37**(4): 334–40.

Neuroendocrine Neoplasm

Primary Neuroendocrine (Merkel Cell, Trabecular) Carcinoma of the Skin

Tumor plaques on cheek and nose

Sheets and clusters of infiltrating cells in the dermis (top right and bottom)

Primary Neuroendocrine (Merkel Cell, Trabecular) Carcinoma of the Skin (Cutaneous APUDoma)

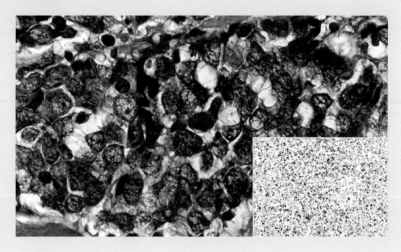

Uniform basophilic cells with granular vesicular nuclei and scant cytoplasm

Inset: CK20 positive tumor cells (paranuclear staining)

APUD (Amine Precursor Uptake and Decarboxylation) cells are endocrine active cells in the epithelia of tissue apart from endocrine organs. Merkel cells are intraepithelial neuroendocrine cells. Most cases of Merkel cell carcinoma have shown integration of Merkel cell polyoma virus (MCPyV) DNA into the tumor genome, suggesting a pathogenetic role. The tumor cells express both features of neuroendocrine and epithelial differentiation. Merkel cell carcinoma has been reported in association with poroma, Bowen, squamous cell carcinoma, basal cell carcinoma, seborrheic and actinic keratosis and other epithelial or adnexal tumors and intraepidermal forms.

Cl: The head and neck of elderly patients are most commonly affected by this rare plaque-like or dome-shaped, rapidly growing, infiltrating and ulcerating tumor, which shows early metastases in regional lymph nodes and visceral organs. Prognosis is bad if not excised early and totally.

Hi:

* Sheets and clusters of infiltrates in occasionally trabecular pattern, in the dermis, extending into the subcutis
* Monomorphous uniform, round basophilic small to medium-sized cells with granular vesicular nuclei and scant cytoplasm
* Numerous mitoses and apoptotic cells
* Occasional focal squamous differentiation
* The Azzopardi phenomenon (basophilic granular nuclear DNA lacing the wall of small vessels), found in small cell carcinoma of the lung, is typically lacking in most cases of cutaneous Merkel cell carcinoma

Immunocytochemistry: Neurofilament, chromogranin, synaptophysin, Cytokeratin 20 (paranuclear dot or membranous staining pattern), BerEP4, neuron-specific enolase. Insulinoma M1 (InsM1) is a new important marker for neuroendokrine differentiation.

Electron microscopy: Neurosecretory granules.

DD: Cutaneous (B-cell) lymphoma, other neuroendocrine carcinomas (lung); sweat gland carcinoma; melanoma.

References

Al-Ahmadie, H.A., Mutasim, D.F., and Mutema, G.K. (2004) A case of intraepidermal Merkel cell carcinoma within squamous cell carcinoma in-situ: Merkel cell carcinoma in-situ? *Am J Dermatopathol* **26**(3): 230–3.

Aljufairi, E. and Alhilli, F. (2017) Merkel cell carcinoma arising in an epidermal cyst. *Am J Dermatopathol* **39**(11): 842–4.

Brown, H.A., Sawyer, D.M., and Woo, T. (2000) Intraepidermal Merkel cell carcinoma with no dermal involvement. *Am J Dermatopathol* **22**(1): 65–9.

Feng, H., Shuda, M., Chang, Y., and Moore, P.S. (2008) Clonal integration of a polyomavirus in human Merkel cell carcinoma. *Science* **319**(5866): 1096–100.

Heath, M., Jaimes, N., Lemos, B., et al. (2008) Clinical characteristics of Merkel cell carcinoma at diagnosis in 195 patients: the AEIOU features. *J Am Acad Dermatol* **58**(3): 375–81.

Hwang, J.H., Alanen, K., Dabbs, K.D., Danyluk, J., and Silverman, S. (2008) Merkel cell carcinoma with squamous and sarcomatous differentiation. *J Cutan Pathol* **35**(10): 955–9.

Jour, G., Aung, P.P., Rozas-Munoz, E., Curry, J.L., Prieto, V., and Ivan, D. (2017) Intraepidermal Merkel cell carcinoma: a case series of a rare entity with clinical follow up. *J Cutan Pathol* **44**(8): 684–91.

Koba, S., Nagase, K., Ikeda, S., Aoki, S., Misago, N., and Narisawa, Y. (2015) Merkel cell carcinoma with glandular differentiation admixed with sweat gland carcinoma and spindle cell carcinoma: histogenesis of merkel cell carcinoma from hair follicle stem cells. *Am J Dermatopathol* **37**(3): e31–6.

Le, M.D., O'Steen, L.H., and Cassarino, D.S. (2017) A rare case of CK20/CK7 double negative merkel cell carcinoma. *Am J Dermatopathol* **39**(3): 208–11.

Llombart, B., Monteagudo, C., Lopez-Guerrero, J.A., et al. (2005) Clinicopathological and immunohistochemical analysis of 20 cases of Merkel cell carcinoma in search of prognostic markers. *Histopathology* **46**(6): 622–34.

McFalls, J., Okon, L., Cannon, S., and Lee, J.B. (2017) Intraepidermal proliferation of Merkel cells within a seborrheic keratosis: Merkel cell carcinoma in situ or Merkel cell hyperplasia? *J Cutan Pathol* **44**(5): 480–5.

Miraflor, A.P., LeBoit, P.E., and Hirschman, S.A. (2016) Intraepidermal Merkel cell carcinoma with pagetoid Bowen's disease. *J Cutan Pathol* **43**(11): 921–6.

Mitteldorf, C., Mertz, K.D., Fernandez-Figueras, M.T., Schmid, M., Tronnier, M., and Kempf, W. (2012) Detection of Merkel cell polyomavirus and human papillomaviruses in Merkel cell carcinoma combined with squamous cell carcinoma in immunocompetent European patients. *Am J Dermatopathol* **34**(5): 506–10.

Papalas, J.A., McKinney, M.S., Kulbacki, E., Dave, S.S., and Wang, E. (2014) Merkel cell carcinoma with partial B-cell blastic immunophenotype: a potential mimic of cutaneous richter transformation in a patient with chronic lymphocytic lymphoma. *Am J Dermatopathol* **36**(2): 148–52.

Sirikanjanapong, S., Melamed, J., and Patel, R.R. (2010) Intraepidermal and dermal Merkel cell carcinoma with squamous cell carcinoma in situ: a case report with review of literature. *J Cutan Pathol* **37**(8): 881–5.

Succaria, F., Radfar, A., and Bhawan, J. (2014) Merkel cell carcinoma (primary neuroendocrine carcinoma of skin) mimicking basal cell carcinoma with review of different histopathologic features. *Am J Dermatopathol* **36**(2): 160–6.

Vazmitel, M., Michal, M., and Kazakov, D.V. (2007) Merkel cell carcinoma and Azzopardi phenomenon. *Am J Dermatopathol* **29**(3): 314–15.

Wick, M.R. and Patterson, J.W. (2007) Reply to Merkel cell carcinoma and Azzopardi phenomenon. *Am J Dermatopathol* **29**(3): 315.

CHAPTER 10

Mast Cells

Atlas of Dermatopathology: Tumors, Nevi, and Cysts, First Edition. Günter Burg, Heinz Kutzner,
Werner Kempf, Josef Feit, and Bruce R. Smoller.
© 2019 John Wiley & Sons Ltd. Published 2019 by John Wiley & Sons Ltd.

Solitary Cutaneous Mast Cell Proliferation

Cutaneous Mastocytoma

Red plaque on the calf of a child (left)

Sign of Darier following rubbing (right)

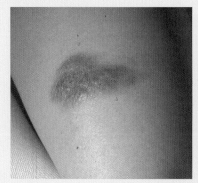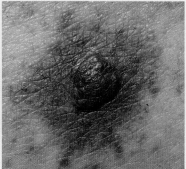

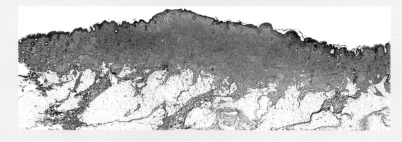

Densely packed mast cells. Hematoxylin-eosin (top) and Giemsa (below)

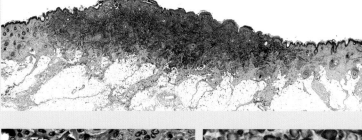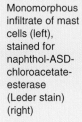

Monomorphous infiltrate of mast cells (left), stained for naphthol-ASD-chloroacetate-esterase (Leder stain) (right)

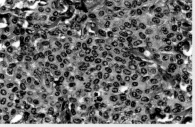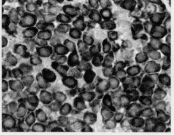

Cl: Red-brown plaques or nodules, which markedly swell or even form blisters upon rubbing or other types of mechanical irritation (Darier's sign).

Hi:

- Cellular diffuse dermal infiltrate
- Monotonous proliferation of round or cuboidal mast cells with granular cytoplasm
- Giemsa, toluidine blue, naphthol-ASD-chloroacetateesterase (Leder) or mast cell tryptase stain allow identification of mast cells
- Immunohistochemical staining for CD117 (c-kit) is the most reliable mast cell stain

DD: Melanocytic nevus; cutaneous (B-cell) lymphoma; Langerhans cell histiocytosis.

References

Ghosn, S., Kurban, M., Kibbi, A.G., and Abbas, O. (2013) Solitary mastocytoma with associated pseudocarcinomatous hyperplasia. *J Cutan Pathol* **40**(3): 351–3.

Kamysz, J.J. and Fretzin, D.F. (1994) Necrobiosis in solitary mastocytoma: coincidence or pathogenesis? *J Cutan Pathol* **21**(2): 179–82.

Ma, D., Stence, A.A., Bossler, A.B., Hackman, J.R., and Bellizzi, A.M. (2014) Identification of KIT activating mutations in paediatric solitary mastocytoma. *Histopathology* **64**(2): 218–25.

Tran, D.T., Jokinen, C.H., and Argenyi, Z.B. (2009) Histiocyte-rich pleomorphic mastocytoma: an uncommon variant mimicking juvenile xanthogranuloma and Langerhans cell histiocytosis. *J Cutan Pathol* **36**(11): 1215–20.

Ueng, S.H. and Kuo, T.T. (2004) An unusual mastocytoma with massive eosinophilic infiltration: identification with immunohistochemistry. *Am J Dermatopathol* **26**(6): 475–7.

Diffuse Cutaneous Mast Cell Proliferations

Urticaria Pigmentosa (Juvenile Maculopapular Mastocytosis)

Telangiectasia Macularis Eruptiva Perstans (Adults)

Urticaria pigmentosa in a child (left). Lesions turning light brown under diaphanoscopy (mid).

Adult telangiectasia macularis eruptiva perstans (right)

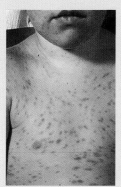
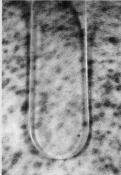
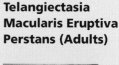
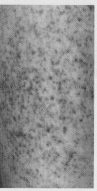

The juvenile form tends to regress spontaneously, whereas in adults the disease persists and frequently involves extracutaneous sites (liver, bone, blood – mast cell leukemia) and may show systemic symptoms such as pruritus, flashing, diarrhea, tachycardia or circulatory collapse due to the release of mediators from activated mast cells (histamin, serotonin, hydroxytryptamine). Check for serum tryptase.

Cl: Hundreds of small red-brown papules, showing light brown color when made anemic under diaphanoscopy. When mediators are released from mast cells by mechanical rubbing or scratching or by medical (non-steroidal antiphlogistics) or alimentary stimuli (banana, alcohol), the lesions become slightly elevated (Darier's sign) or may show blister formation. Palms, soles, and face usually are spared

Hi: In some cases, the increased number of mast cells between collagen bundles of the dermis is not conspicuous and cannot be detected without special stains: Giemsa, toluidine blue or naphthol-ASD-chloroacetateesterase (Leder) stain, CD117 (c-kit).

- Upper and mid dermis
- Sleeve-like accumulation of monomorphous mast cells preferentially around vessels
- Dilated vessels
- Scattered eosinophils may be present, which should not be confused with bone marrow-derived mast cell precursors with eosinophilic cytoplasm, lacking the lobated nucleus typical for eosinophils
- Pigment in the basal layer

DD: Multiple leiomyomas; multiple adnexal tumors; Langerhans cell histiocytosis; myelomonocytic leukemia.

References

Fett, N.M., Teng, J., and Longley, B.J. (2013) Familial urticaria pigmentosa: report of a family and review of the role of KIT mutations. *Am J Dermatopathol* **35**(1): 113–16.

Hu, S., Kuo, T.T., and Hong, H.S. (2002) Mast cells with bilobed or multilobed nuclei in a nodular lesion of a patient with urticaria pigmentosa. *Am J Dermatopathol* **24**(6): 490–2.

Sweet, W.L. and Smoller, B.R. (1996) Perivascular mast cells in urticaria pigmentosa. *J Cutan Pathol* **23**(3): 247–53.

Urticaria Pigmentosa and Telangiectasia Macularis Eruptiva Perstans (TMEP) (Adults)

Sleeve-like perivascular infiltrates of mast cells with overlying hyperpigmented epidermis

Perivascular accumulation of mast cells (left). Blistering following rubbing (right)

Urticaria Pigmentosa

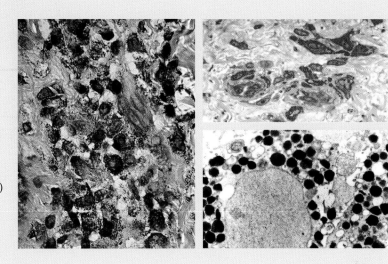

Mast cells with typical granules. Giemsa (left). Semithin section (right top) and electron microscopy (right bottom)

TMEP is nosologically closely related to urticaria pigmentosa, with similar clinical and histopathological presentation. The clinical setting is much more obvious to the eye than the subtle histopathological changes ("invisible dermatosis") for the pathologist. **Cl**: Mostly in adults, multiple distinct or confluent small red-brown macules, patches or papules with telangiectases.

Hi:
- Hyperpigmentation of the basal layer
- No increase of melanocytes
- Subepidermal scant splaying of mast cells
- Accompanying telangiectasias
- Eosinophils
- Mast cells positive for CD117 (c-kit)

DD: See urticaria pigmentosa.

Systemic Mast Cell Proliferation

Involvement of Skin and Bone Marrow

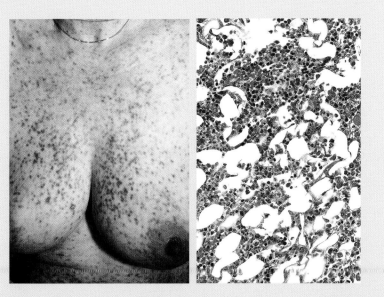

Red papules disseminated on the trunk (left). Proliferation of mast cells in the bone marrow (right)

For more detailed clinical and histomorphological description, see the following references.

References

Berezowska, S., Flaig, M.J., Rueff, F., et al. (2014) Adult-onset mastocytosis in the skin is highly suggestive of systemic mastocytosis. *Mod Pathol* **27**(1): 19–29.

Fusco, N., Bonometti, A., Augello, C., et al. (2017) Clonal reticulohistiocytosis of the skin and bone marrow associated with systemic mastocytosis and acute myeloid leukaemia. *Histopathology* **70**(6): 1000–8.

Krahl, J., Baldauf, P., and Stoermer, D. (1999) [Systemic congenital mastocytosis with universal skin involvement] *Hautarzt* **50**(12): 893–6.

Lange, M., Zawrocki, A., Nedoszytko, B., et al. (2014) Does the aberrant expression of CD2 and CD25 by skin mast cells truly correlate with systemic involvement in patients presenting with mastocytosis in the skin? *Int Arch Allergy Immunol* **165**(2): 104–10.

van Doormaal, J.J., van der Veer, E., van Voorst Vader, P.C., et al. (2012) Tryptase and histamine metabolites as diagnostic indicators of indolent systemic mastocytosis without skin lesions. *Allergy* **67**(5): 683–90.

Zink, A., Bohner, A., Schuch, A., Biedermann, T., and Brockow, K. (2017) Systemic mastocytosis with generalised skin involvement. *Lancet* **389**(10072): 940.

CHAPTER 11

Histiocytes

Atlas of Dermatopathology: Tumors, Nevi, and Cysts, First Edition. Günter Burg, Heinz Kutzner,
Werner Kempf, Josef Feit, and Bruce R. Smoller.
© 2019 John Wiley & Sons Ltd. Published 2019 by John Wiley & Sons Ltd.

PRECURSORS

Langerhans Cell Histiocytoses (LCH)

Langerhans cell histiocytoses are proliferative disorders of Langerhans cells, presenting with a wide spectrum of cutaneous and extracutaneous manifestations.

Precursors of Langerhans Cell Histiocytoses

The Langerhans cell (LHC) usually presents with characteristic morphological features: polygonal (histocytoid) silhouette, pale ample cytoplasm,

"coffee bean"-shaped nucleus; at the ultrastructural level, tennis racket-shaped Birbeck granules within the cytoplasm. Immunohistochemically, Langerhans cells express S100, CD1a, and Langerin (CD207). The latter is highly distinctive for Langerhans cells and allows differentiation from so-called indeterminate or veiled cells that are S100 positive, CD1a positive, Langerin (CD207) negative, and lack Birbeck granules.

Congenital Self-healing Reticulohistiocytosis (Hashimoto–Pritzker)

Nodule on the heel of a baby* (left)

Dense granulomatous infiltrate (top mid and right)

Large histiocytic cells (bottom mid)

Concentric intracytoplasmic lamellar bodies (bottom right)

*copyright: Bonifazi, E., R. Caputo, et al. (1982)

Cl: In newborns, multiple papules and nodules are found on the trunk, head, palms, and soles, occasionally with central ulceration. The children are otherwise healthy. As the lesions involute, they leave behind hypo- or hyperpigmented macules or patches.

Hi: Dense proliferation of large histiocytic cells, which show characteristic intracellular concentric lamellae under the electron microscope. No Birbeck granules.

Indeterminate Cell Histiocytosis

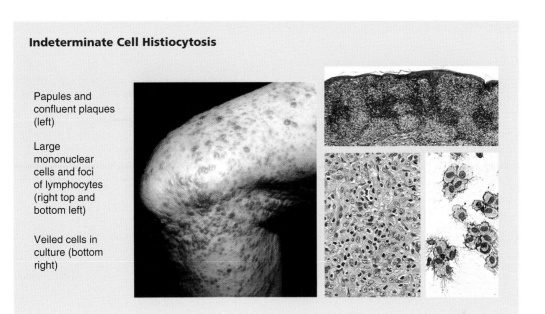

Papules and confluent plaques (left)

Large mononuclear cells and foci of lymphocytes (right top and bottom left)

Veiled cells in culture (bottom right)

Indeterminate cell histiocytosis (ICH) is a rare neoplastic disorder typified by the proliferation of indeterminate histiocytic cells, which are morphologically and immunophenotypically (CD1a+, S-100+) related to Langerhans cells but possess no Birbeck granules and are negative for Langerin (CD207).

Cl: Multiple asymptomatic red-brown papules and plaques on the trunk and limbs of adults.

Hi: Non-epidermotropic dermal infiltrate composed of mononuclear cells with abundant cytoplasm and prominent nuclei. These cells are so-called veiled cells (S100+, CD1a+, Langerin negative). Concomitant lymphocytic infiltrate may simulate a pseudofollicular pattern under low power.

Langerhans Cell Histiocytoses (Histiocytosis X)

Class I: S100 positive, CD1a positive, Langerin (CD207) positive, Birbeck granules positive.

Occurs in several forms: proliferative (malignant Letterer–Siwe), storing (Hand–Schüller–Christian), granulomatous (eosinophilic granuloma). Affects various organs, including the skin.

Table 11.1 Langerhans cell histiocytoses and their characteristics.

Disease	Age	Skin involvement	Clinical features	Course	Prognosis
Letterer–Siwe	First years of life	~90–100%	Fever, weight loss, lymphadenopathy, hepatosplenomegaly, pancytopenia, bone lesions	Acute	Mortality rate: 50–66%
Hand–Schüller–Christian	Children, adults	~30%	Osteolytic bone lesions, diabetes insipidus, exophthalmos, otitis	Subacute to chronic	Mortality rate: <50%
Eosinophilic granuloma	Mainly adults	<10%	Solitary bone or skin lesions	Chronic	Favorable

Source: Kazakov, D., Burg, G., and Kempf, W. (2005) Langerhans cell histiocytosis (histiocytosis X). In: Burg, G. and Kempf, W. (eds) *Cutaneous Lymphomas*. Boca Raton: CRC Press.

References

Bhattacharjee, P. and Glusac, E.J. (2007) Langerhans cell hyperplasia in scabies: a mimic of Langerhans cell histiocytosis. *J Cutan Pathol* **34**(9): 716–20.

Billings, T.L., Barr, R., and Dyson, S. (2008) Langerhans cell histiocytosis mimicking malignant melanoma: a diagnostic pitfall. *Am J Dermatopathol* **30**(5): 497–9.

Bouloc, A., Boulland, M.L., Geissmann, F., et al. (2000) CD101 expression by Langerhans cell histiocytosis cells. *Histopathology* **36**(3): 229–32.

Burg, G. and Kempf, W. (eds) (2005) *Cutaneous Lymphomas.* Boca Raton: CRC Press.

Favara, B.E. and Jaffe, R. (1994) The histopathology of Langerhans cell histiocytosis. *Br J Cancer* **23**(Suppl): S17–23.

Grace, S.A., Sutton, A.M., Armbrecht, E.S., Vidal, C.I., Rosman, I.S., and Hurley, M.Y. (2017) p53 is a helpful marker in distinguishing Langerhans cell histiocytosis from Langerhans cell hyperplasia. *Am J Dermatopathol* **39**(10): 726–30.

Kalen, J.E., Shokeen, D., Mislankar, M., Wangia, M., and Motaparthi, K. (2017) Langerhans cell histiocytosis with clinical and histologic features of hidradenitis suppurativa: brief report and review. *Am J Dermatopathol* Sept 11, doi: 10.1097 [epub ahead of print].

Kim, H.K., Park, C.J., Jang, S., et al. (2014) Bone marrow involvement of Langerhans cell histiocytosis: immunohistochemical evaluation of bone marrow for CD1a, Langerin, and S100 expression. *Histopathology* **65**(6): 742–8.

Kim, S.H., Kim, D.H., and Lee, K.G. (2007) Prominent Langerhans' cell migration in the arthropod bite reactions simulating Langerhans' cell histiocytosis. *J Cutan Pathol* **34**(12): 899–902.

Petersen, B.L., Rengtved, P., Bank, M.I., and Carstensen, H. (2003) High expression of markers of apoptosis in Langerhans cell histiocytosis. *Histopathology* **42**(2): 186–93.

Wheller, L., Carman, N., and Butler, G. (2013) Unilesional self-limited Langerhans cell histiocytosis: a case report and review of the literature. *J Cutan Pathol* **40**(6): 595–9.

Congenital Langerhans Cell Histiocytosis (Letterer–Siwe Disease)

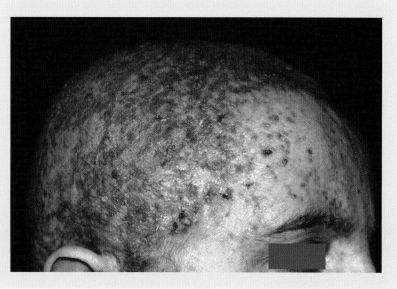

Scaly crusty lesions in a child

Congenital Langerhans Cell Histiocytosis (Letterer–Siwe Disease)

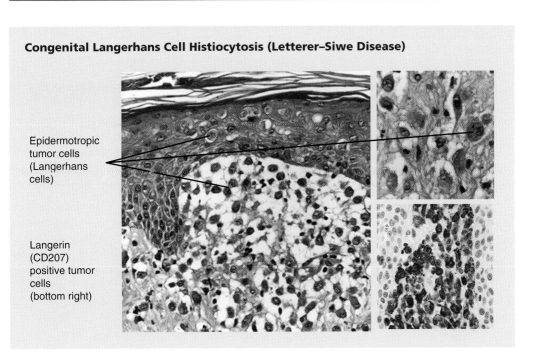

Epidermotropic tumor cells (Langerhans cells)

Langerin (CD207) positive tumor cells (bottom right)

Cl: Skin lesions occur during the first year of life and are composed of tiny rose-pink or brownish-red, translucent papules and patches, which become scaly and crusted and may coalesce into plaques. Petechial and purpuric lesions, pustules, and vesicles as well as small erosions can also be seen. Predilection sites are the scalp and seborrheic sites such as the postauricular area, nasolabial folds, perioral region, and upper trunk. Additional symptoms include fever, weight loss, rash, lymphadenopathy, hepatosplenomegaly, pancytopenia, and purpura.

Hi:

- Superficial erosion and scale crust
- In the papillary dermis, band-like pale cell infiltrate with epidermotropism
- In the epidermis, prominent pagetoid spread of single cells or accumulation of Pautrier abscess-like intraepidermal cellular clusters
- Hallmark cell type: Langerhans cell with abundant amphophilic cytoplasm and coffee bean-shaped nucleus. Cells often have histiocytoid morphology
- Variable number of lymphocytes, plasma cells, eosinophils

- Immunohistochemical expression of S100, CD1a, Langerin (CD207)

Electron microscopy: Tennis racket-shaped Birbeck granules.

DD: Seborrheic dermatitis; other eczematous lesions; other forms of LCH.

References

Abdelatif, O.M., Chandler, F.W., Pantazis, C.G., and McGuire, B.S. (1990) Enhanced expression of c-myc and H-ras oncogenes in Letterer-Siwe disease. A sequential study using colorimetric in situ hybridization. *Arch Pathol Lab Med* **114**(12): 1254–60.

Ferreira, L.M., Emerich, P.S., Diniz, L.M., Lage, L., and Redighieri, I. (2009) [Langerhans cell histiocytosis: Letterer-Siwe disease – the importance of dermatological diagnosis in two cases] *An Bras Dermatol* **84**(4): 405–9.

Pant, C., Madonia, P., Bahna, S.L., Bass, P.F., and Jeroudi, M. (2009) Langerhans cell histiocytosis, a case of Letterer Siwe disease. *J La State Med Soc* **161**(4): 211–12.

Zhou, H.M., Zeng, X., and Chen, Q.M. (2007) [Clinical and pathologic features of Letterer–Siwe disease: a case report and review] *Hua Xi Kou Qiang Yi Xue Za Zhi* **25**(5): 517–19.

Hand–Schüller–Christian Adult LHC Histiocytosis

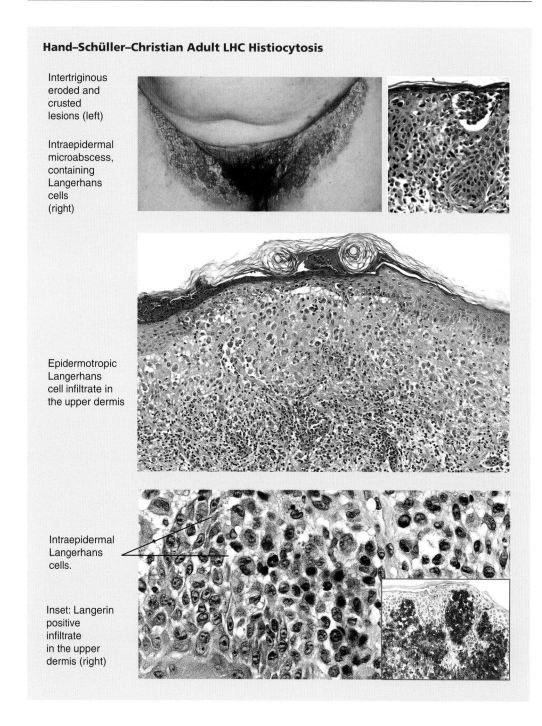

Intertriginous eroded and crusted lesions (left)

Intraepidermal microabscess, containing Langerhans cells (right)

Epidermotropic Langerhans cell infiltrate in the upper dermis

Intraepidermal Langerhans cells.

Inset: Langerin positive infiltrate in the upper dermis (right)

Cl: Skin lesions occur in about 30% of cases, preferentially in the large skinfolds in the perianal and inguinal area. The typical triad includes osteolytic skull lesions (100%), diabetes insipidus (50%), and exophthalmos (10%). Otitis media, generalized lymphadenopathy, hepatosplenomegaly, and pulmonary disease may be additional findings.

Hi: The histological features are identical with those of Letterer–Siwe disease. In addition, some foamy cells may be present.

DD: Psoriasis; intertriginous eczema; candida mycosis.

References

Miura, A.B. (1993) [Hand–Schueller–Christian disease and eosinophilic granuloma] *Nihon Rinsho* **51**(Suppl): 1101–6.

Zabucchi, G., Soranzo, M.R., Menegazzi, R., et al. (1991) Eosinophilic granuloma of the bone in Hand–Schuller–Christian disease: extensive in vivo eosinophil degranulation and subsequent binding of released eosinophil peroxidase (EPO) to other inflammatory cells. *J Pathol* **163**(3): 225–31.

Solitary Langerhans Cell Tumor (Eosinophilic Granuloma)

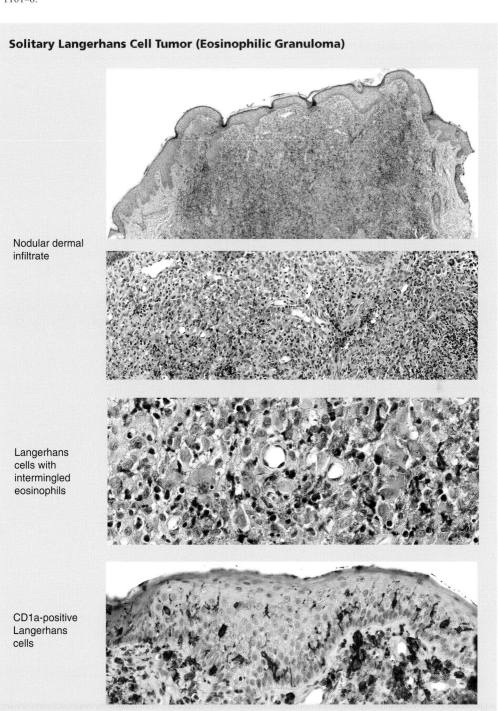

Nodular dermal infiltrate

Langerhans cells with intermingled eosinophils

CD1a-positive Langerhans cells

PROLIFERATIVE

Cl: The most common site of involvement is bone. Skin lesions are uncommon and present as deep dermal or subcutaneous nodules which are not clinically distinct.

Hi: Cellular mixed granulomatous infiltrate without necrosis, composed of large mononuclear cells with amphophilic eosinophilic cytoplasm (Langerhans cells), histiocytes, lymphocytes, and many eosinophils.

DD: Lesions with predominant eosinophilic infiltration: lymphomatoid papulosis; granuloma faciale; insect bite reaction; Wells syndrome.

References

Cambazard, F., Dezutter-Dambuyant, C., Staquet, M.J., Schmitt, D., and Thivolet, J. (1991) Eosinophilic granuloma of bone and biochemical demonstration of 49-kDa CD1a molecule expression by Langerhans-cell histiocytosis. *Clin Exp Dermatol* **16**(5): 377–82.

Garcia Muret, M.P., Fernandez-Figueras, M.T., Gonzalez, M.J., and de Moragas, J.M. (1995) [Congenital spontaneously regressive cutaneous Langerhans cell histiocytosis with bone involvement (eosinophilic granuloma)] *Ann Dermatol Venereol* **122**(9): 612–14.

Non-Langerhans Cell Histiocytoses

Class II: CD1a negative, Langerin (CD207) negative, Birbeck granule negative, S100 and histiocytic monocytic markers with variable expression (CD14, CD64, CD68, CD163).

Proliferative

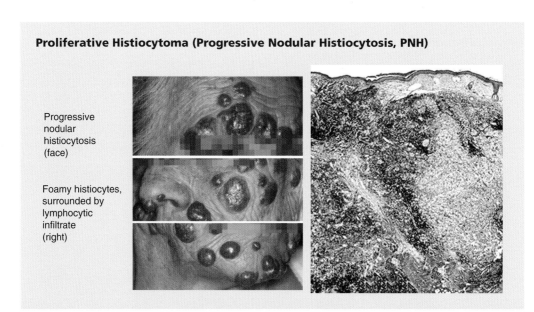

Proliferative Histiocytoma (Progressive Nodular Histiocytosis, PNH)

Progressive nodular histiocytosis (face)

Foamy histiocytes, surrounded by lymphocytic infiltrate (right)

Cl: Multiple, slowly growing red-brown nodules with smooth surface in adults, preferentially involving the face and neck, increasing in number over time. No systemic or lymph node involvement.

Hi:
- Dermal infiltrates of foamy histiocytes
- Variants with spindled cells and large histiocytes with ample cytoplasm
- Lymphocytic infiltrate in the adjacent dermis

Immunohistochemistry: Histiomonocytic markers mostly positive (CD14, CD64, CD68, CD163).

DD: Cutaneous B-cell lymphoma; sinus histiocytosis.

References

Caputo, R., Brezzi, A., Vaccari, G., Cavicchini, S., and Gianotti, R. (2002) Progressive histiocytosis: description of a case of slow-course non-Langerhans cell histiocytosis. *Dermatology* **205**(3): 293–7;discussion 296–7.

Glavin, F.L., Chhatwall, H., and Karimi, K. (2009) Progressive nodular histiocytosis: a case report with literature review and discussion of differential

PROLIFERATIVE

diagnosis and classification. *J Cutan Pathol* **36**(12): 1286–92.

Hilker, O., Kovneristy, A., Varga, R., et al. (2013) Progressive nodular histiocytosis. *J Dtsch Dermatol Ges* **11**(4): 301–7.

Luftl, M., Seybold, H., Simon, M. Jr, and Burgdorf, W. (2006) [Progressive nodular histiocytosis – rare variant of cutaneous non-Langerhans cell histiocytosis] *J Dtsch Dermatol Ges* **4**(3): 236–8.

Benign Cephalic Histiocytosis

Flat papules in the face, simulating flat warts

Histiocytes and multinucleated giant cells intermingled with lymphocytes (right)

Cl: Benign, self-healing, non-Langerhans cell proliferation of unknown cause affecting infants and children, which presents with multiple asymptomatic flat yellow to red-brown papules, confined to the head and neck area. Spontaneous regression after months and years.

Hi:

- The histological features are very similar to those seen in juvenile xanthogranuloma
- Large histiocytes with eosinophilic cytoplasm and multinucleated giant cells with lymphocytes in between
- Three variants:
  - papillary dermal
  - lichenoid
  - diffuse

Immunohistochemistry: S100 positive; CD1a negative.

Electron microscopy: No Birbeck granules.

DD: Plane warts; multiple juvenile xanthogranulomas; generalized eruptive histiocytomas.

References

D'Auria, A.A., de Clerck, B., and Kim, G. (2011) Benign cephalic histiocytosis with S-100 protein positivity. *J Cutan Pathol* **38**(10): 842–3.

Gianotti, R., Alessi, E., and Caputo, R. (1993) Benign cephalic histiocytosis: a distinct entity or a part of a wide spectrum of histiocytic proliferative disorders of children? A histopathological study. *Am J Dermatopathol* **15**(4): 315–19.

Rodriguez-Jurado, R., Duran-McKinster, C., and Ruiz-Maldonado, R. (2000) Benign cephalic histiocytosis progressing into juvenile xanthogranuloma: a non-Langerhans cell histiocytosis transforming under the influence of a virus? *Am J Dermatopathol* **22**(1): 70–4.

PROLIFERATIVE

Multicentric Reticulohistiocytosis (Lipoid Dermatoarthritis) (Solitary Reticulohistiocytoma)

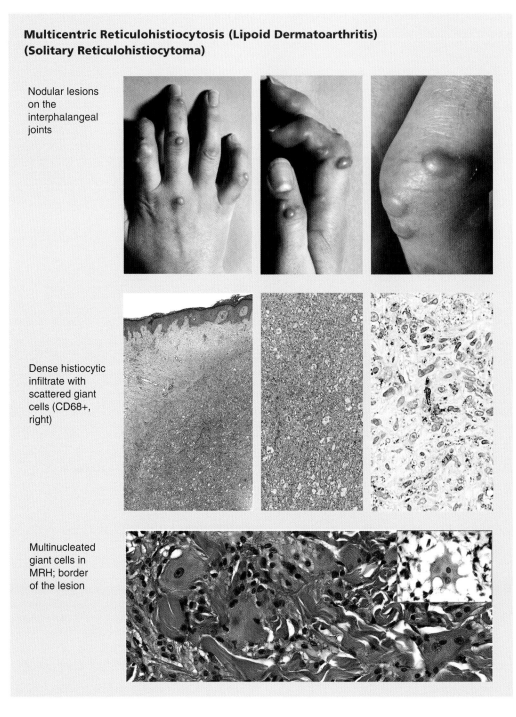

Nodular lesions on the interphalangeal joints

Dense histiocytic infiltrate with scattered giant cells (CD68+, right)

Multinucleated giant cells in MRH; border of the lesion

Cl: The disease typically affects women in their fourth or fifth decade. Small firm red-brown papules with smooth surface on the distal interphalangeal joints of the hands and on the ears. Rings of papules along the nailfolds. Mucosal involvement in 50% of patients. Association with arthritis, immunological disorders, and malignancies.

Hi:
- Diffuse dermal infiltrate of oncocytic histiocytes with ample eosinophilic, finely granular ("ground-glass") cytoplasm and small round nuclei

PROLIFERATIVE

- Foamy histiocytes and lymphocytes
- Sudan black B fat stain and oil red O are positive
- Fibrosis in older lesions

DD: Reticulohistiocytosis; rheumatoid arthritis; gout; lipogranulomatosis of Farber.

References

Perrin, C., Lacour, J.P., Michiels, J.F., Flory, P., Ziegler, G., and Ortonne, J.P. (1992) Multicentric reticulohistiocytosis. Immunohistological and ultrastructural study: a pathology of dendritic cell lineage. *Am J Dermatopathol* **14**(5): 418–25.

Perrin, C., Lacour, J.P., Michiels, J.F., and Ortonne, J.P. (1995) Reticulohistiocytomas versus multicentric reticulohistiocytosis. *Am J Dermatopathol* **17**(6): 625–6.

Tan, B.H., Barry, C.I., Wick, M.R., et al. (2011) Multicentric reticulohistiocytosis and urologic carcinomas: a possible paraneoplastic association. *J Cutan Pathol* **38**(1): 43–8.

Zelger, B., Cerio, R., Soyer, H.P., Misch, K., Orchard, G., and Wilson-Jones, E. (1994) Reticulohistiocytoma and multicentric reticulohistiocytosis. Histopathologic and immunophenotypic distinct entities. *Am J Dermatopathol* **16**(6): 577–84.

Sinus Histiocytosis With Massive Lymphadenopathy

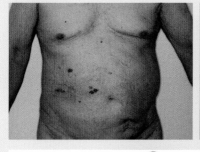
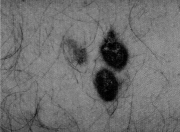

Small nodular lesions on the trunk

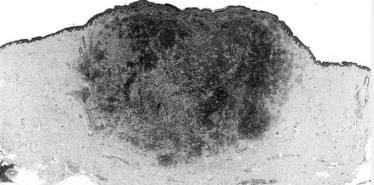

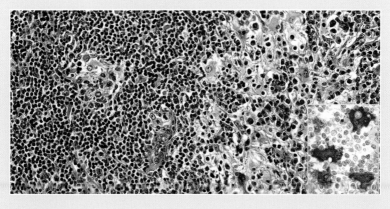

Strands and patches of dense lymphocytic infiltrate with scattered macrophages (mid and bottom). Inset: S100+ macrophages with phagocytosed lymphocytes (emperipolesis; beanbag sign)

GRANULOMATOUS STORING

Cl: Solitary or multiple cutaneous nodules imitating nevi or dermatofibromas. The lymph nodes are spared. The term *sinus histiocytosis with massive lymphadenopathy* is a misnomer which reflects the identical histomorphology of a probably unrelated reactive disorder in the lymph nodes (Rosai–Dorfman type of sinus histiocytosis). Cutaneous lesions generally are regarded to represent specific morphological variants of a histiocytic disorder.

Hi:
- Lymphoma-like diffuse cellular mixed infiltrate in the upper and mid dermis
- Mostly lymphocytes and plasma cells
- Hallmark cells are very large interspersed histiocytic cells ("fried eggs") with ample cytoplasm and large vesicular nucleus. Within the cytoplasm, there are one or more phagocytosed (emperipolesis) lymphocytes or plasma cells
- Immunohistochemically, these cells are strongly positive for S100
- There may be intratumoral dilated lymphatics filled with lymphocytes and plasma cells

Granulomatous Storing

Juvenile Xanthogranuloma (Nevoxanthoendothelioma; Xanthoma Multiplex; Juvenile Giant Cell Granuloma)

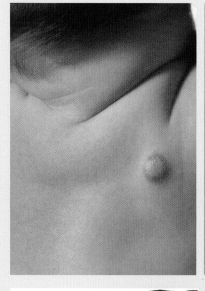
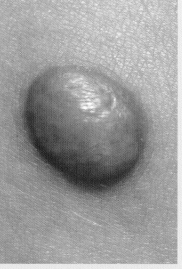

Slightly red early lesion (left)

Yellowish mature nodule (right)

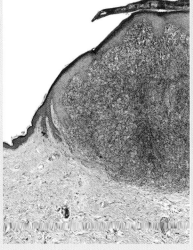
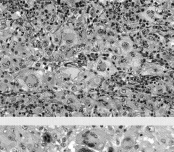
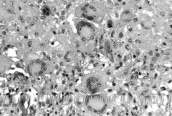

Histiocytic nodular infiltrate without grenz zone ("touching the epidermis") (left)

Foamy histiocytes and macrophages (top right)

Touton giant cells (bottom right)

GRANULOMATOUS STORING

Juvenile xanthogranuloma (JXG) is a benign, self-limited histiocytic disorder of unknown cause, predominantly affecting infants and children, but also seen in adults.

Cl: Solitary, sometimes multiple yellow-brown papules with smooth surface, preferentially in the head and neck area of white children, with a tendency to spontaneous regression over a period of months or years. Extracutaneous involvement affects the eye and internal organs.

Hi:

- Early lesion: moderately dense perivascular and interstitial infiltrate composed mainly of medium-sized histiocytes with oval or irregular nuclei and eosinophilic, granular cytoplasm
- Fully evolved lesion:
  - Well-circumscribed nodular dermal infiltrate
  - The infiltrate lacks a grenz zone and completely fills the papillary dermis, even in early stages of the lesion
  - Histiocytes with foamy, eosinophilic or vacuolated cytoplasm
  - Multinucleated giant cells of the Touton type
  - Concomitant mixed inflammatory infiltrate of lymphocytes and eosinophils
  - Spindle cell variants and morphological overlap with dermatofibroma exist
  - Fibrosis in resolving lesions

Immunohistochemistry: Variable expression of CD14, CD64, CD68, and CD163. S100 protein often positive, particularly in lesions rich in phagocytosing cells and neutrophils; CD1a negative.

DD: Xanthoma (disseminatum); mastocytoma; Spitz nevus; eruptive histiocytoma.

References

Fernandez-Flores, A., Nicklaus, I., Browne, F., and Colmenero, I. (2017) Hemosiderotic juvenile xanthogranuloma. *Am J Dermatopathol* **39**(10): 773–5.

Kraus, M.D., Haley, J.C., Ruiz, R., Essary, L., Moran, C.A., and Fletcher, C.D. (2001) "Juvenile" xanthogranuloma: an immunophenotypic study with a reappraisal of histogenesis. *Am J Dermatopathol* **23**(2): 104–11.

Sanchez Yus, E., Requena, L., Villegas, C., and Valle, P. (1995) Subcutaneous juvenile xanthogranuloma. *J Cutan Pathol* **22**(5): 460–5.

Sangueza, O.P., Salmon, J.K., White, C.R. Jr, and Beckstead, J.H. (1995) Juvenile xanthogranuloma: a clinical, histopathologic and immunohistochemical study. *J Cutan Pathol* **22**(4): 327–35.

Tran, D.T., Wolgamot, G.M., Olerud, J., Hurst, S., and Argenyi, Z. (2008). An 'eruptive' variant of juvenile xanthogranuloma associated with langerhans cell histiocytosis. *J Cutan Pathol* **35**(Suppl 1): 50–4.

Xanthoma Disseminatum

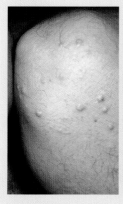 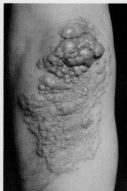 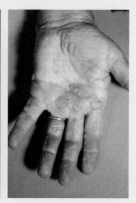

Eruptive xanthomas   Nodular xanthomas   Tendinous xanthomas

GRANULOMATOUS STORING

Xanthoma Disseminatum

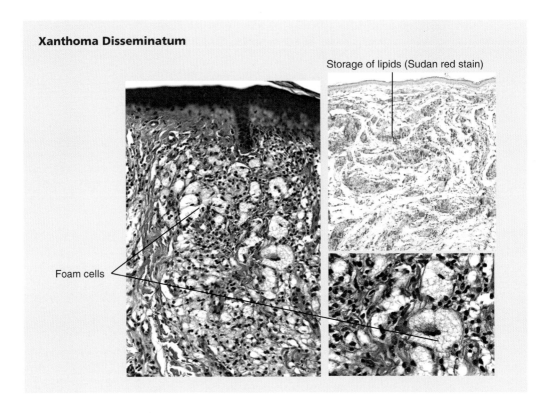

Storage of lipids (Sudan red stain)

Foam cells

Cl: Multiple yellowish papules and plaques are found on the eyelids, joints, and flexural areas of the extremities, axillae, groin, face (eyelids), perianal region, and trunk. Frequent association with diabetes insipidus and hyperlipoproteinemia.

Hi:
- Foamy histiocytes amidst a monocytic-histiocytic infiltrate in the reticular dermis
- Characteristic granuloma annulare-like pattern with foamy histiocytes near the center
- Histiocytes show broad, pale, foamy, fat-containing cytoplasm (Sudan red stain) and small, roundish, regular nuclei
- Concomitant inflammatory infiltrate with lymphocytes, neutrophils, and eosinophils

Immunohistochemistry: Expression of histiocytic markers (CD14, CD68, CD163); S100 and CD1a negative. Hallmark marker is adipophilin which detects intracytoplasmic lipids.

DD: Juvenile xanthogranuloma; eruptive histiocytoma; benign cephalic histiocytosis.

References

Kuligowski, M., Gorkiewicz-Petkow, A., and Jablonska, S. (1992) Xanthoma disseminatum. *Int J Dermatol* **31**(4): 281–3.

Nanda, A., Kanwar, A.J., Kapoor, M.M., Radotra, B.D., and Kaur, S. (1990) Xanthoma disseminatum. *Int J Dermatol* **29**(10): 727–8.

Park, M., Boone, B., and Devos, S. (2014) Xanthoma disseminatum: case report and mini-review of the literature. *Acta Dermatovenerol Croat* **22**(2): 150–4.

Pinto, M.E., Escalaya, G.R., Escalaya, M.E., Pinto, J.L., and Chian, C.A. (2010) Xanthoma disseminatum: case report and literature review. *Endocr Pract* **16**(6): 1003–6.

Rupec, R.A. and Schaller, M. (2002) Xanthoma disseminatum. *Int J Dermatol* **41**(12): 911–13.

Zelger, B., Cerio, R., Orchard, G., Fritsch, P., and Wilson-Jones, E. (1992) Histologic and immunohistochemical study comparing xanthoma disseminatum and histiocytosis X. *Arch Dermatol* **128**(9): 1207–12.

GRANULOMATOUS STORING

Xanthelasma Palpebrarum

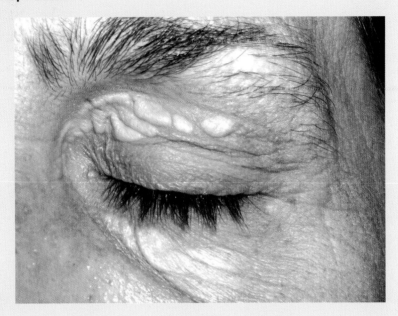

Yellow plaques

Foam cells

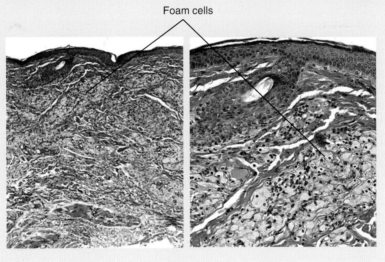

Cl: Yellowish plaques, preferentially on the eyelids.
Hi: In the reticular dermis there are lobular aggregates of foam cells, which are macrophages filled with lipids.
DD: Xanthoma.

References

Bergman, R., Kasif, Y., Aviram, M., et al. (1996) Normolipidemic xanthelasma palpebrarum: lipid composition, cholesterol metabolism in monocyte-derived macrophages, and plasma lipid peroxidation. *Acta Derm Venereol* **76**(2): 107–10.

Kavoussi, H., Ebrahimi, A., Rezaei, M., Ramezani, M., Najafi, B., and Kavoussi, R. (2016) Serum lipid profile and clinical characteristics of patients with xanthelasma palpebrarum. *An Bras Dermatol* **91**(4): 468–71.

Singla, A. (2006) Normolipemic papular xanthoma with xanthelasma. *Dermatol Online J* **12**(3): 19.

GRANULOMATOUS STORING

Verruciform Xanthoma

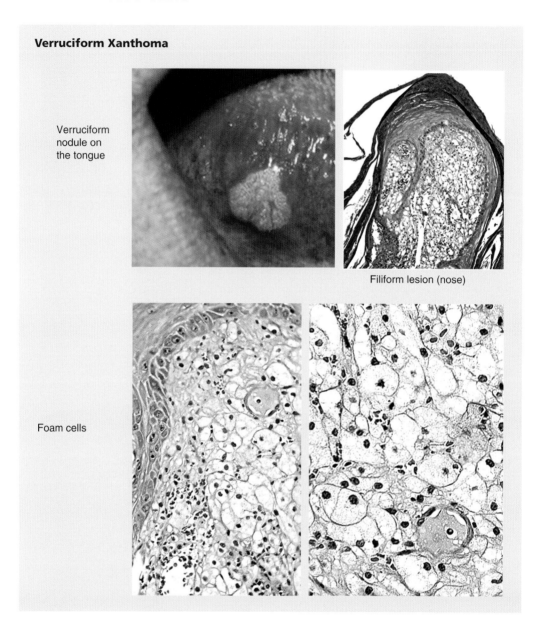

Verruciform nodule on the tongue

Filiform lesion (nose)

Foam cells

Cl: Typical localisation is the oral mucosa but anogenital, nasal mucosa and other sites may be involved, showing a yellow-red filiform or papillomatous lesion. Much larger and confluent lesions with identical histomorphology may be encountered in CHILD nevus (females) and CHILD mosaicism (males), the latter lesions being much smaller and wart-like.

Hi:
- Verrucous and markedly acanthotic epithelial hyperplasia with elongation of the rete ridges
- Multifocal funnel-shaped eosinophilic keratinous columns within the epidermis ("wart on fire")
- Accumulation of foamy histiocytes and macrophages loaded with lipids, filling the papillary dermis
- Fat-storing histiocytes strongly express adipophilin and histiocytic markers

DD: Verruca vulgaris; squamous cell carcinoma.

References

Agarwal-Antal, N., Zimmermann, J., Scholz, T., Noyes, R.D., and Leachman, S.A. (2002) A giant verruciform xanthoma. *J Cutan Pathol* **29**(2): 119–24.

de Andrade, B.A., Agostini, M., Pires, F.R., et al. (2015) Oral verruciform xanthoma: a clinicopathologic and immunohistochemical study of 20 cases. *J Cutan Pathol* **42**(7): 489–95.

Helm, T.N., Richards, P., Lin, L., and Helm, K.F. (2012) Verruciform xanthoma with porokeratosis-like features but no clinically apparent lymphedema. *J Cutan Pathol* **39**(9): 887–8.

Khaskhely, N.M., Uezato, H., Kamiyama, T., et al. (2000) Association of human papillomavirus type 6 with a verruciform xanthoma. *Am J Dermatopathol* **22**(5): 447–52.

Val-Bernal, J.F., Argueta, L., Val, D., Gonzalez-Vela, M.C., and Garijo, M.F. (2012) Verruciform xanthoma is another condition associated with pseudoepitheliomatous hyperplasia. *Am J Dermatopathol* **34**(3): 341–2.

Wu, Y.H., Hsiao, P.F., and Lin, Y.C. (2006) Verruciform xanthoma-like phenomenon in seborrheic keratosis. *J Cutan Pathol* **33**(5): 373–7.

Necrobiotic Xanthogranuloma (with Paraproteinemia)

Infiltrated plaques on the trunk (left) and suborbital (right)

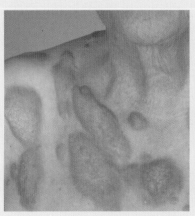
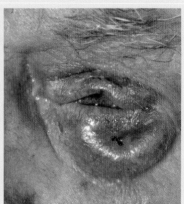

Foam cells (mid) with Touton giant cells (bottom right)

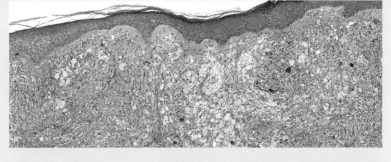

Palisading pattern with granulomatous border around necrosis and cholesterol deposits (left)

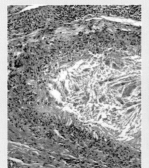
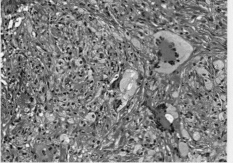

Cl: Yellow-red indurated nodules or plaques preferentially in the periorbital region and upper trunk. Often central depression. Association with paraproteinemia.

Hi:

- Early: dense histiocytic infiltrate with many plasma cells, often imitating diffuse type of granuloma annulare
- Late: large palisaded granulomatous lesion ("giant granuloma annulare")
- Large focal necrosis with stellate cholesterol clefts
- Foamy macrophages and exceedingly large multinucleate Touton-type giant cells
- Many plasma cells
- Sometimes marked lymphocytic infiltrate with germinal centers

DD: Xanthelasma; diffuse normolipemic plane xanthoma; granuloma annulare; necrobiosis lipoidica; sarcoidosis.

References

Fortson, J.S. and Schroeter, A.L. (1990) Necrobiotic xanthogranuloma with IgA paraproteinemia and extracutaneous involvement. *Am J Dermatopathol* **12**(6): 579–84.

Gergen, N., Biebl, K., Berg, B.C., and Suwattee, P. (2011) Slowly growing yellow nodules: challenge. Necrobiotic xanthogranuloma. *Am J Dermatopathol* **33**(1): 92–3, 103–4.

Kossard, S., Chow, E., Wilkinson, B., and Killingsworth, M. (2000) Lipid and giant cell poor necrobiotic xanthogranuloma. *J Cutan Pathol* **27**(7): 374–8.

Naghashpour, M., Setoodeh, R., Moscinski, L., et al. (2011) Nonnecrobiotic necrobiotic xanthogranuloma as an initial manifestation of paraproteinemia and small lymphocytic lymphoma in a patient with Sjogren syndrome. *Am J Dermatopathol* **33**(8): 855–7.

Stork, J., Kodetova, D., Vosmik, F., and Krejca, M. (2000) Necrobiotic xanthogranuloma presenting as a solitary tumor. *Am J Dermatopathol* **22**(5): 453–6.

Ziemer, M., Norgauer, J., Simon, J.C., and Koehler, M.J. (2012) An unusual histologic variant of necrobiotic xanthogranuloma. *Am J Dermatopathol* **34**(2): e22–6.

Hereditary Progressive Mucinous Histiocytosis

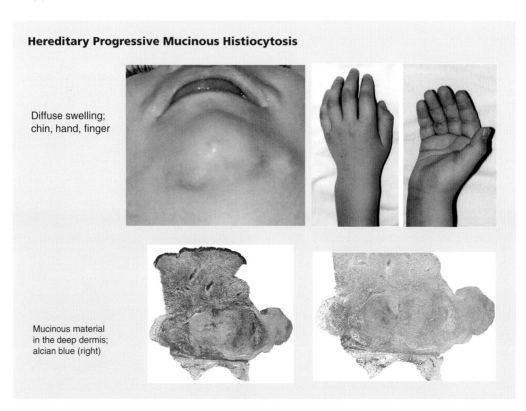

Diffuse swelling; chin, hand, finger

Mucinous material in the deep dermis; alcian blue (right)

Hereditary Progressive Mucinous Histiocytosis

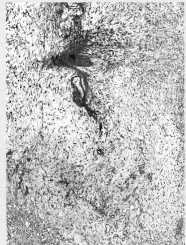 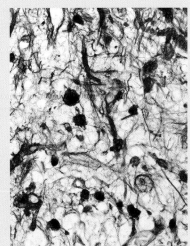

Mucinous stroma
(left) with large
histiocytes (right)

* Courtesy of L Requena, Madrid

This disease is considered to be a rare familial form of eruptive histiocytoma with prominent mucinosis.

Cl: Slowly progressive inherited disease presenting with plaques or papules, mostly starting in childhood or young adulthood. Temporary spontaneous regression. No extracutaneous involvement. No involvement of mucous membranes.

Hi:

- Epidermis not affected
- Well-circumscribed unencapsulated aggregates of histiocytes with abundant mucin (alcian blue) in the mid or deep dermis
- Scattered large epithelioid histiocytes with bizarre nuclei (CD68 and lysozyme positive; S100/CD1a and F XIIIa negative)
- No inflammation
- Few mast cells

Electron microscopy: Myelin bodies and zebra bodies but no Birbeck granules.

References

Bork, K. (1994) Hereditary progressive mucinous histiocytosis. Immunohistochemical and ultrastructural studies in an additional family. *Arch Dermatol* **130**(10): 1300–4.

Bork, K. and Hoede, N. (1988) Hereditary progressive mucinous histiocytosis in women. Report of three members in a family. *Arch Dermatol* **124**(8): 1225–9.

Hemmati, I., McLeod, W.A., and Crawford, R.I. (2010) Progressive mucinous histiocytosis: importance of electron microscopy to confirm diagnosis. *J Cutan Med Surg* **14**(5): 245–8.

Mizushima, J., Nogita, T., Higaki, Y., and Kawashima, M. (1997) Hereditary progressive mucinous histiocytosis. *Int J Dermatol* **36**(12): 958–60.

Nguyen, N.V., Prok, L., Burgos, A., and Bruckner, A.L. (2015) Hereditary progressive mucinous histiocytosis: new insights into a rare disease. *Pediatr Dermatol* **32**(6): e273–6.

Schroder, K., Hettmannsperger, U., Schmuth, M., Orfanos, C.E., and Goerdt, S. (1996) Hereditary progressive mucinous histiocytosis. *J Am Acad Dermatol* **35**(2 Pt 2): 298–303.

Wong, D., Killingsworth, M., Crosland, G., and Kossard, S. (1999) Hereditary progressive mucinous histiocytosis. *Br J Dermatol* **141**(6): 1101–5.

Hemophagocytic
Familial Hemophagocytic Lymphohistiocytosis

Extremely rare fatal disease showing macrophagocytic infiltrates with hemophagocytosis in several organs and rarely also involving the skin.

HEMOPHAGOCYTIC

References

Hesse, C., Hansmann, M.L., Janka-Schaub, G.E., Rontogianni, D., Radzun, H.J., and Fischer, R. (1991) [Familial hemophagocytic lymphohistiocytosis] *Verh Dtsch Ges Pathol* **75**: 200–4.

Kakkar, N., Vasishta, R.K., Banerjee, A.K., Marwaha, R.K., and Thapa, B.R. (2003) Familial hemophagocytic lymphohistiocytosis: an autopsy study. *Pediatr Pathol Mol Med* **22**(3): 229–42.

Histiocytic Cytophagic Panniculitis

Lobular panniculitis

Necrobiosis and macrophages containing phagocytised cells ("beanbag cells"). Karyorrhexis

Cl: Clinical aspect of deep-seated panniculitis with moderate overlying erythema. May occur at any site.

Hi:
- Mostly lobular cellular panniculitis, with infiltrate spilling over into the septa
- Mixed infiltrate, containing many histiocytes, macrophages, and multinucleate cells

- Hallmark cells are large histiocytic phagocytosing multinucleate cells (bean-bag cells) with intracytoplasmic lymphocytes
- No "rimming" of CD8-positive T-suppressor cells
- Immunophenotypically, histiocytes (CD68, CD163) predominate
- Negative for CD30 and CD56

CHAPTER 12

Hematopoietic Disorders

Some disorders formerly referred to as malignant proliferations of "histiocytes" or "mononuclear phagocytes" in fact turned out to be large cell lymphoproliferative disorders and will be discussed in this chapter.

Lymphoid Skin Infiltrates

The skin provides distinct homing conditions for lymphoid cells, which depend on the homing behavior of the cells themselves due to different surface molecules and cytokines released on one side and the composition and structure of target tissue where the cells tend to settle and proliferate. Lymphocytic infiltrates can be distinguished by their growth pattern, the cytomorphology of the neoplastic cells and their phenotypes.

In routine hematoxylin-eosin staining, small T-cell and B-cell infiltrates and their subtypes can be roughly differentiated due to the distinct cytomorphology of cells and the histological compartment of skin, presenting as T-cell and B-cell patterns respectively. A *diffuse growth pattern* extending between collagen bundles is found in large T-cell or B-cell lymphomas. Pseudolymphomatous infiltrates also may present a distinct pattern (see Pseudolymphomas, below). An *interstitial growth* is very typical for myelomonocytic skin infiltrates. These prototypes of growth pattern of hematopoietic cells in the skin can provide preliminary cyto- and histogenetic information which must be supplemented and confirmed by additional clinical, immunological, and molecular findings.

Atlas of Dermatopathology: Tumors, Nevi, and Cysts, First Edition. Günter Burg, Heinz Kutzner,
Werner Kempf, Josef Feit, and Bruce R. Smoller.
© 2019 John Wiley & Sons Ltd. Published 2019 by John Wiley & Sons Ltd.

CYTOMORPHOLOGY

Cytomorphology, Major Cell Types

T-Cells

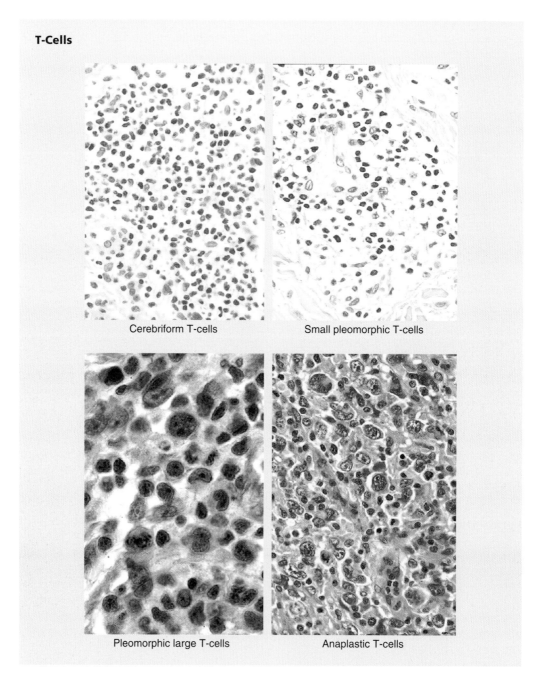

Cerebriform T-cells

Small pleomorphic T-cells

Pleomorphic large T-cells

Anaplastic T-cells

- Small cerebriform T-cells
- Small pleomorphic T-cells

- Pleomorphic large T-cells
- Anaplastic T-cells

CYTOMORPHOLOGY

B-Cells

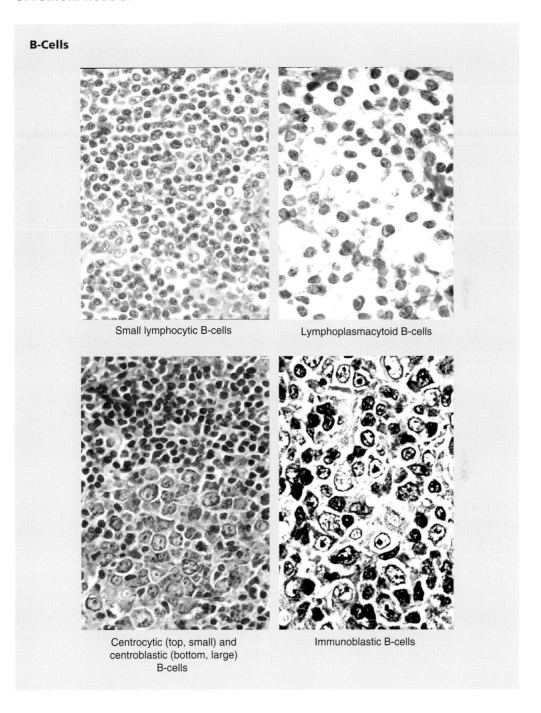

Small lymphocytic B-cells

Lymphoplasmacytoid B-cells

Centrocytic (top, small) and
centroblastic (bottom, large)
B-cells

Immunoblastic B-cells

- Small lymphocytic B-cells
- Small lymphoplasmacytoid B-cells
- Small/medium-sized cleaved follicle center cells (centrocytes)
- Large non-cleaved follicle center cells (centroblasts)
- Large immunoblastic B-cells

PATTERN

Pattern of Small Cell Lymphocytic Infiltrates

T-Cell Pattern

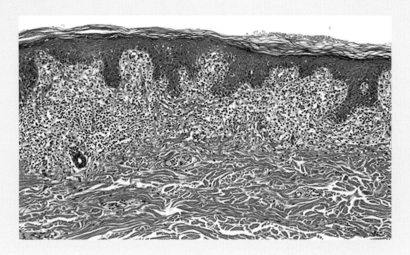

- Upper dermis
- Band-like epidermotropic infiltrate with single cells or clusters of lymphoid cells in the epidermis (Pautrier microabscesses)
- Infiltrate in the papillary dermis; cells are loosely packed due to edema in the dermis

- Edema in the papillary dermis, sometimes simulating a free "grenz zone," transforming into fibrosis
- Infiltration along adnexal structures
- Prominent postcapillary venules

B-Cell Pattern

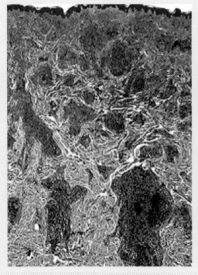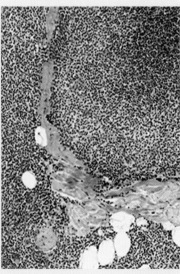

NODULAR B-CELL PL

- Mid and deep dermis, perivascular rather than periadnexal
- Nodular, compact, well-circumscribed lymphocytic infiltrates
- Well-defined concave borders of the infiltrates
- Cells are densely packed without intercellular edema
- "Grenz zone"; no epidermotropism

References

Burg, G. and Braun-Falco, O. (1983) *Cutaneous Lymphomas, Pseudolymphomas and Related Disorders.* Berlin: Springer-Verlag.

Burg, G., Kadin, M.E., and Kempf, W. (2005) Growth patterns of lympho- and myeloproliferative infiltrates of the skin. In: Burg, G. and Kempf, W. (eds) *Cutaneous Lymphomas.* Boca Raton: CRC Press.

Burg, G., Hoffmann, F.G., Rodt, H., and Schmoeckel, C. (1978) Patterns of cutaneous lymphomas. Histological, enzyme cytochemical, and immunological typing of lymphoreticular proliferations in the skin. *Dermatologica* **157**(5): 282–91.

Kummermehr, J.B.G. (1982) Audioradiographic pattern of cell proliferation in cutaneous malignant lymphoma. In: *Lymphoproliferative Diseases of the Skin.* Berlin: Springer.

Pseudolymphoma (PL)

Nodular B-Cell PL

Lymphadenosis Cutis Benigna (Lymphocytoma Cutis)

Pseudolympho-
matous swelling
of the concha of
the ear (left)

"Follicular"
infiltrates (right)

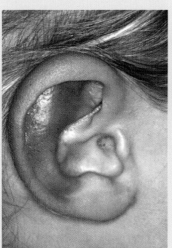
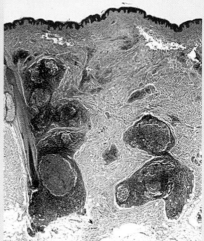

Germinal center
formation (left)
with starry sky
macrophages
(right)

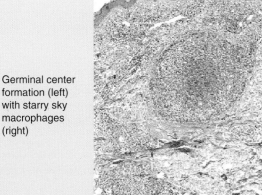
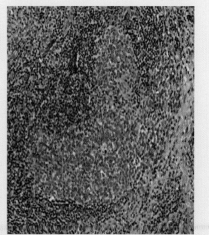

NODULAR B-CELL PL

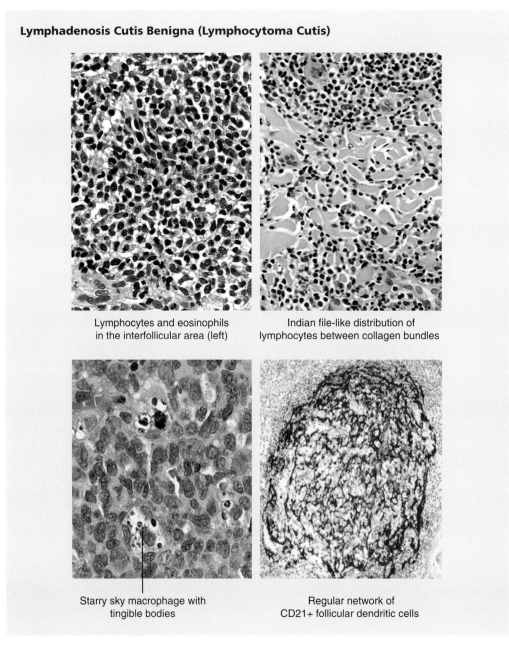

Lymphadenosis Cutis Benigna (Lymphocytoma Cutis)

Lymphocytes and eosinophils
in the interfollicular area (left)

Indian file-like distribution of
lymphocytes between collagen bundles

Starry sky macrophage with
tingible bodies

Regular network of
CD21+ follicular dendritic cells

In Europe, this is most commonly caused by infection with *Borrelia burgdorferi* after a tick bite (*Ixodes ricinus*), but also by other microbiological, physical or chemical agents. In the United States and other parts of the world, *Borrelia burgdorferi* DNA in cutaneous B-cell lymphomas or pseudolymphomas is absent.

Giant follicular forms of lymphadenosis benigna cutis with "inverted follicular pattern" (dark chromatin in the center and clear border zone) today are regarded as marginal zone B-cell lymphomas.

Cl: Mostly solitary, rarely multiple, disseminated soft red nodules on the head, preferentially on the ear lobes. Other predilections are the nose, nipples, inguinal area, and scrotum.

Hi:
- Nodular dermal infiltrates, located in the upper and mid dermis, but may extend into the deep dermis
- Reactive lymph follicles with macrophages containing ingested nuclear material (Fleming's tingible body macrophages) within the follicles, producing a "starry sky" pattern

- Small lymphocytes surrounding the reactive lymph follicles and large follicle center cells (centroblasts)
- Interfollicular area composed of small B-cells, loosely arranged small T-cells, histiocytes and some eosinophils and plasma cells, spreading between collagen bundles and rendering the border less well demarcated than in cutaneous B-cell lymphoma, in which the border is convex and sharply demarcated

Immunophenotype: Polyclonal B-lymphocytic infiltrate (CD20; CD79a) without immunoglobulin (Ig) heavy or light chain restriction; however, monotypic expression of kappa or lambda chains can be identified in some cases. Regular and sharply demarcated network of CD21+ follicular dendritic cells in the reactive lymph follicles. Lymphocytes expressing T-cell markers in the interfollicular areas.

DD: Marginal zone lymphoma and follicle center lymphoma.

Differentiation between B-Pseudolymphoma (PL) and Cutaneous B-Cell Lymphoma (CBCL)

	CBCL	PL
Clinical features		
Number of lesions	Solitary or multiple	Usually solitary
Extracutaneous involvement	Possible	Absent
Recurrences	Likely	Unusual
Survival time	Affected	Not affected
Histological features		
Pattern of infiltrate	Diffuse or nodular, "bottom-heavy"	Nodular (>90%), "top-heavy"
Additional cells	Usually absent	Eosinophils, plasma cells
Transformation	May occur	Never occurs
Border of the infiltrate	Sharply demarcated, concave	Lacerated, convex
Immunophenotype		
Immunoglobulin light chains	Monotypic	Polytypic expression (kappa or lambda)
B-cell marker expressing cells	>50% cells	≤50% cells
T-cell marker expressing cells	Few	>50% cells
CD21-positive dendritic cells	Mostly absent or grossly irregular pattern	Mostly present, regular pattern
Genotype		
Ig heavy chain rearrangement	Present in most cases	Absent in most cases

References

Baefverstedt, B. (1944) Ueber lymphadenosis benigna cutis.Eine klinische pathologisch-anatomische Studie. *Acta Derm Venereol (Suppl XI) (Stockh)* **24**: 1–102.

Buechner, S.A., Lautenschlager, S., Itin, P., Bircher, A., and Erb, P. (1995) Lymphoproliferative responses to Borrelia burgdorferi in patients with erythema migrans, acrodermatitis chronica atrophicans, lymphadenosis benigna cutis, and morphea. *Arch Dermatol* **131**(6): 673–7.

Colli, C., Leinweber, B., Mullegger, R., Chott, A., Kerl, H., and Cerroni, L. (2004) Borrelia burgdorferi-associated lymphocytoma cutis: clinicopathologic, immunophenotypic, and molecular study of 106 cases. *J Cutan Pathol* **31**(3): 232–40.

Duncan, S.C., Evans, H.L., and Winkelmann, R.K. (1980) Large cell lymphocytoma. *Arch Dermatol* **116**(10): 1142–6.

Falco, O.B. and Burg, G. (1975) [Lymphoreticular proliferations in the skin. Cytochemical and immunocytological studies in lymphadenosis benigna cutis] *Hautarzt* **26**(3): 124–32.

Moulonguet, I., Ghnassia, M., Molina, T., and Fraitag, S. (2012) Miliarial-type perifollicular B-cell pseudolymphoma (lymphocytoma cutis): a misleading eruption in two women. *J Cutan Pathol* **39**(11): 1016–21.

Nakayama, H., Mihara, M., and Shimao, S. (1987) Malignant transformation of lymphadenosis benigna cutis: a possibly transformed case and B-cell lymphoma. *J Dermatol* **14**(3): 266–9.

Rijlaarsdam, J.U., Meijer, C.J., and Willemze, R. (1990) Differentiation between lymphadenosis benigna cutis and primary cutaneous follicular center cell lymphomas. A comparative clinicopathologic study of 57 patients. *Cancer* **65**(10): 2301–6.

NODULAR T-CELL PL

Schmoeckel, C., Burg, G., Wolf, H.H., and Braun, F.O. (1977) The ultrastructure of lymphadenosis benigna cutis (pseudolymphoma cutis). *Arch Dermatol Res* **258**(2): 161–7.

Watanabe, R., Nanko, H., and Fukuda, S. (2006) Lymphocytoma cutis due to pierced earrings. *J Cutan Pathol* **33**(Suppl 2): 16–19.

Wood, G.S., Kamath, N.V., Guitart, J., et al. (2001) Absence of Borrelia burgdorferi DNA in cutaneous B-cell lymphomas from the United States. *J Cutan Pathol* **28**(10): 502–7.

Nodular T-Cell PL

CD30+ Pseudolymphoma in Scabies

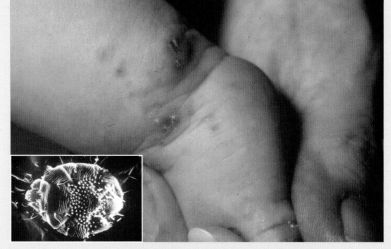

Scabies in a child. Inset: mite

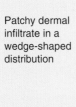

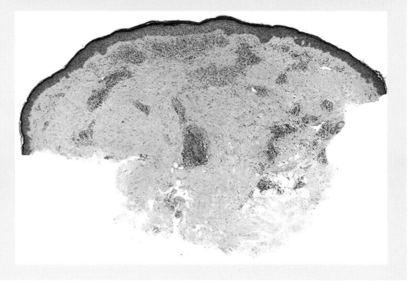

Patchy dermal infiltrate in a wedge-shaped distribution

NODULAR T-CELL PL

CD30+ Pseudolymphoma in Scabies

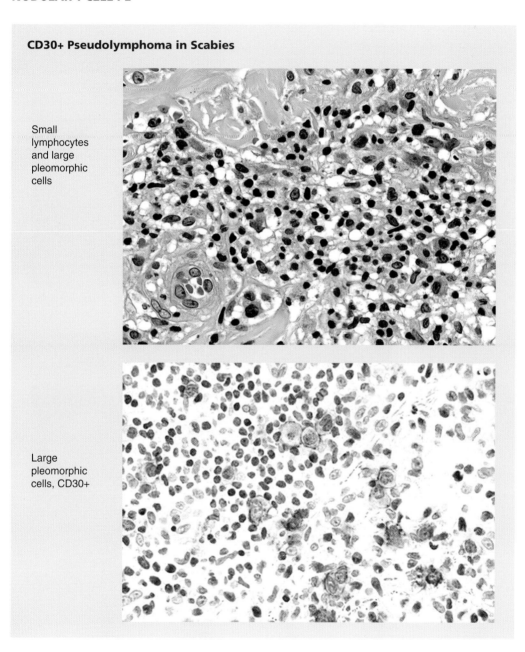

Small lymphocytes and large pleomorphic cells

Large pleomorphic cells, CD30+

Cl: Nodular lesion at the site of a tick bite,
Hi: Wedge-shaped infiltrate composed of activated polyclonal T helper cells (CD3+, CD4+) and admixture of a few medium-sized to large activated CD30+ T-cells; some eosinophils.

References

Gallardo, F., Barranco, C., Toll, A., and Pujol, R.M. (2002) CD30 antigen expression in cutaneous inflammatory infiltrates of scabies: a dynamic immunophenotypic pattern that should be distinguished from lymphomatoid papulosis. *J Cutan Pathol* **29**(6): 368–73.

Guitart, J. and Hurt, M.A. (1999).Pleomorphic T-cell infiltrate associated with molluscum contagiosum. *Am J Dermatopathol* **21**(2): 178–80.

Kempf, W. (2006) CD30+ lymphoproliferative disorders: histopathology, differential diagnosis, new variants, and simulators. *J Cutan Pathol* **33**(Suppl 1): 58–70.

McCalmont, T.H. and LeBoit, P.E. (2000) A lymphomatoid papule, but not lymphomatoid papulosis! *Am J Dermatopathol* **22**(2): 188–90.

NODULAR T-CELL PL

Papular (Secondary) Syphilis

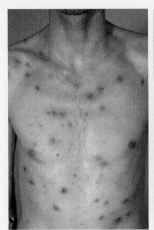
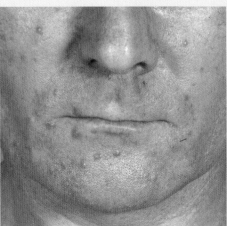

Papulosqua-
mous lesions
on the trunk
and in the face

Dense infiltrate
in the papillary
dermis

Lymphohistio-
cytic dermal
perivascular
Infiltrate (left)

Treponema
pallidum
immunostaining
(inset)

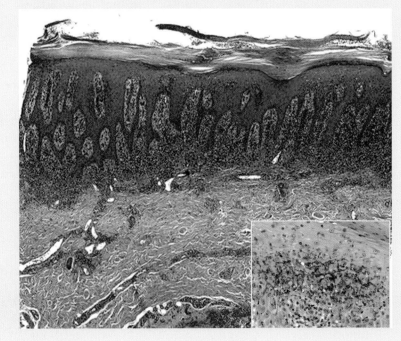

Cl: In late-stage secondary syphilis (>2 years after infection, without treatment), disseminated small papules and papulosquamous lesions may appear on head, trunk, and extremities, including mucous membranes, presenting as plaques and patches on the palms and soles or as condyloma-like lesions in the anogenital region.

Hi:
- Interface dermatitis
- Superficial and deep perivascular and interstitial infiltrate
- Lymphocytes and histiocytes with scattered eosinophils and many plasma cells
- Occasionally granulomatous features
- In early stages of secondary syphilis, spirochetes may be detected using Warthin–Starry stain

DD: Lymphomatoid papulosis; tick bites.

PSEUDO-MYCOSIS FUNGOIDES (MYCOSIS FUNGOIDES SIMULATORS)

References

Hoang, M.P., High, W.A., and Molberg, K.H. (2004) Secondary syphilis: a histologic and immunohistochemical evaluation. *J Cutan Pathol* **31**(9): 595–9.

Park, J.H. and Kım, Y.C. (2013) Secondary syphilis with numerous eosinophils. *J Cutan Pathol* **40**(12): 1063–4.

Pichardo, R.O., Lu, D., Sangueza, O.P., and Tucker, R. (2002) What is your diagnosis? Secondary syphilis. *Am J Dermatopathol* **24**(6): 503–4.

Rysgaard, C., Alexander, E., and Swick, B.L. (2014) Nodular secondary syphilis with associated granulomatous inflammation: case report and literature review. *J Cutan Pathol* **41**(4): 370–9.

Pseudo-Mycosis Fungoides (Mycosis Fungoides Simulators)

Reference

Massone, C., Kodama, K., Kerl, H., and Cerroni, L. (2005).Histopathologic features of early (patch) lesions of mycosis fungoides: a morphologic study on 745 biopsy specimens from 427 patients. *Am J Surg Pathol* **29**(4): 550–60.

Lymphomatoid Contact Dermatitis

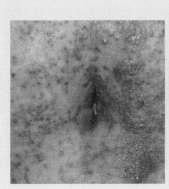
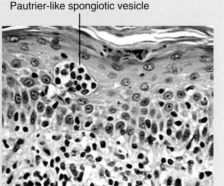

Contact dermatitis against nickel (left)

Pautrier-like spongiotic vesicle

Cl: Red macules and papules in the area of contact with the allergen (chromium, nickel, other) and surroundings.

Hi:

- Acanthosis, spongiosis
- Lymphohistiocytic infiltrate in the upper dermis

- Epidermotropism of single cells or of clusters of lymphocytes, forming Pautrier-like intraepidermal microabscesses
- Eosinophils may be present
- Edema, followed by fibrosis in the upper dermis
- Prominent postcapillary venules

Lichen Planus

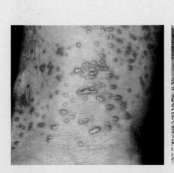
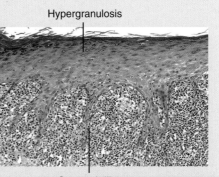

Flat papules (left)

Hypergranulosis

Sawtooth-like elongation of rete ridges

PSEUDO-MYCOSIS FUNGOIDES (MYCOSIS FUNGOIDES SIMULATORS)

Cl: Small papules with whitish smooth surface and Wickham stripes preferentially on the wrist of the arm.

Hi:
- Interface dermatitis
- Acanthosis, sawtooth-like elongation of rete ridges
- V-shaped hypergranulosis, hyperkeratosis

- Subepidermal band-like lymphocytic infiltrate
- *Caveat*: rare cases may harbor clonal T-cells

Reference

Schiller, P.I., Flaig, M.J., Puchta, U., Kind, P., and Sander, C.A. (2000) Detection of clonal T cells in lichen planus. *Arch Dermatol Res* **292**(11): 568–9.

Drug Reactions

Red-bluish well circumscribed plaques (left)

Apoptotic keratinocytes

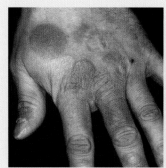
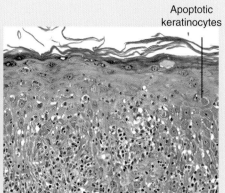

Lichenoid interface dermatitis

Cl: Fixed drug reactions present as well-circumscribed red-brown macular lesion(s).

Hi:
- Very similar to lichen planus, but usually larger number of eosinophils
- Apoptotic keratinocytes
- Extravasation of erythrocytes

Early Vitiligo

Band-like subepidermal infiltrate, simulating patch-stage mycosis fungoides, may be found at the active border of vitiligo.

Lichen Sclerosus et Atrophicus

Whitish atrophic plaques on the trunk (left)

Epidermal atrophy. Band-like lymphocytic infiltrate in the upper dermis (right)

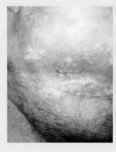
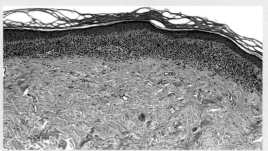

PSEUDO-MYCOSIS FUNGOIDES (MYCOSIS FUNGOIDES SIMULATORS)

Cl: Whitish atrophic plaques; occasional intracutaneous bleeding, especially in the genital area.
Hi: In early lesions, there is interface dermatitis and lymphocytic infiltrate in the papillary dermis. Later lesions develop prominent subepidermal edema and hyalinized connective tissue overlying the lymphocytic infiltrate.

Reference

Citarella, L., Massone, C., Kerl, H., and Cerroni, L. (2003) Lichen sclerosus with histopathologic features simulating early mycosis fungoides. *Am J Dermatopathol* **25**(6): 463–5.

Pityriasis Lichenoides Chronica

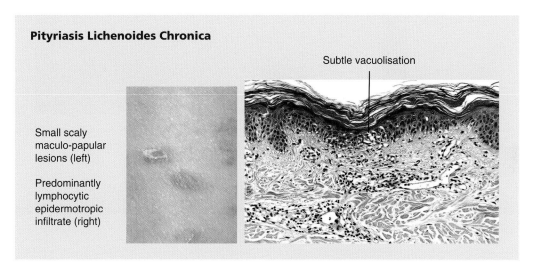

Subtle vacuolisation

Small scaly maculo-papular lesions (left)

Predominantly lymphocytic epidermotropic infiltrate (right)

Cl: Disseminated red scaly maculopapular lesions.
Hi: Focal vacuolisation, spongiosis, hyperparakeratosis with inclusions of neutrophils, wedge-shaped superficial and deep predominant perivascular lymphocytic infiltrate.

Graft Versus Host Reaction (Acute)

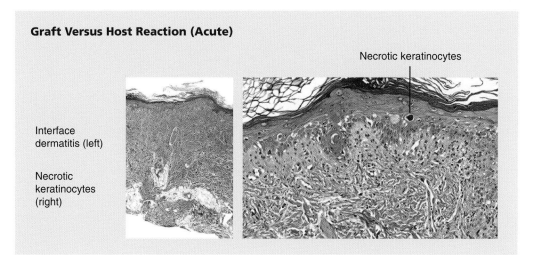

Necrotic keratinocytes

Interface dermatitis (left)

Necrotic keratinocytes (right)

Cl: Maculopapular exanthema.
Hi: Similar to toxic epidermolytic necrolysis (TEN).
- Thinned epidermis
- Numerous apoptotic keratinocytes
- Satellite cell necrosis
- Vacuolar change at the dermoepidermal junction
- Scattered lymphocytic infiltrate in the papillary dermis

PSEUDO-MYCOSIS FUNGOIDES (MYCOSIS FUNGOIDES SIMULATORS)

Pityriasis Lichenoides et Varioliformis Acuta (PLEVA)

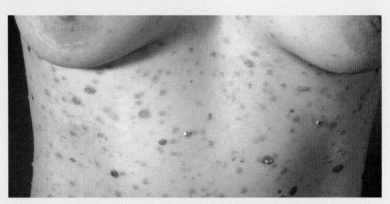

Maculopapular lesions with necrotic crusted center, covered by small scales

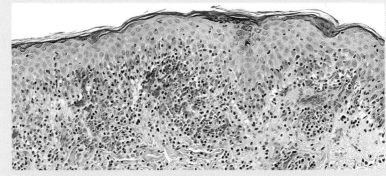

Interface dermatitis and extravasation of erythrocytes (mid and bottom)

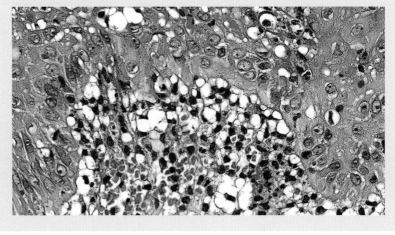

Cl: Preferentially in children, disseminated red scaly maculopapular lesions with necrotic center and crust formation are found. The disease regresses spontaneously within two years or earlier.

Hi:
- Necrotic keratinocytes
- Interface dermatitis, edema
- Lymphocytes in the papillary dermis, some showing epidermotropism
- Erythrocyte extravasation and erythrocytes in the epidermis

PSEUDO-MYCOSIS FUNGOIDES (MYCOSIS FUNGOIDES SIMULATORS)

Pigmented Purpuric Dermatitis (Lichen Aureus)

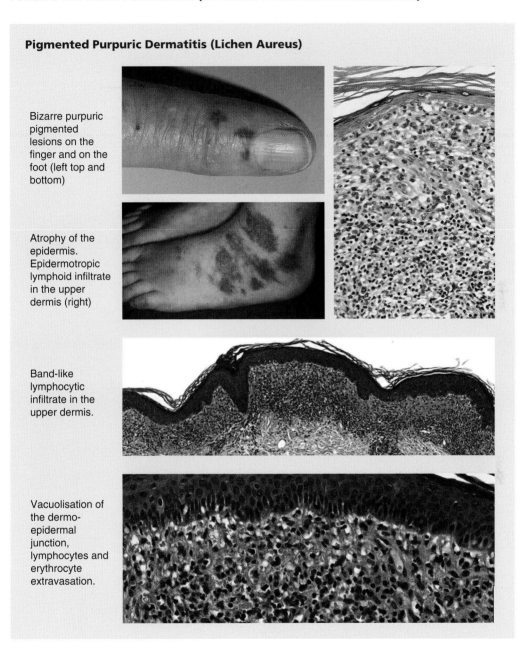

Bizarre purpuric pigmented lesions on the finger and on the foot (left top and bottom)

Atrophy of the epidermis. Epidermotropic lymphoid infiltrate in the upper dermis (right)

Band-like lymphocytic infiltrate in the upper dermis.

Vacuolisation of the dermo-epidermal junction, lymphocytes and erythrocyte extravasation.

Cl: Red-brown macular lesion(s).

Hi:

- Band-like infiltrate
- vacuolisation of the dermoepidermal junction
- Extravasated erythrocytes
- Deposits of hemosiderin (iron stain)

DD: Kaposi's sarcoma (clinically); cutaneous T-cell lymphoma; lichen planus.

PSEUDO-MYCOSIS FUNGOIDES (MYCOSIS FUNGOIDES SIMULATORS)

References

Macquarrie, E.K., Pasternak, S., Torok, M., Veerassamy, S., and Walsh, N.M. (2011) Persistent pigmented purpuric dermatitis: granulomatous variant. *J Cutan Pathol* **38**(12): 979–83.

Smoller, B.R. and Kamel, O.W. (1991) Pigmented purpuric eruptions: immunopathologic studies supportive of a common immunophenotype. *J Cutan Pathol* **18**(6): 423–7.

Toro, J.R., Sander, C.A., and LeBoit, P.E. (1997) Persistent pigmented purpuric dermatitis and mycosis fungoides: simulant, precursor, or both? A study by light microscopy and molecular methods. *Am J Dermatopathol* **19**(2): 108–18.

Lymphocytic Infiltration Jessner–Kanof

Perivascular and periadnexial lymphocytic infiltrates in the upper and mid dermis

Inset: Erythematous swelling suborbital

Patchy lymphocytic Infiltrates with CD 123-positive plasmacytoid dendritic cells

Although the original presentation by Jessner and Kanof emphasized that the eruption is not due to drugs, most cases seem to be induced by drugs or food ingredients.

CI: According to the original description, the lesions are "flat, discoid, more or less elevated, pinkish to reddish brown ... sometimes showing a circinate arrangement ... They disappear without sequelae and may return ... These cases must be distinguished particularly from ... drug eruption ... the face is the area of predilection.

MYCOSIS FUNGOIDES

Hi:
- Normal epidermis
- Patchy well-circumscribed polyclonal lympho-cytic infiltrates in the upper and mid dermis, perivascular and periadnexal
- Predominantly T-cells but B-cells are also present

DD: Other pseudolymphomatous reactions; lupus erythematosus; acute contact dermatitis.

References

Facchetti, F., Boden, G., de Wolf-Peeters, C., Vandaele, R., Degreef, H., and Desmet, V.J. (1990) Plasmacytoid monocytes in Jessner's lymphocytic infiltration of the skin. *Am J Dermatopathol* **12**(4): 363–9.

Jessner, M. and Kanof, N.B. (1953) Lymphocytic infil-tration of the skin. *Arch Dermatol* **68**: 447–9.

Kuo, T.T., Lo, S.K., and Chan, H.L. (1994) Immunohistochemical analysis of dermal mononu-clear cell infiltrates in cutaneous lupus erythemato-sus, polymorphous light eruption, lymphocytic infiltration of Jessner, and cutaneous lymphoid hyperplasia: a comparative differential study. *J Cutan Pathol* **21**(5): 430–6.

Toonstra, J., and van der Putte, S.C. (1991) Plasmacytoid monocytes in Jessner's lymphocytic infiltration of the skin. A valuable clue for the diagnosis. *Am J Dermatopathol* **13**(4): 321–8.

Weyers, W., Bonczkowitz, M., and Weyers, I. (1998) LE or not LE – that is the question: an unsuccessful attempt to separate lymphocytic infiltration from the spectrum of discoid lupus erythematosus. *Am J Dermatopathol* **20**(3): 225–32.

Cutaneous Mature T-Cell Lymphoid Neoplasms (CTCL)

Mycosis Fungoides, Classic Alibert–Bazin Type

Mycosis fungoides (MF) is the most common peripheral cutaneous T-cell lymphoma, initially and preferentially presenting in the skin and showing distinct clinical, histological (except in early stages), immunophenotypical, and geno-typical features. It is slowly progressive over years and decades, developing stepwise through three clinical stages: patch stage, plaque stage, and tumor stage. Transformation into large cell lymphoma and extracutaneous spread may occur in the final stage of the disease. Besides the classic form of MF, there are many variants, presenting as erythrodermic, hypo- and hyper-pigmented, follicular, granulomatous, bullous, hyperkeratotic, palmoplantar, ichthyosiform, and other forms.

Reference

Kazakov, D.V., Burg, G., and Kempf, W. (2004) Clinicopathological spectrum of mycosis fungoides. *J Eur Acad Dermatol Venereol* **18**(4): 397–415.

Mycosis Fungoides Patch Stage I

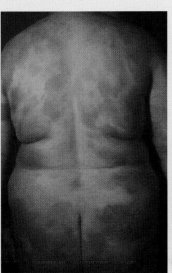
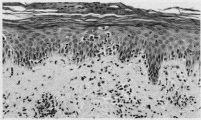
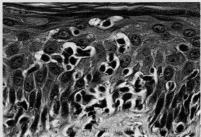

Patches on the trunk (left)

Epidermotropic infiltrate (right top and bottom)

MYCOSIS FUNGOIDES

Mycosis Fungoides Patch Stage I

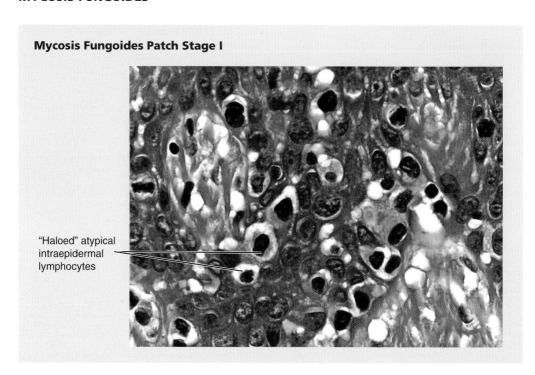

"Haloed" atypical intraepidermal lymphocytes

The diagnosis of mycosis fungoides in early patch stage is one of the most challenging difficulties in dermatopathology. Many inflammatory conditions showing interface dermatitis, epidermotropism of lymphoid cells and prominent postcapillary venules can simulate patch-stage MF. Additional clinical and/or molecular information and long-term clinical follow-up are needed to make a correct diagnosis.

Cl: Multiple non-specific eczematous patches with no or subtle scaling, resembling chronic eczema, chronic superficial dermatitis ("parapsoriasis") or tinea corporis.

Hi: Differentiation of the non-specific lesions from superficial dermatitis may be difficult or impossible.

- Epidermis normal or slightly hyperkeratotic; no spongiosis
- Slight edema and small lymphocytes in the papillary dermis
- Lymphocytes (more than three in a row) in the basal layer of the epidermis, especially at the tips of the rete ridges

DD: Chronic (atopic) dermatitis; parapsoriasis; superficial fungal infection.

References

Massone, C., Kodama, K., Kerl, H., and Cerroni, L. (2005) Histopathologic features of early (patch) lesions of mycosis fungoides: a morphologic study on 745 biopsy specimens from 427 patients. *Am J Surg Pathol* **29**(4): 550–60.

Pimpinelli, N., Olsen, E.A., Santucci, M., et al. (2005) Defining early mycosis fungoides. *J Am Acad Dermatol* **53**(6): 1053–63.

Santucci, M., Biggeri, A., Feller, A.C., Massi, D., and Burg, G. (2000) Efficacy of histologic criteria for diagnosing early mycosis fungoides: an EORTC cutaneous lymphoma study group investigation. European Organization for Research and Treatment of Cancer. *Am J Surg Pathol* **24**(1): 40–50.

MYCOSIS FUNGOIDES

Mycosis Fungoides Plaque Stage II (CD4+; CD8–)

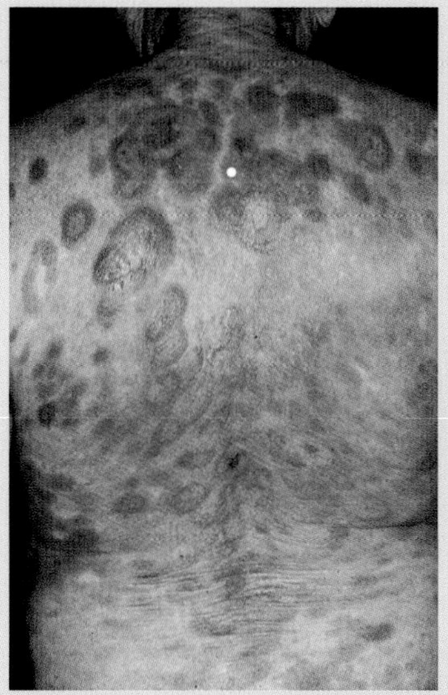

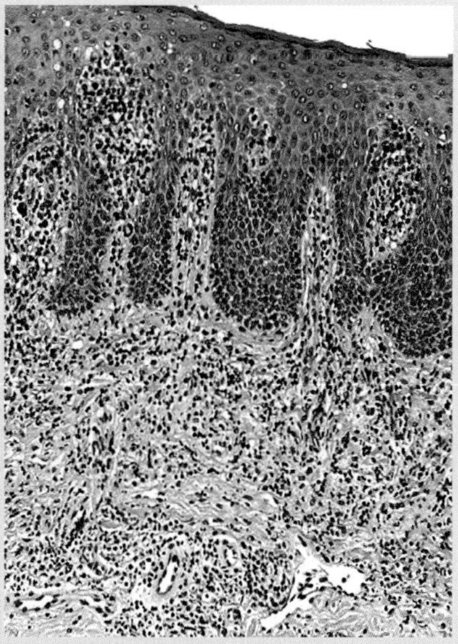

Plaques on the trunk (left)

Acanthosis, papillomatosis, band-like infiltrate in the upper dermis (right)

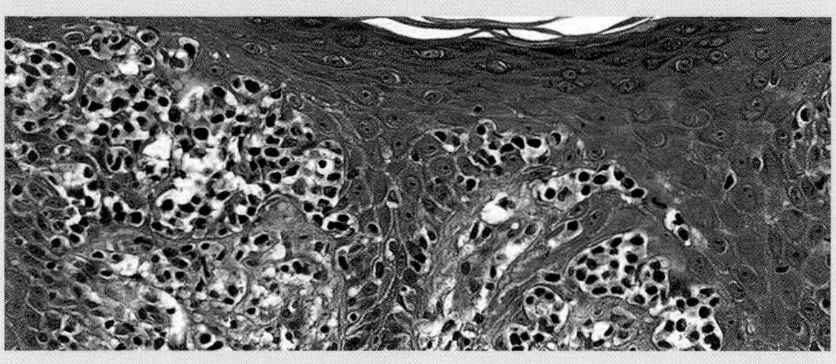

Epidermotropic infiltrate

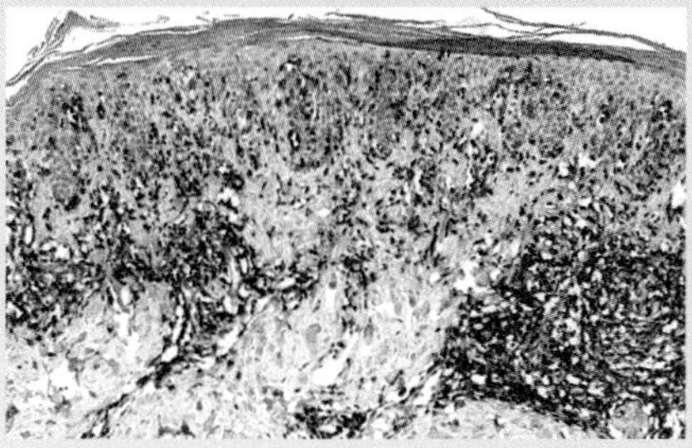

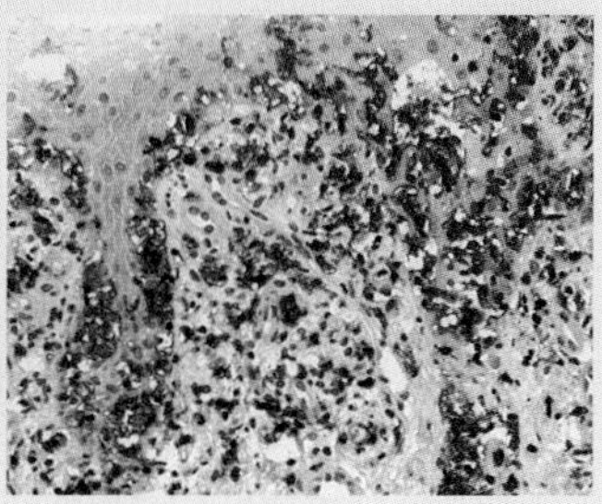

CD4+ (left). Variant: CD8+ (right)

MYCOSIS FUNGOIDES

Mycosis Fungoides Plaque Stage II, Planta

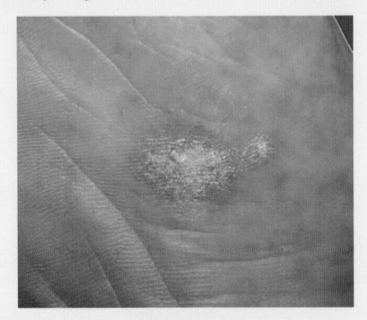

Plantar hyperkeratotic plaque

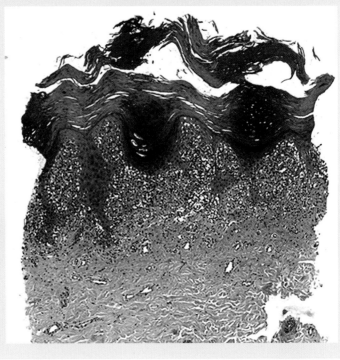

Plantar hyperkeratosis and acanthosis. Band-like subepidermal infiltrate

Cl: After some years or even decades, patches transform into infiltrated, sometimes itchy plaques. **Hi**: In this stage of the disease, the diagnosis can be made due to typical histopathological features.

- Variable hyperkeratosis

- Acanthosis and papillomatosis of the epidermis with elongation of the rete ridges
- Edema in the papillary dermis
- Band-like infiltrate of small lymphocytes with cerebriform nuclei in the upper dermis

MYCOSIS FUNGOIDES

- Epidermotropism of lymphocytes:
  - Single cells in the basal layer, especially on the tips of rete ridges
  - Small intraepidermal clusters (Pautrier microabscesses)
  - Intraepidermal lymphocytes have a halo and appear larger than small lymphocytes in the dermis
- Eosinophils and plasma cells present
- Prominent postcapillary (high endothelial) venules in the upper and mid dermis. This is commonly seen in all cutaneous T-cell infiltrates and is not specific for cutaneous T-cell lymphomas

Variant: CD8+ Mycosis Fungoides

Cl: Corresponds to the classic CD4+ type of mycosis fungoides. Good prognosis.

Hi:
- Superficial band-like infiltrate
- Epidermotropism of lymphocytes
- Absence of apoptotic keratinocytes. No necrosis
- Small lymphocytes. Subtle nuclear atypia
- Intraepidermal CD8+ T-cell clone, occasionally pagetoid infiltration into the epidermis as seen in pagetoid reticulosis (see below)

Immunophenotype: CD2−, CD3+, CD4−, CD5−, CD8+, TIA-1+, CD7+.

Reference

Nikolaou, V.A., Papadavid, E., Katsambas, A., et al. (2009) Clinical characteristics and course of CD8+ cytotoxic variant of mycosis fungoides: a case series of seven patients. *Br J Dermatol* **161**(4): 826–30.

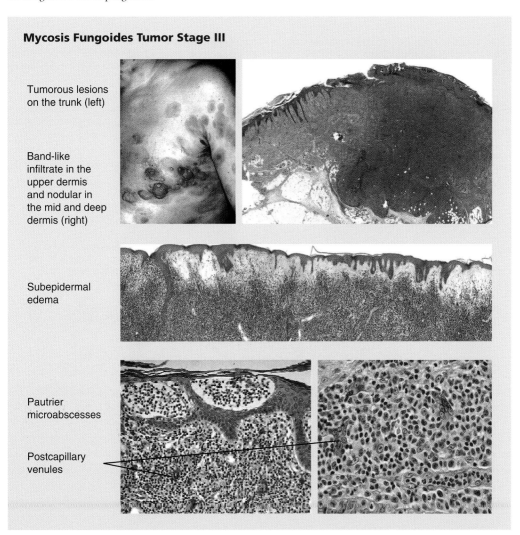

Mycosis Fungoides Tumor Stage III

Tumorous lesions on the trunk (left)

Band-like infiltrate in the upper dermis and nodular in the mid and deep dermis (right)

Subepidermal edema

Pautrier microabscesses

Postcapillary venules

MYCOSIS FUNGOIDES

Cl: Soft tumors, developing either on normal-looking skin (d'emblé) or on pre-existing plaques. Surface mostly ulcerated.

Hi:

- Nodular and diffuse infiltrate, covering all layers of the dermis
- Epidermotropism may be lost
- In addition to a predominant population of small cerebriform cells, there is a variable admixture of immunoblasts, lymphoblasts, and medium-sized or large pleomorphic or anaplastic cells
- When transformation into higher malignancy occurs, large atypical CD30+ cells appear and may even predominate

Immunohistochemistry: The typical phenotype of the neoplastic cell is CD2+, CD3+, CD5+, CD4+, CD45RO+, beta-F1+, CD8−. In rare cases expression of CD30 is found in the patch or plaque stage. In tumor stage, expression of CD30 by a variable number of large tumor cells is observed. In rare cases, expression of CD8 and TCRdelta can occur. As the disease progresses, an aberrant phenotype with loss of mature T-cell antigens is a common finding.

Reference

Smoller, B.R. (1997) The role of immunohistochemistry in the diagnosis of cutaneous lymphoma. *Adv Dermatol* **13**: 207–34.

Comment: Functionally, the neoplastic cells in MF express TH2 phenotype, which accounts for many systemic changes associated with MF due to the production of a TH2-specific cytokine pattern (IL-4, IL-5, IL-10, and others) leading to eosinophilia, increase of IgE or IgA, impaired delayed type reactivity, and itching.

References

Dummer, R. and Schwarz, T. (1994) Cytokines as regulatory proteins in lymphoproliferative skin infiltrates. *Dermatol Clin* **12**(2): 283–94.

Vowels, B.R., Lessin, S.R., Cassin, M., et al. (1994) Th2 cytokine mRNA expression in skin in cutaneous T-cell lymphoma. *J Invest Dermatol* **103**(5): 669–73.

Molecular biology: TCR beta or gamma chain genes are clonally rearranged in most cases of mycosis fungoides.

References

Bergman, R. (1999) How useful are T-cell receptor gene rearrangement studies as an adjunct to the histopathologic diagnosis of mycosis fungoides? *Am J Dermatopathol* **21**(5): 498–502.

Guitart, J. and Kaul, K. (1999) A new polymerase chain reaction-based method for the detection of T- cell clonality in patients with possible cutaneous T-cell lymphoma [see comments]. *Arch Dermatol* **135**(2): 158–62.

Large Cell Transformation

Small and large atypical lymphoid cells (left)

CD30+ cells (right)

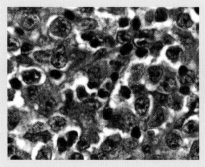
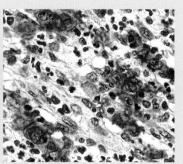

Cl: Plaques or tumors may show sudden progression, different from the indolent course in past years. Involvement of mucous membranes, which usually are unaffected in "classic" mycosis fungoides, may occur.

Hi:

- Loss of epidermotropism

- The hallmark is the appearance of large atypical cells with pleomorphic nuclei and abundant cytoplasm within the infiltrate of predominantly small cerebriform lymphocytes. These large cells express the CD30 antigen

SIMULATORS AND VARIANTS OF MYCOSIS FUNGOIDES

Simulators and Variants of Mycosis Fungoides: "Parapsoriasis"

The term *parapsoriasis* is confusing. It encompasses a number of different pathological states clinically manifested by chronic recalcitrant erythematous scaling lesions.

In the context of mycosis fungoides, three types have to be differentiated.

- "Parapsoriasis en gouttes" (guttate parapsoriasis; pityriasis lichenoides chronica; parapsoriasis guttata of Jadassohn and Juliusberg). Nosologically, it is completely unrelated to mycosis fungoides
- "Parapsoriasis lichenoides," featuring a poikilodermatous appearance
- "Parapsoriasis en plaques" (Brocq's disease), referred to as small plaque parapsoriasis

The common features of the subgroups described by Brocq are:

- Long duration of the disease
- Good general health
- Absence of itching
- Erythema and pityriasiform scaling
- Control of disease without cure by topical treatment
- Round cell infiltrate in the papillary dermis

References

Brocq, L. (1902) Les parapsoriasis. *Ann Dermatol Syphilol* **3**: 433–68.

Burg, G., Kempf, W., Dummer, R., and Kazakov, D.V. (2005) Parapsoriasis. In: Burg, G. and Kempf, W. (eds) *Cutaneous Lymphomas*. Boca Raton: CRC Press.

Simulator: Small Plaque Parapsoriasis (SPP) (Brocq's Disease, Digitate Dermatosis)

Small macules along the tension lines on the trunk (left)

Scattered lymphocytes in the papillary dermis (right)

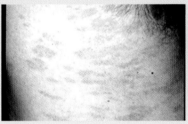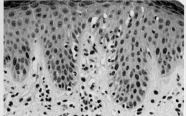

Cl: Round or oval well-circumscribed macules preferentially on the trunk along the tension lines of the skin. This disease shares some features with early patch-stage mycosis fungoides. However, the clinical, histological, and prognostic characteristics favor a nosological disease, whereas large plaque parapsoriasis (see below) is identical with early patch-stage mycosis fungoides.

Hi: Simulates normal skin.

- Epidermis normal or slightly acanthotic
- Some scattered lymphocytes in the dermis
- No marked epidermotropism, in contrast to early lesions in MF
- No edema in the papillary dermis

References

Ackerman, A.B. (1996) If small plaque (digitate) parapsoriasis is a cutaneous T-cell lymphoma, even an 'abortive' one, it must be mycosis fungoides! *Arch Dermatol* **132**(5): 562–6.

Burg, G. and Dummer, R. (1995) Small plaque (digitate) parapsoriasis is an 'abortive cutaneous T-cell lymphoma' and is not mycosis fungoides. *Arch Dermatol* **131**(3): 336–8.

Burg, G., Dummer, R., Nestle, F.O., Doebbeling, U., and Haeffner, A. (1996) Cutaneous lymphomas consist of a spectrum of nosologically different entities including mycosis fungoides and small plaque parapsoriasis. *Arch Dermatol* **132**(5): 567–72.

Burg, G., Kempf, W., Dummer, R., and Kazakov, D.V. (2005) Small plaque parapsoriasis. In: Burg, G. and Kempf, W. (eds) *Cutaneous Lymphomas*. Boca Raton: CRC Press.

King, I.D. and Ackerman, A.B. (1992) Guttate parapsoriasis/digitate dermatosis (small plaque parapsoriasis) is mycosis fungoides [see comments]. *Am J Dermatopathol* **14**(6): 518–30.

Schmoeckel, C., Burg, G., and Braun, F.O. (1979) Quantitative analysis of lymphoid cells in mycosis fungoides, Sezary's syndrome and parapsoriasis en plaques. *Arch Dermatol Res* **264**(1): 17–28.

SIMULATORS AND VARIANTS OF MYCOSIS FUNGOIDES

Large Plaque Parapsoriasis (LPP)

Large plaques
on the trunk
(left)

Epidermotropic
infiltrate (right)

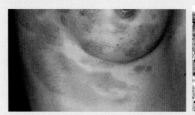
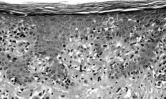

Variant: Large Plaque Parapsoriasis with Poikiloderma

Poikiloderma
(left)

Atrophy of the
epidermis (right)

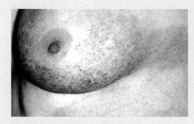
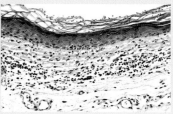

Large plaque parapsoriasis is an indolent form of early patch-stage mycosis fungoides, showing no or only slow progression over years or decades. This distinct favorable prognosis has an impact on therapy, which should be conservative and topical rather than aggressive and systemic.

Cl: Preferentially on the trunk there are large (>10 cm), fairly demarcated, irregularly shaped erythematous patches with pityriasiform scaling. *Poikiloderma atrophicans vasculare* is a special variant occurring in light protected areas and showing a reticular network of hyperpigmentation, atrophy, and telangiectasia. Transformation into the plaque and tumor stages of mycosis fungoides may occur after decades.

Hi:

- Epidermis is normal or slightly acanthotic. The poikilodermatous variant shows atrophy of the epidermis
- Scarce lymphocytic infiltrate in the papillary dermis
- Single cell epidermotropism with arrangement of lymphocytes along the basal layer
- Spongiosis usually is absent
- Intraepidermal lymphocytes are often larger than those seen in the dermal infiltrate

Immunophenotype and Genetic Features: CD4+, CD8−, CD45RO+, beta-F1 +.

Genotype: Clonal T-cell receptor rearrangement in about 50% of cases.

Reference

Burg, G., Kempf, W., Dummer, R., and Kazakov, D.V. (2005) Large plaque parapsoriasis with and wthout poikiloderma. In: Burg, G. and Kempf, W. (eds) *Cutaneous Lymphomas*. Boca Raton: CRC Press.

Pigmented Purpuric Mycosis Fungoides

Cl: Hyperpigmented, mostly macular lesions.

Hi: Erythrocyte extravasation. Hemosiderin in macrophages of the upper dermis.

DD: Lichenoid pigmented purpuric dermatitis of Gougerot–Blum.

Reference

Lor, P., Krueger, U., Kempf, W., Burg, G., and Nestle, F.O. (2002) Monoclonal rearrangement of the T cell receptor gamma-chain in lichenoid pigmented purpuric dermatitis of gougerot-blum responding to topical corticosteroid therapy. *Dermatology* **205**(2): 191–3.

Erythrodermic Mycosis Fungoides

Cl: In primary erythroderma, as seen in Sézary syndrome (see below), 100% of the skin is involved from the beginning of the disease. Due to local tissue pressure (skinfolds), clinically some areas may seem to be uninvolved ("deck-chair sign"). Erythroderma in mycosis fungoides

SIMULATORS AND VARIANTS OF MYCOSIS FUNGOIDES

may result from secondary confluence of patches and plaques, leaving non-erythematous islands of uninvolved skin in between, showing at least 80% of skin surface involved. Besides erythema, there usually is pityriasiform scaling and itching.

Hi: Corresponds to the patch or plaque stage of the disease.

Folliculotropic (Pilotropic) Mycosis Fungoides

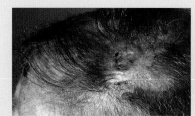

Flat ulcerated nodule on the capillitium

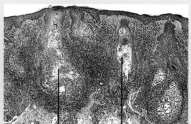

Follicular mucinosis

DD of Folliculotropic MF: Idiopathic Mucinosis Follicularis

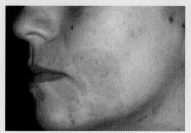

Circumscribed flat plaque in the face

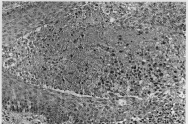

Mucin deposits

Cl: Folliculotropic MF and MF-associated follicular mucinosis belong to a spectrum of MF with a predilection for hair follicles. It presents as erythematous patches or plaques with follicular hyperkeratosis producing comedo-like plugs and often hair loss. Two prognostic subgroups are distinguished: early and advanced disease. The prognosis of the advanced form is worse than in non-follicular variants of MF.

Hi:

- Variably dense lymphocytic infiltrates surrounding and infiltrating the hair follicles and sparing more or less interfollicular skin
- Small to medium-sized lymphocytes with irregular nuclei
- Exocytosis of lymphocytes into the follicular epithelium
- Cystic dilation of the follicles, cornified plugging
- Mucin deposition in the hair follicle epithelia in 50–70% of cases

DD: Idiopathic mucinosis follicularis (Pinkus) showing mucin deposits in the hair follicles without association with cutaneous lymphoma; other forms of mycosis fungoides.

References

Amitay-Laish, I., Feinmesser, M., Ben-Amitai, D., Fenig, E., Sorin, D., and Hodak, E. (2016) Unilesional folliculotropic mycosis fungoides: a unique variant of cutaneous lymphoma. *J Eur Acad Dermatol Venereol* **30**(1): 25–9.

Flaig, M.J., Cerroni, L., Schuhmann, K., et al. (2001) Follicular mycosis fungoides. A histopathologic analysis of nine cases. *J Cutan Pathol* **28**(10): 525–30.

Hodak, E., Amitay-Laish, I., Atzmony, L., et al. (2016) New insights into folliculotropic mycosis fungoides (FMF): a single-center experience. *J Am Acad Dermatol* **75**(2): 347–55.

Kamo, S., Niizuma, K., Machida, S., et al. (1984) Follicular mucinosis developing into cutaneous

SIMULATORS AND VARIANTS OF MYCOSIS FUNGOIDES

lymphoma. Report of two cases and review of literature and 64 cases in Japan. *Acta Derm Venereol Stockh* **64**(1): 86–8.

Pinkus, H. (1957) Alopecia mucinosa. Inflammatory plaques with alopecia characterized by rooth-sheath mucinosis. *Arch Dermatol* **76**: 419–26.

van Doorn, R., Scheffer, E., and Willemze, R. (2002) Follicular mycosis fungoides, a distinct disease entity with or without associated follicular mucinosis: a clinicopathologic and follow-up study of 51 patients. *Arch Dermatol* **138**(2): 191–8.

van Santen, S., Roach, R.E., van Doorn, R., et al. (2016) Clinical staging and prognostic factors in folliculotropic mycosis fungoides. *JAMA Dermatol* **152**(9): 992–1000.

Syringotropic Mycosis Fungoides (Syringolymphoid Hyperplasia with Alopecia)

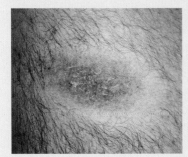

Hairless plaque on the trunk (left)

Lymphocytes in and around hyperplastic glandular structure (right)

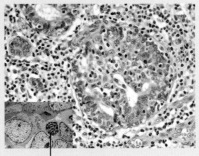

Electron microscopy: cerebriform lymphocyte between glandular epithelial cells

Cl: Male preponderance. Red-brown slightly infiltrated scaling flat plaque. Anhidrosis and hair loss in the affected areas are common.

Hi:

- Proliferation of small eccrine epithelial islands
- Small cerebriform lymphocytes invading both the secretory and ductal portions of hyperplastic eccrine glands
- Epidermotropism is not a prominent feature
- Destruction of hair follicles by the neoplastic infiltrate
- Mucinous degeneration is typically lacking

Immunohistochemistry: CD3+, CD4+, CD8–.

DD: Idiopathic syringolymphoid hyperplasia.

References

Burg, G. and Schmockel, C. (1992) Syringolymphoid hyperplasia with alopecia – a syringotropic cutaneous T-cell lymphoma? *Dermatology* **184**(4): 306–7.

Esche, C., Sander, C.A., Zumdick, M., et al. (1998) Further evidence that syringolymphoid hyperplasia with alopecia is a cutaneous T-cell lymphoma. *Arch Dermatol* **134**(6): 753–4.

Haller, A., Elzubi, E., and Petzelbauer, P. (2001) Localized syringolymphoid hyperplasia with alopecia and anhidrosis. *J Am Acad Dermatol* **45**(1): 127–30.

Hobbs, J.L., Chaffins, M.L., and Douglass, M.C. (2003) Syringolymphoid hyperplasia with alopecia: two case reports and review of the literature. *J Am Acad Dermatol* **49**(6): 1177–80.

Tannous, Z., Baldassano, M.F., Li, V.W., Kvedar, J., and Duncan, L.M. (1999) Syringolymphoid hyperplasia and follicular mucinosis in a patient with cutaneous T-cell lymphoma. *J Am Acad Dermatol* **41**(2 Pt 2): 303–8.

Tomaszewski, M.M., Lupton, G.P., Krishnan, J., Welch, M., and James, W.D. (1994) Syringolymphoid hyperplasia with alopecia. A case report. *J Cutan Pathol* **21**(6): 520–6.

Vijayashree, R., Kumar, A., Nott, A., and Rao, R. (2011) Syringolymphoid hyperplasia with alopecia and anhidrosis in a 12-year-old boy: a case report from rural south India. *Int J Dermatol* **50**(12): 1552–4.

Zelger, B., Sepp, N., Weyrer, K., Grunewald, K., and Zelger, B. (1994) Syringotropic cutaneous T-cell lymphoma: a variant of mycosis fungoides? *Br J Dermatol* **130**(6): 765–9.

GRANULOMATOUS SLACK SKIN

Granulomatous Mycosis Fungoides

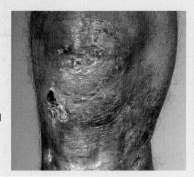
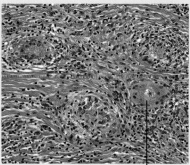

Hyperpigmented crusted patches and plaques on the leg (left)

Fibrosis and focal granulomas with multinucleated giant cells (right)

Asteroid body

Granulomatous changes are frequently seen in cutaneous T-cell lymphomas. The granulomatous process may represent a local tissue response to the infiltrating malignant cells. The influence of granulomatous features on the prognosis is debated but most studies indicate an impaired prognosis.

Cl: Hyperpigmented patches and plaques.

Hi:

- Granulomatous infiltrates, composed of histiocytes, macrophages, and multinucleated giant cells, sometimes hiding the underlying mycosis fungoides
- Small lymphocytes with only subtle nuclear atypia
- Epidermotropism is lacking in 50% of cases

Immunophenotype: CD 3+, CD4+, CD8+/−.

Genotype: Clonal T-cell receptor rearrangement.

DD: Cutaneous sarcoidosis; deep fungal infection.

References

Ackerman, A.B. and Flaxman, B.A. (1970) Granulomatous mycosis fungoides. *Br J Dermatol* **82**(4): 397–401.

Dabski, K. and Stoll, H.L. Jr (1987) Granulomatous reactions in mycosis fungoides. *J Surg Oncol* **34**(4): 217–29.

Kempf, W., Ostheeren-Michaelis, S., Paulli, M., et al. (2008) Granulomatous mycosis fungoides and granulomatous slack skin: a multicenter study of the Cutaneous Lymphoma Histopathology Task Force Group of the European Organization For Research and Treatment of Cancer (EORTC). *Arch Dermatol* **144**(12): 1609–17.

van Haselen, C.W., Toonstra, J., van der Putte, S.J., et al. (1998) Granulomatous slack skin. Report of three patients with an updated review of the literature. *Dermatology* **196**(4): 382–91.

Granulomatous Slack Skin

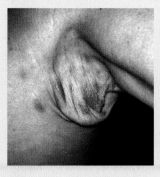
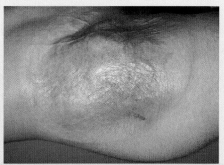

"Slack" skin in the axillary fold (left) and on the hip of the (lying) patient (right)

GRANULOMATOUS SLACK SKIN

Granulomatous Slack Skin

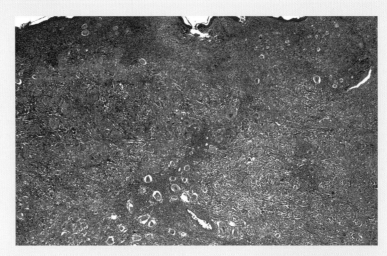

Multinucleated giant cells in a background of lymphoid infiltrate

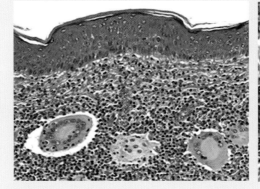

Multinucleated giant cells with phagozytosed lymphocytes (emperipolesis)

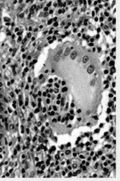

Emperipolesis

Cl: Intertriginous areas, especially the axillary and inguinal areas show "slack" skinfolds due to bulky lymphoid infiltrates and loss of elastic fibers. In non-intertriginous areas, the folding of the slack skin is less obvious and presents as lax skin, resembling cutis laxa.

Hi:

- Loosely distributed, single-layer multinucleated histiocytic giant cells, containing 20–30 nuclei located at the periphery of the abundant eosinophilic cytoplasm within a dense infiltrate of small lymphocytes
- Giant cells contain remnants of elastic fibers and engulfed lymphoid cells. This phenomenon is referred to as *emperipolesis*
- Background of mycosis fungoides showing small cerebriform lymphocytes with variable epidermotropism

- Loss of elastic fibers at the sites of the infiltrate

DD: Cutis laxa.

References

Ackerman, A. (1978) Granulomatous slack skin. In: *Histologic Diagnosis of Inflammatory Skin Diseases.* Philadelphia: Lea and Febiger.

Balus, L., Manente, L., Remotti, D., Grammatico, P., and Bellocci, M. (1996) Granulomatous slack skin. Report of a case and review of the literature. *Am J Dermatopathol* **18**(2): 199–206.

Bazex, A., Dupre, A., and Christol, B. (1968) [Chalazodermic Besnier–Boeck–Schaumann disease?] *Bull Soc Fr Dermatol Syphiligr* **75**(4): 448–9.

Benton, E.C., Morris, S.L., Robson, A., and Whittaker, S.J. (2008) An unusual case of granulomatous slack skin disease with necrobiosis. *Am J Dermatopathol* **30**(5): 462–5.

PAGETOID RETICULOSIS

Camacho, F.M., Burg, G., Moreno, J.C., Campora, R.G., and Villar, J.L. (1997) Granulomatous slack skin in childhood. *Pediatr Dermatol* **14**(3): 204–8.

Convit, J., Kerdel, F., Goihman, M., Rondon, A.J., and Soto, J.M. (1973) Progressive, atrophying, chronic granulomatous dermohypodermitis. Autoimmune disease? *Arch Dermatol* **107**(2): 271–4.

Echeverria, B., Vitiello, M., Milikowski, C., and Kerdel, F. (2015) Granulomatous slack skin-like clinical findings in Sezary syndrome. *J Cutan Pathol* Aug 12. doi: 10.1111/cup.12592 [epub ahead of print].

Ferrara, G. and Stefanato, C.M. (2013) Mycosis fungoides with reactive lymphoid follicles may represent an early histopathologic picture of granulomatous slack skin. *J Cutan Pathol* **40**(6): 611–13.

LeBoit, P.E., Beckstead, J.H., Bond, B., Epstein, W.L., Frieden, I.J., and Parslow, T.G. (1987) Granulomatous slack skin: clonal rearrangement of the T-cell receptor beta gene is evidence for the lymphoproliferative nature of a cutaneous elastolytic disorder. *J Invest Dermatol* **89**(2): 183–6.

Metzler, G., Schlagenhauff, B., Krober, S.M., Kaiserling, E., Schaumburg-Lever, G., and Lischka, G. (1999) Granulomatous mycosis fungoides: report of a case with some histopathologic features of granulomatous slack skin. *Am J Dermatopathol* **21**(2): 156–60.

Tronnier, M. (2009) Foreign-body-associated granulomatous slack skin in folliculotropic mycosis fungoides of childhood. *J Cutan Pathol* **36**(5): 578–81.

Tsang, W.Y., Chan, J.K., Loo, K.T., Wong, K.F., and Lee, A.W. (1994) Granulomatous slack skin. *Histopathology* **25**(1): 49–55.

Pagetoid Reticulosis (PR), Unilesional (Woringer–Kolopp)

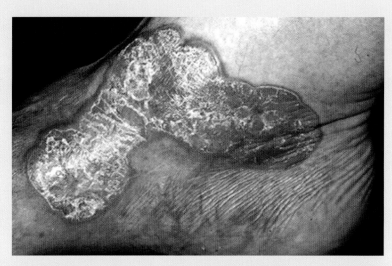

Well demarcated psoriasiform lesion

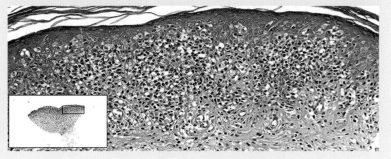

Epidermotropic band-like infiltrate in the epidermis and the upper dermis

SÉZARY SYNDROME (SS)

Pagetoid Reticulosis (PR), Unilesional (Woringer–Kolopp)

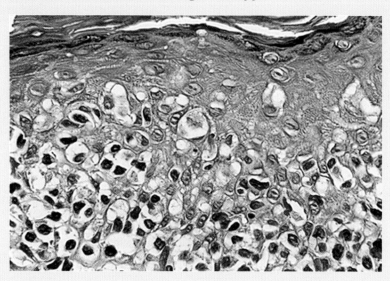

Sponge-like disaggregation of keratino-cytes by lymphoid cells with abundant cytoplasm

The term *pagetoid reticulosis*, proposed by Braun-Falco, should be used to designate only the unilesional Woringer–Kolopp type. The term *disseminated Ketron and Goodman type* is no longer used since it represents other forms of CTCL.

Cl: Solitary psoriasiform or bowenoid erythematous, scaling or crusty centrifugally growing plaque with preferential acral localisation.

Hi:
- Marked psoriasiform hyperplasia of the epidermis with para- and orthohyperkeratosis

- Sponge-like disaggregation of the acanthotic epidermis by medium-sized to large atypical lymphoid cells with vacuolated, abundant cytoplasm, singly or arranged in clusters
- Single cells and small clusters of tumor cells can also be observed within the epithelia of adnexal structures

Sézary Syndrome (SS)

Erythroderma, swelling of, lymph nodes, scaling (left)

"Nappes claires" (right top) and palmar hyperkeratosis (right bottom)

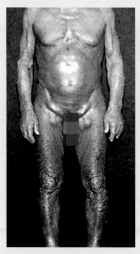
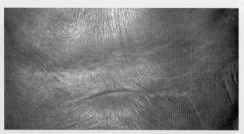
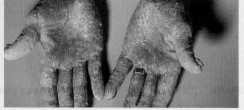

SÉZARY SYNDROME (SS)

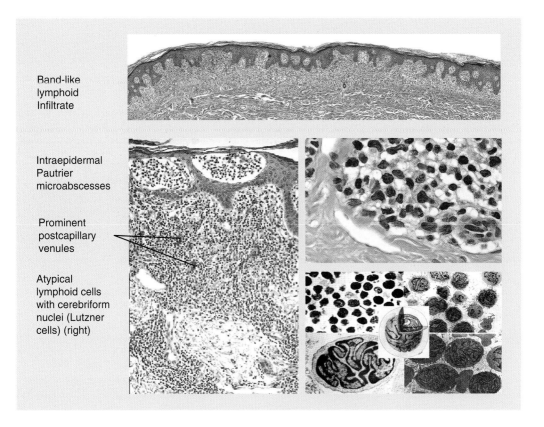

Band-like lymphoid Infiltrate

Intraepidermal Pautrier microabscesses

Prominent postcapillary venules

Atypical lymphoid cells with cerebriform nuclei (Lutzner cells) (right)

Cl: (Primary) edematous erythroderma with scaling and "nappes claires" ("deck-chair sign"; non-erythematous skinfolds), generalized lymphadenopathy, intense pruritus, palmoplantar hyperkeratosis, diffuse alopecia, onychodystrophy, leukemic spread of tumor cells with atypical cerebriform nuclei (Lutzner cells).

Hi:

- Psoriasiform acanthosis of the epidermis
- Lichenoid subepidermal perivascular or band-like infiltrate composed of predominantly small lymphocytes with or without nuclear atypia
- Epidermotropism and lining up of lymphocytes with cerebriform nuclei
- Pautrier microabscesses not regularly present
- Edema in the upper dermis, followed by fibrosis

Lymph nodes show dermatopathic changes in early stages of the disease, whereas effacement of normal architecture by a dense, diffuse, and monotonous infiltration of small lymphoid cells is found in later stages with specific involvement.

Immunophenotype : CD 2+, CD 3+, CD4+, CD 5+, CD 45RO+, CD 30−. Expression of PD-1 and TOX by more than 50% of the lymphocytes.

Genotype: Clonal T-cell receptor rearrangement.

DD: The so-called red man syndrome encompasses cases of erythroderma which cannot be assigned to any other underlying disease such as atopic dermatitis, psoriasis, and pityriasis rubra pilaris.

References

Bernengo, M.G., Novelli, M., Quaglino, P., et al. (2001) The relevance of the CD4+ CD26- subset in the identification of circulating Sezary cells. *Br J Dermatol* **144**(1): 125–35.

Imai, S., Burg, G., and Braun-Falco, O. (1986) Mycosis fungoides and Sezary's syndrome show distinct histomorphological features. *Dermatologica* **173**(3): 131–5.

Lutzner, M.A. and Jordan, H.W. (1968) The ultrastructure of an abnormal cell in Sezary's syndrome. *Blood* **31**(6): 719–26.

Marti, R.M., Pujol, R.M., Servitje, O., et al. (2003) Sezary syndrome and related variants of classic cutaneous T-cell lymphoma. A descriptive and prognostic clinicopathologic study of 29 cases. *Leuk Lymphoma* **44**(1): 59–69.

SÉZARY SYNDROME (SS)

Thestrup-Petersen, K., Halkier-Sorensen, L., Sogaard, H., and Zachariae, H. (1988) The red man syndrome. Exfoliative dermatitis of unknown etiology: a description and follow up of 38 patients. *J Am Acad Dermatol* **18**: 1307–12.

Vonderheid, E.C., Bigler, R.D., Kotecha, A., et al. (2001) Variable CD7 expression on T cells in the leukemic phase of cutaneous T cell lymphoma (Sezary syndrome). *J Invest Dermatol* **117**(3): 654–62.

Vonderheid, E.C., Bernengo, M.G., Burg, G., et al. (2002) Update on erythrodermic cutaneous T-cell lymphoma: report of the International Society for Cutaneous Lymphomas. *J Am Acad Dermatol* **46**(1): 95–106.

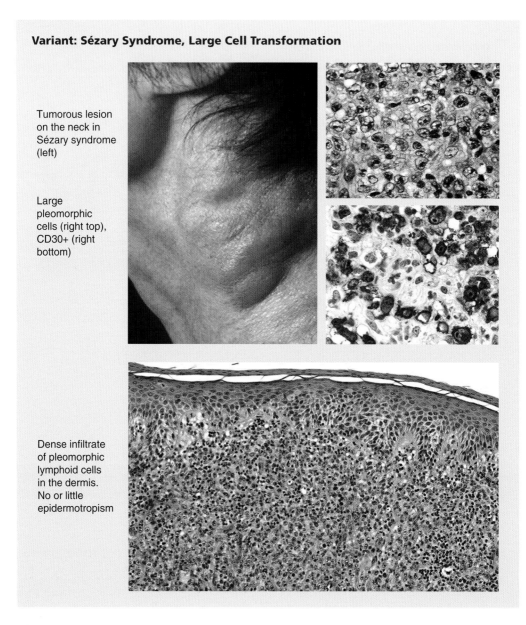

Variant: Sézary Syndrome, Large Cell Transformation

Tumorous lesion on the neck in Sézary syndrome (left)

Large pleomorphic cells (right top), CD30+ (right bottom)

Dense infiltrate of pleomorphic lymphoid cells in the dermis. No or little epidermotropism

Cl: Development of nodules and tumors against the background of erythroderma.

SÉZARY SYNDROME (SS)

DD of SS: Erythrodermic Atopic Dermatitis

White
dermographism
in a patient with
atopic
erythroderma

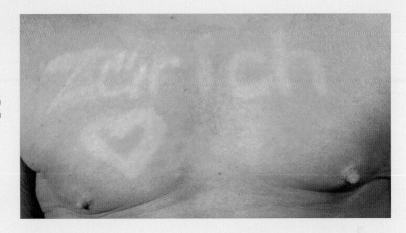

Broad acanthosis and
papillomatosis

Predominantly
lymphocytic
inflammatory
infiltrate in the
upper dermis,
without epider-
motropism
or edema

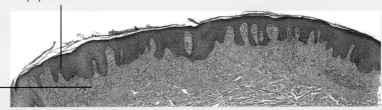

Predominantly
lymphocytic
inflammatory
infiltrate

Scattered
eosinophils

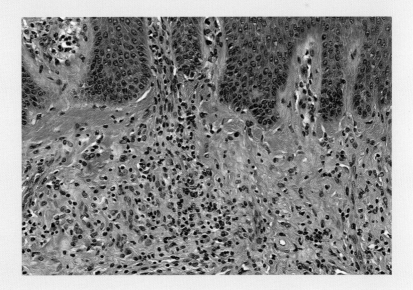

SÉZARY SYNDROME (SS)

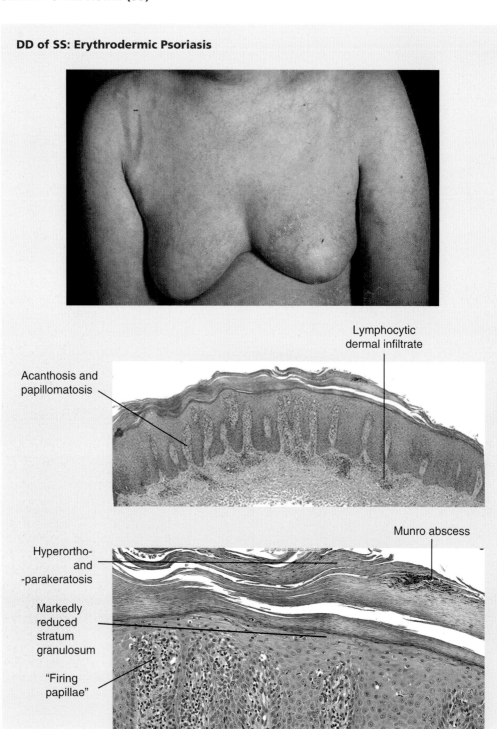

DD of SS: Erythrodermic Psoriasis

SÉZARY SYNDROME (SS)

DD of SS: Pityriasis Rubra Pilaris

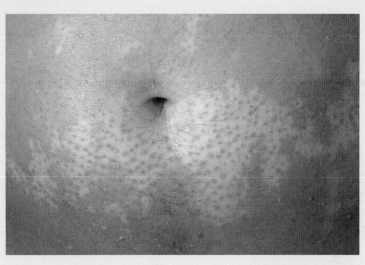

Erythematous patches and follicle-bound infiltrates

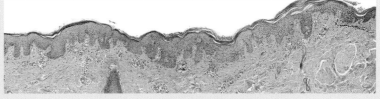

Plump acanthosis and papillomatosis (mid and bottom)

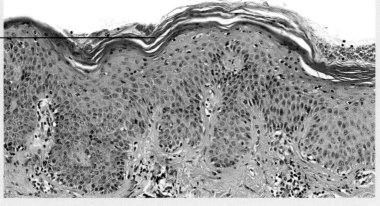

Horizontally and vertically alternating ortho- and parahyper-keratosis

Sparse inflammatory infiltrate in the upper dermis

Hi:

- Large pleomorphic cells, sometimes CD30+
- Epidermotropism may be lost

References

Michaelis, S., Kazakov, D.V., Burg, G., Dummer, R., and Kempf, W. (2006) Extracutaneous transformation into a high-grade lymphoma: a potential pitfall in the management of patients with Sezary syndrome. *Int J Dermatol* **45**(3): 277–9.

Schmoeckel, C., Burg, G., Braun-Falco, O., and Klingmuller, G. (1981) [High-grade malignant mycosis fungoides with cytological transformation (author's transl)] *Ann Dermatol Venereol* **108**(3): 231–6, 239–41.

CD30-Positive Lymphoproliferative Disorders (LPD) of the Skin

CD30-positive T-cell lymphoproliferative disorders of the skin (CD30+ LPD) comprise a clinical and morphological spectrum of diseases including

CD30-POSITIVE LYMPHOPROLIFERATIVE DISORDERS (LPD)

lymphomatoid papulosis (LyP), primary cutaneous CD30+ large T-cell lymphoma (CD30+ LTCL) as well as so-called borderline cases. The hallmark of the tumor cells is the expression of CD30, a cytokine receptor belonging to the tumor necrosis factor receptor (TNFR) superfamily.

References

Drews, R., Samel, A., and Kadin, M.E. (2000) Lymphomatoid papulosis and anaplastic large cell lymphomas of the skin. *Semin Cutan Med Surg* **19**(2): 109–17.

Kaudewitz, P. and Burg, G. (1991) Lymphomatoid papulosis and Ki-1 (CD30)-positive cutaneous large cell lymphomas. *Semin Diagn Pathol* **8**(2): 117–24.

Kempf, W. (2014) Cutaneous CD30-positive lymphoproliferative disorders. *Surg Pathol Clin* **7**(2): 203–28.

Paulli, M., Berti, E., Rosso, R., et al. (1995) CD30/Ki-1-positive lymphoproliferative disorders of the skin – clinicopathologic correlation and statistical analysis of 86 cases: a multicentric study from the European Organization for Research and Treatment of Cancer Cutaneous Lymphoma Project Group. *J Clin Oncol* **13**(6): 1343–54.

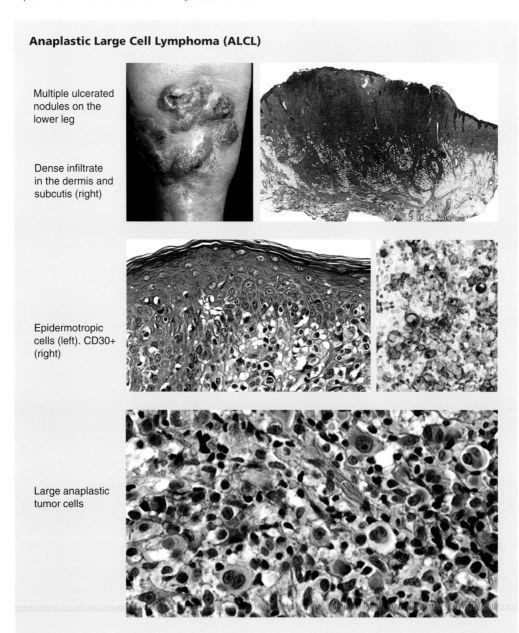

Anaplastic Large Cell Lymphoma (ALCL)

Multiple ulcerated nodules on the lower leg

Dense infiltrate in the dermis and subcutis (right)

Epidermotropic cells (left). CD30+ (right)

Large anaplastic tumor cells

CD30-POSITIVE LYMPHOPROLIFERATIVE DISORDERS (LPD)

Cl: Asymptomatic, mostly solitary, in 20% of cases multiple, firm, and often ulcerated nodules, which grow rapidly and are preferentially located on the extremities or the head. Most patients have a favorable prognosis.

Hi:

- Diffuse dense nodular infiltrate composed of cohesive sheets of atypical large lymphoid cells
- All levels of the dermis and also the subcutis are involved
- Epidermotropism usually is lacking
- The morphologic hallmark are large, pleomorphic (anaplastic) cells:
  - Irregularly shaped nuclei
  - Sometimes multinucleated
  - One or multiple nucleoli
  - Abundant, clear or eosinophilic cytoplasm
- Many mitoses
- Clusters of small reactive lymphocytes within and around the tumor
- Eosinophils, plasma cells, and accessory dendritic cells usually are not prominent

Immunochemistry: CD30+, CD2+, CD3+, CD4+, and CD45RO+, and activation markers such as CD25 (IL-2R), CD71, and HLA-DR. Translocation t(2;5)(p23;q35) and expression of anaplastic lymphoma kinase (ALK), usually found in nodal ALCL, are not found in primary cutaneous CD30+ LPD.

DD: Undifferentiated epithelial, mesenchymal, and melanocytic tumors with anaplastic morphology.

References

Assaf, C., Hirsch, B., Wagner, F., et al. (2007) Differential expression of TRAF1 aids in the distinction of cutaneous CD30-positive lymphoproliferations. *J Invest Dermatol* **127**(8): 1898–904.

Bekkenk, M.W., Geelen, F.A., van Voorst Vader, P.C., et al. (2000) Primary and secondary cutaneous CD30(+) lymphoproliferative disorders: a report from the Dutch Cutaneous Lymphoma Group on the long-term follow-up data of 219 patients and guidelines for diagnosis and treatment. *Blood* **95**(12): 3653–61.

Beljaards, R.C., Kaudewitz, P., Berti, E., et al. (1993) Primary cutaneous CD30-positive large cell lymphoma: definition of a new type of cutaneous lymphoma with a favorable prognosis. A European Multicenter Study of 47 patients. *Cancer* **71**(6): 2097–104.

de Bruin, P.C., Beljaards, R.C., van Heerde, P., et al. (1993) Differences in clinical behaviour and immunophenotype between primary cutaneous and primary nodal anaplastic large cell lymphoma of T-cell or null cell phenotype. *Histopathology* **23**(2): 127–35.

Kadin, M.E. (1990) The spectrum of Ki-1+ cutaneous lymphomas. *Curr Probl Dermatol* **19**(132): 132–43.

Kaudewitz, P., Burg, G., and Stein, H. (1990) Ki-1 (CD30) positive cutaneous anaplastic large cell lymphomas. *Curr Probl Dermatol* **19**(150): 150–6.

Kaudewitz, P., Stein, H., Dallenbach, F., et al. (1989) Primary and secondary cutaneous Ki-1+ (CD30+) anaplastic large cell lymphomas. Morphologic, immunohistologic, and clinical-characteristics. *Am J Pathol* **135**(2): 359–67.

Kempf, W. (2014) Cutaneous CD30-positive lymphoproliferative disorders. *Surg Pathol Clin* **7**(2): 203–28.

Liu, H.L., Hoppe, R.T., Kohler, S., Harvell, J.D., Reddy, S., and Kim, Y.H. (2003) CD30+ cutaneous lymphoproliferative disorders: the Stanford experience in lymphomatoid papulosis and primary cutaneous anaplastic large cell lymphoma. *J Am Acad Dermatol* **49**(6): 1049–58.

Stein, H., Foss, H.D., Durkop, H., et al. (2000) CD30(+) anaplastic large cell lymphoma: a review of its histopathologic, genetic, and clinical features. *Blood* **96**(12): 3681–95.

CD30-POSITIVE LYMPHOPROLIFERATIVE DISORDERS (LPD)

Neutrophil-Rich (Pyogenic) Anaplastic Large Cell Lymphoma

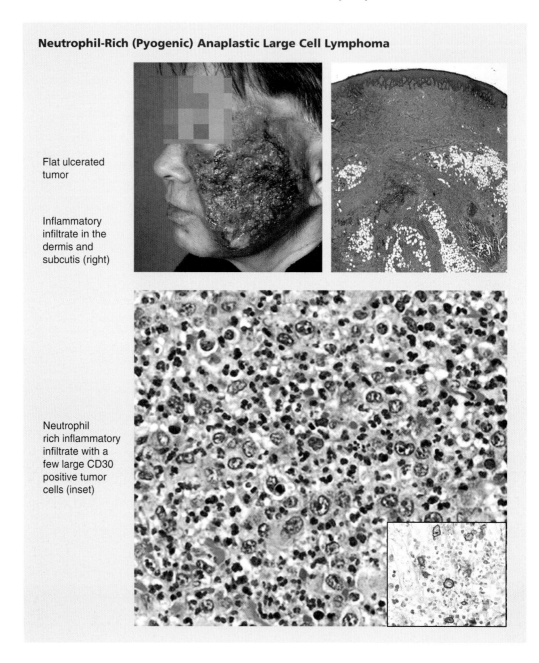

Flat ulcerated tumor

Inflammatory infiltrate in the dermis and subcutis (right)

Neutrophil rich inflammatory infiltrate with a few large CD30 positive tumor cells (inset)

Cl: Nodular tumor(s) preferentially in the face, ulcerated and abscess-forming, simulating pyoderma gangrenosum or deep vegetating fungus infection. Soft nodules may also appear on the trunk and extremities. High amounts of IL-8 produced by a few CD30+ tumor cells are responsible for the neutrophil-rich inflammatory infiltrate.

Hi:
- Abscess-like inflammatory infiltrate, predominantly composed of neutrophils
- Loosely distributed, large atypical cells, CD30+

DD: Pyoderma gangrenosum; abscess; deep fungal infection.

CD30-POSITIVE LYMPHOPROLIFERATIVE DISORDERS (LPD)

References

Burg, G., Kempf, W., Kazakov, D.V., et al. (2003) Pyogenic lymphoma of the skin: a peculiar variant of primary cutaneous neutrophil-rich CD30+ anaplastic large-cell lymphoma. Clinicopathological study of four cases and review of the literature. *Br J Dermatol* **148**(3): 580–6.

Mann, K.P., Hall, B., Kamino, H., Borowitz, M.J., and Ratech, H. (1995) Neutrophil-rich, Ki-1-positive anaplastic large-cell malignant lymphoma. *Am J Surg Pathol* **19**(4): 407–16.

McCluggage, W.G., Walsh, M.Y., and Bharucha, H. (1998) Anaplastic large cell malignant lymphoma with extensive eosinophilic or neutrophilic infiltration. *Histopathology* **32**(2): 110–15.

Lymphomatoid Papulosis

Papules in various stages of development (left)

Early (bottom left) and healed lesion with scar formation (bottom right)

Dense wedge-shaped infiltrate in the dermis (right)

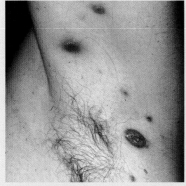
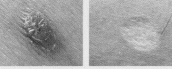
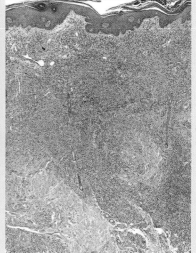

Mixed cellular infiltrate consisting of lymphocytes, eosinophils and scattered large atypical cells (left)

Scattered CD30+ cells in LYP type A (right and inset)

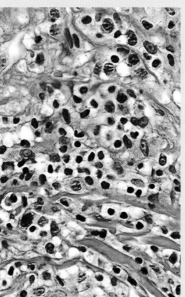
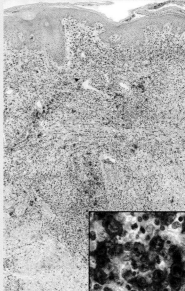

CD30-POSITIVE LYMPHOPROLIFERATIVE DISORDERS (LPD)

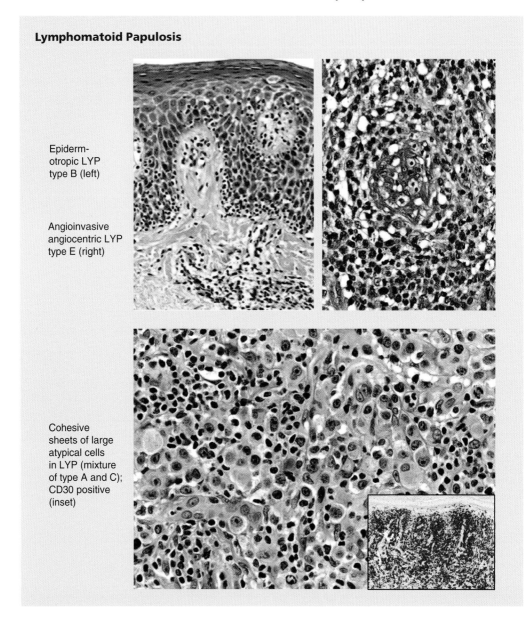

Lymphomatoid Papulosis

Epiderm-
otropic LYP
type B (left)

Angioinvasive
angiocentric LYP
type E (right)

Cohesive
sheets of large
atypical cells
in LYP (mixture
of type A and C);
CD30 positive
(inset)

In 1968, Macaulay described a chronic recurrent, self-healing, papulonodular skin eruption with histological features of a high-grade lymphoma.
Cl: Disseminated papules and/or small nodules, which within days or a few weeks become red-brown, hemorrhagic or pustular and finally undergo ulceration, followed by complete spontaneous regression of the lesion, occasionally leaving behind hyper- or hypopigmented varioliform scars.
Hi: Broad spectrum with variably dense infiltrates of medium-sized to large atypical pleomorphic CD30+ cells are the hallmarks of the disease. Depending on the lesion's stage of evolution, the histological presentation is different. In fresh lesions, there is a wedge-shaped infiltrate of tumor cells with ulceration.

Various subtypes have been differentiated.
- Type A: scattered CD30+ cells
- Type B: epidermotropic, small CD30–/+ cells
- Type C: cohesive large CD30+ cells
- Type D: epidermotropic, small CD30+, CD8+ cells
- Type E: angioinvasive, medium/large CD30+, CD8+ cells
- Type 6p25.3 rearrangement (*DUSP22-IRF4 fusion gene*)

Immunophenotype: CD3+, CD4+/−, CD8−/+, CD25+, CD30+, TIA-1+, granzyme B+, CD56−/+ [10%].

Genotype: Clonal T-cell receptor rearrangement in 50% of cases.

DD: Anaplastic large cell lymphoma.

References

Bekkenk, M.W., Kluin, P.M., Jansen, P.M., Meijer, C.J., and Willemze, R. (2001) Lymphomatoid papulosis with a natural killer-cell phenotype. *Br J Dermatol* **145**(2): 318–22.

El Shabrawi-Caelen, L., Kerl, H., and Cerroni, L. (2004) Lymphomatoid papulosis: reappraisal of clinicopathologic presentation and classification into subtypes A, B, and C. *Arch Dermatol* **140**(4): 441–7.

Kadin, M.E. (1985) Common activated helper-T-cell origin for lymphomatoid papulosis, mycosis fungoides, and some types of Hodgkin's disease. *Lancet* **2**(8460): 864–5.

Kadin, M., Nasu, K., Sako, D., Said, J., and Vonderheid, E. (1985) Lymphomatoid papulosis. A cutaneous proliferation of activated helper T cells expressing Hodgkin's disease-associated antigens. *Am J Pathol* **119**(2): 315–25.

Karai, L.J., Kadin, M.E., Hsi, E.D., et al. (2013) Chromosomal rearrangements of 6p25.3 define a new subtype of lymphomatoid papulosis. *Am J Surg Pathol* **37**(8): 1173–81.

Kaudewitz, P. and Burg, G. (1991) Lymphomatoid papulosis and Ki-1 (CD30)-positive cutaneous large cell lymphomas. *Semin Diagn Pathol* **8**(2): 117–24.

Kaudewitz, P., Stein, H., Burg, G., Mason, M., and Braun-Falco, O. (1984) Detection of Sternberg-Reed and Hodgkin cell specific antigen on atypical cells in lymphomatoid papulosis. Poster presentation at the Second International Conference on Malignant Lymphoma, Lugano, June 13–16.

Kaudewitz, P., Stein, H., Burg, G., Mason, D.Y., and Braun, F.O. (1986) Atypical cells in lymphomatoid papulosis express the Hodgkin cell-associated antigen Ki-1. *J Invest Dermatol* **86**(4): 350–4.

Kaudewitz, P., Stein, H., Plewig, G., et al. (1990) Hodgkin's disease followed by lymphomatoid papulosis. Immunophenotypic evidence for a close relationship between lymphomatoid papulosis and Hodgkin's disease. *J Am Acad Dermatol* **22**(6 Pt 1): 999–1006.

Kempf, W. (2017) A new era for cutaneous CD30-positive T-cell lymphoproliferative disorders. *Semin Diagn Pathol* **34**(1): 22–35.

Macaulay, W.L. (1968) Lymphomatoid papulosis. A continuing self-healing eruption, clinically benign, histologically malignant. *Arch Dermatol* **97**(1): 23–30.

Willemze, R. and Beljaards, R.C. (1993) Spectrum of primary cutaneous CD30 (Ki-1)-positive lymphoproliferative disorders. A proposal for classification and guidelines for management and treatment. *J Am Acad Dermatol* **28**(6): 973–80.

Differential Diagnosis: Hodgkin's Lymphoma, Lymphocyte Predominance

Nodules on the arm (left) and nodular infiltrate in the dermis (right) in "primary" cutaneous HD

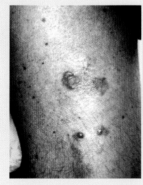
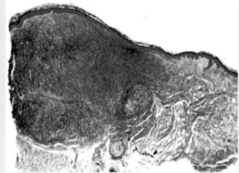

CD30-POSITIVE LYMPHOPROLIFERATIVE DISORDERS (LPD)

Differential Diagnosis: Hodgkin's Lymphoma, Lymphocyte Predominance

Hodgkin cells and Sternberg-Reed cells (left), CD30+ (right)

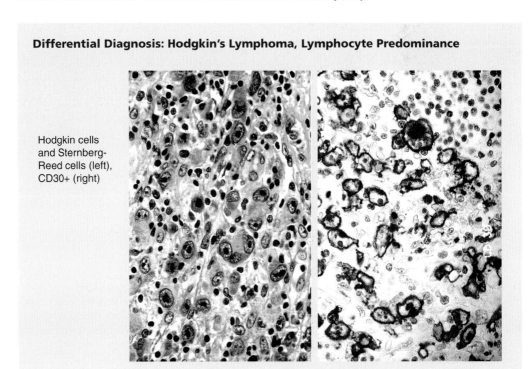

Cl: There have been reports on primary cutaneous Hodgkin's disease, but its existence is very questionable, and most probably these lesions are CD30+ anaplastic large cell lymphomas. However, they may represent retrograde lymphatic spread of Hodgkin's disease from affected lymph nodes or result from extension per continuitatem.

Hi: Mixed cellularity: Reed–Sternberg cells, Hodgkin cells, eosinophils, neutrophils, small lymphocytes. T- or B-cell phenotype.

Immunophenotype: Reed–Sternberg cells express CD15, CD30, and MUM-1.

DD: Anaplastic large cell lymphoma; lymphomatoid papulosis.

References

Cho, R.J., McCalmont, T.H., Ai, W.Z., Fox, L.P., Treseler, P., and Pincus, L.B. (2012) Use of an expanded immunohistochemical panel to distinguish cutaneous Hodgkin lymphoma from histopathologic imitators. *J Cutan Pathol* **39**(6): 651–8.

Eberle, F.C., Song, J.Y., Xi, L., et al. (2012) Nodal involvement by cutaneous CD30-positive T-cell lymphoma mimicking classical Hodgkin lymphoma. *Am J Surg Pathol* **36**(5): 716–25.

Huhn, D., Burg, G., and Mempel, W. (1973) [Specific cutaneous changes in Hodgkin's disease (author's transl)] *Dtsch Med Wochenschr* **98**(52): 2469–72.

Huong, G., Olson, L.C., Rippis, G.E., and Magro, C.M. (2016) An index case of cutaneous hodgkin lymphoma and review of the literature. *Am J Dermatopathol* **38**(10): 739–43.

Khawandanah, M., Kraus, T., and Cherry, M. (2014) Refractory classical Hodgkin lymphoma presenting with atypical cutaneous involvement and diagnosis of ZZ phenotype alpha-1 antitrypsin deficiency. *Case Rep Hematol* **2014**: 642868.

Pranteda, G., Osti, M.F., Cox, M.C., et al. (2010) Primary cutaneous Hodgkin lymphoma. *J Am Acad Dermatol* **63**(2): e52–3.

SUBCUTANEOUS PANNICULITIS-LIKE LYMPHOMA

Subcutaneous Panniculitis-Like Lymphoma

Subcutaneous (Panniculitis-Like; Alpha/Beta) T-Cell Lymphoma

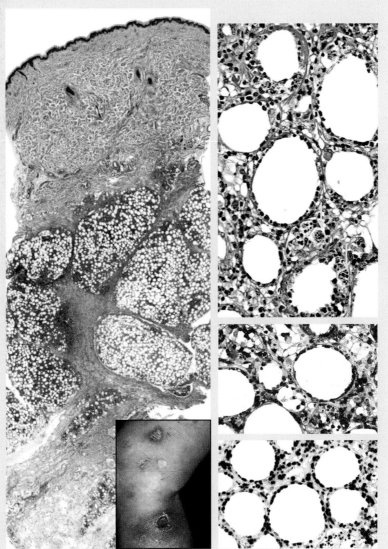

Predominantly lobular infiltrate in the subcutis with septal fibrosis (left)

Inset: panniculitis-like lesions on the leg with necrosis

Lymphoid infiltrate rimming around fat vacuoles (upper right); hemophagocytosis (arrows)

CD8 (mid right) and Ki67/MIB-1 (bottom right) positive tumor cells

Cl: Subcutaneous nodules, simulating panniculitis; usually no ulceration.

Hi:

- Subcutaneous lobular infiltrates
- Small, medium-sized to large pleomorphic lymphocytes
- Lymphocyte-rimming of adipocytes (not specific!)
- Karyorrhexis and phagocytosis of nuclear debris

Immunophenotype: CD3+, CD4–, CD8+, CD56–, TIA-1+, granzyme B+, perforin+, EBER–, LMP-1–, beta-F1+ (TCR alpha/beta). Demonstration of expression of TCR alpha/beta is essential as it is the defining criterion for this lymphoma.

Genotype: Clonal rearrangement of alpha/beta T-cell receptor.

DD: Panniculitis; subcutaneous gamma/delta lymphoma.

SUBCUTANEOUS PANNICULITIS-LIKE LYMPHOMA

References

Gallardo, F. and Pujol, R. M. (2008) Subcutaneous panniculitic-like T-cell lymphoma and other primary cutaneous lymphomas with prominent subcutaneous tissue involvement. *Dermatol Clin* **26**(4): 529–40, viii.

Massone, C., Chott, A., Metze, D., et al. (2004) Subcutaneous, blastic natural killer (NK), NK/T-cell, and other cytotoxic lymphomas of the skin: a morphologic, immunophenotypic, and molecular study of 50 patients. *Am J Surg Pathol* **28**(6): 719–35.

Springinsfeld, G., Guillaume, J.C., Boeckler, P., Tortel, M.C., and Cribier, B. (2009) [Two cases of subcutaneous panniculitis-like T-cell lymphoma (CD4– CD8+ CD56–)] *Ann Dermatol Venereol* **136**(3): 264–8.

Willemze, R., Jansen, P.M., Cerroni, L., et al. (2008) Subcutaneous panniculitis-like T-cell lymphoma: definition, classification, and prognostic factors: an EORTC Cutaneous Lymphoma Group Study of 83 cases. *Blood* **111**(2): 838–45.

Differential Diagnosis: Subcutaneous (Panniculitis-Like) Gamma/Delta Lymphoma

Panniculitis-like lesions on the leg (left)

Panniculitis-like septal and lobular infiltrate in the subcutaneous tissue (left)

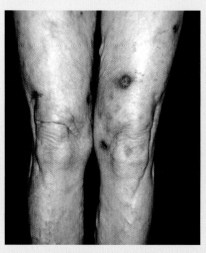
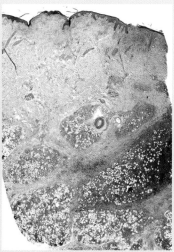

Rimming of tumor cells around fat vacuoles (left)

Scattered large atypical cells (right)

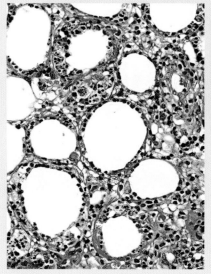
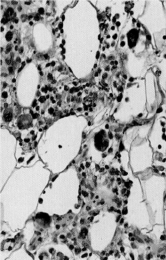

SUBCUTANEOUS PANNICULITIS-LIKE LYMPHOMA

Cl: Subcutaneous nodular infiltrate. Usually aggressive, rapidly progressive course. However, less aggressive variants producing high levels of interferon gamma have been reported.

Hi:

- Lobular panniculitis-like infiltrate in the subcutis. In addition, dermal and epidermotropic infiltrates can be present
- Small and medium-sized lymphocytes with chromatin-dense atypical nuclei
- Rimming around fat cells
- Scattered large atypical lymphoblasts
- Karyorrhexis and phagocytosis of nuclear debris

Immunophenotype: CD3+, CD4−, CD8−, CD56+, TIA-1+, granzyme B+, beta-F1−, TCR gamma (or delta)+.

Genotype: Clonal rearrangement of the T-cell receptor.

DD: Panniculitis; subcutaneous panniculitis-like alpha/beta T-cell lymphoma.

References

Burg, G., Dummer, R., Wilhelm, M., et al. (1991) A subcutaneous delta positive T-cell lymphoma that produces interferon gamma. *N Engl J Med* **325**: 1078–81.

Massone, C., Chott, A., Metze, D., et al. (2004) Subcutaneous, blastic natural killer (NK), NK/T-cell, and other cytotoxic lymphomas of the skin: a morphologic, immunophenotypic, and molecular study of 50 patients. *Am J Surg Pathol* **28**(6): 719–35.

Salhany, K.E., Macon, W.R., Choi, J.K., et al. (1998) Subcutaneous panniculitis-like T-cell lymphoma: clinicopathologic, immunophenotypic, and genotypic analysis of alpha/beta and gamma/delta subtypes. *Am J Surg Pathol* **22**(7): 881–93.

Differential Diagnosis: Lupus Panniculitis (Lupus Profundus)

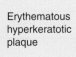

Erythematous hyperkeratotic plaque

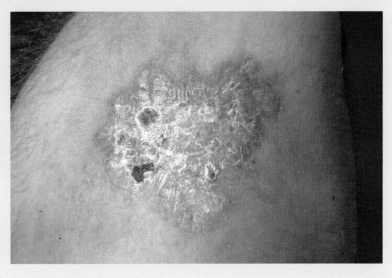

SUBCUTANEOUS PANNICULITIS-LIKE LYMPHOMA

Differential Diagnosis: Lupus Panniculitis (Lupus Profundus)

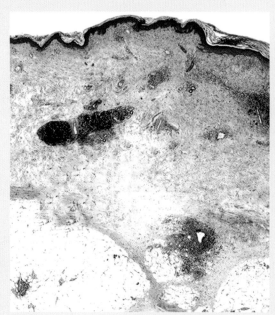
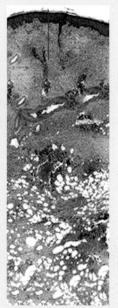

Nodular dense lymphocytic infiltrates (left)

Septal and lobular panniculitis (left and right)

Cl: Slightly elevated subcutaneous nodular lesion or plaque. The overlying epidermis is normal or retracted and sometimes may show involvement with erythema and firm hyperkeratosis. Ulceration may occur. Association with systemic or cutaneous lupus erythematosus possible.

Hi: Infiltrates in the deep dermis and in septa and lobules of the subcutaneous fat tissue. Mucin and admixture of plasma cells. Clusters of CD123-positive plasmacytoid dendritic cells.

References

LeBlanc, R.E., Tavallaee, M., Kim, Y.H., and Kim, J. (2016) Useful parameters for distinguishing subcutaneous panniculitis-like t-cell lymphoma from lupus erythematosus panniculitis. *Am J Surg Pathol* **40**(6): 745–54.

Liau, J.Y., Chuang, S.S., Chu, C.Y., Ku, W.H., Tsai, J.H., and Shih, T.F. (2013) The presence of clusters of plasmacytoid dendritic cells is a helpful feature for differentiating lupus panniculitis from subcutaneous panniculitis-like T-cell lymphoma. *Histopathology* **62**(7): 1057–66.

Ma, L., Bandarchi, B., and Glusac, E.J. (2005) Fatal subcutaneous panniculitis-like T-cell lymphoma with interface change and dermal mucin, a dead ringer for lupus erythematosus. *J Cutan Pathol* **32**(5): 360–5.

Magro, C.M., Crowson, A.N., Kovatich, A.J., and Burns, F. (2001) Lupus profundus, indeterminate lymphocytic lobular panniculitis and subcutaneous T-cell lymphoma: a spectrum of subcuticular T-cell lymphoid dyscrasia. *J Cutan Pathol* **28**(5): 235–47.

Massone, C., Kodama, K., Salmhofer, W., et al. (2005) Lupus erythematosus panniculitis (lupus profundus): clinical, histopathological, and molecular analysis of nine cases. *J Cutan Pathol* **32**(6): 396–404.

Park, H.S., Choi, J.W., Kim, B.K., and Cho, K.H. (2010) Lupus erythematosus panniculitis: clinicopathological, immunophenotypic, and molecular studies. *Am J Dermatopathol* **32**(1): 24–30.

Pincus, L.B., LeBoit, P.E., McCalmont, T.H., et al. (2009) Subcutaneous panniculitis-like T-cell lymphoma with overlapping clinicopathologic features of lupus erythematosus: coexistence of 2 entities? *Am J Dermatopathol* **31**(6): 520–6.

Primary Cutaneous Peripheral Lymphoma (PTL), Unspecified (NOS)

A heterogeneous group of cutaneous T-cell lymphomas that do not fit into one of the well-defined subtypes of T-cell lymphoma/leukaemia. It includes the following entities: (1) cutaneous gamma-delta T-cell lymphoma; (2) primary cutaneous small-medium CD4+ T-cell lymphoproliferative disorder (provisional); (3) primary cutaneous aggressive epidermotropic CD8+ cyto toxic T-cell lymphoma (provisional).

PRIMARY CUTANEOUS PERIPHERAL LYMPHOMA (PTL), UNSPECIFIED (NOS)

Reference

Ralfkiaer, E., Willemze, R., Meijer, C.J.L.M., et al. (2006) Primary cutaneous peripheral T-cell lymphoma, unspecified. In: LeBoit, P.E., Burg, G., Weedon, D., and Sarasin, A. (eds) *World Health Organization Classification of Tumors: Pathology and Genetics: Skin Tumours*. Oxford: Oxford University Press.

Primary Cutaneous CD4-positive (Acral) Small/Medium-Sized T-Cell Lymphoproliferative Disorder

Papules on the hand (left)

Nodular dermal infiltrate (right)

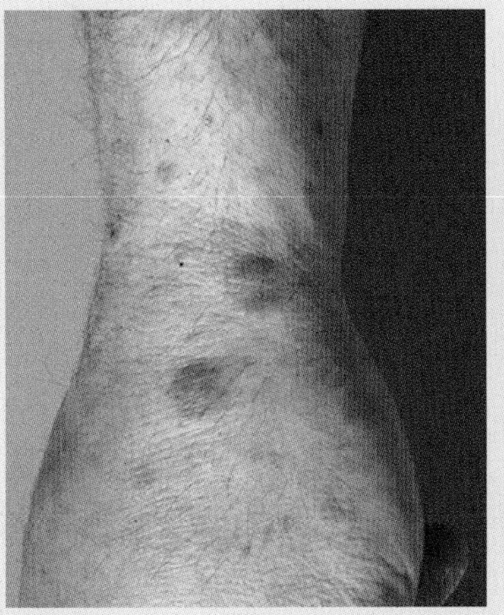

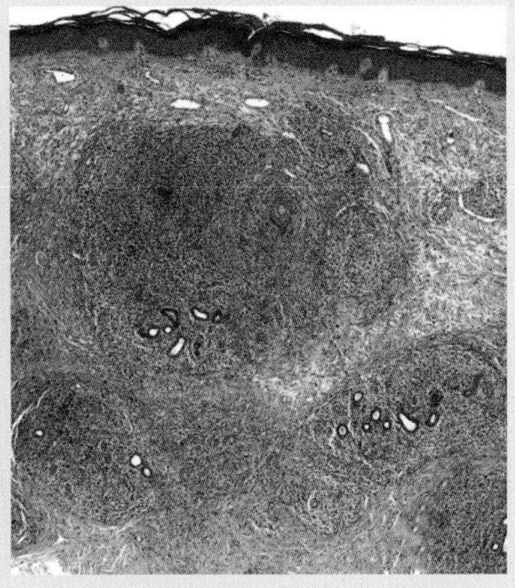

Small to medium-sized pleomorphic lymphoid cells

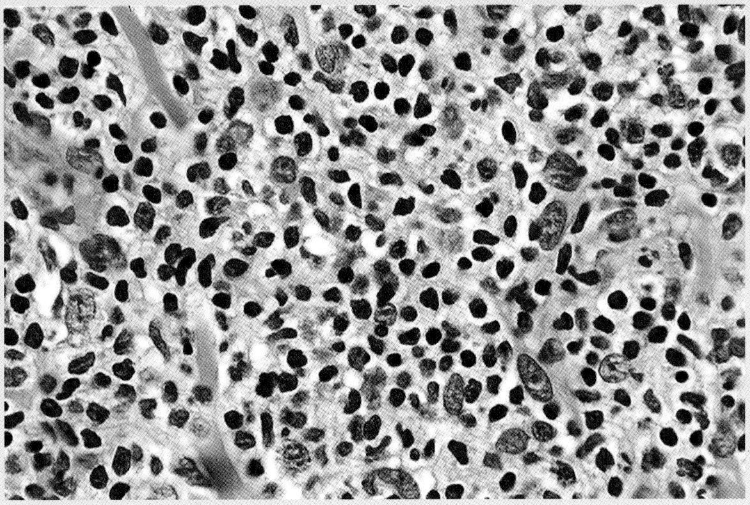

Cl: Circumscribed nodular lesion predominantly on the head and neck region, showing an indolent course with excellent prognosis.

Hi:
- Nodular dermal infiltrates
- No epidermotropism
- Small to medium-sized pleomorphic lymphoid cells
- Eosinophils
- Sometimes clusters of plasma cells

Immunophenotype: CD3+, CD4+, CD8−, CD30-, beta-F1+, PD-1+ (20–30% of the infiltrate).

Genotype: Monoclonal rearrangement of T-cell receptor in approximately 60% of cases.

DD: T-cell pseudolymphoma; primary cutaneous peripheral lymphoma (PTL), unspecified (NOS).

PRIMARY CUTANEOUS PERIPHERAL LYMPHOMA (PTL), UNSPECIFIED (NOS)

References

Beltraminelli, H., Leinweber, B., Kerl, H., and Cerroni, L. (2009) Primary cutaneous CD4+ small-/medium-sized pleomorphic T-cell lymphoma: a cutaneous nodular proliferation of pleomorphic T lymphocytes of undetermined significance? A study of 136 cases. *Am J Dermatopathol* **31**(4): 317–22.

Friedmann, D., Wechsler, J., Delfau, M.H., et al. (1995) Primary cutaneous pleomorphic small T-cell lymphoma. A review of 11 cases. The French Study Group on Cutaneous Lymphomas. *Arch Dermatol* **131**(9): 1009–15.

von den Driesch, P. and Coors, E.A. (2002) Localized cutaneous small to medium-sized pleomorphic T-cell lymphoma: a report of 3 cases stable for years. *J Am Acad Dermatol* **46**(4): 531–5.

Cutaneous Aggressive Epidermotropic CD8-positive T-Cell Lymphoma (Berti)

Plaques in the groin (left). CD8+ cells in the epidermis (right)

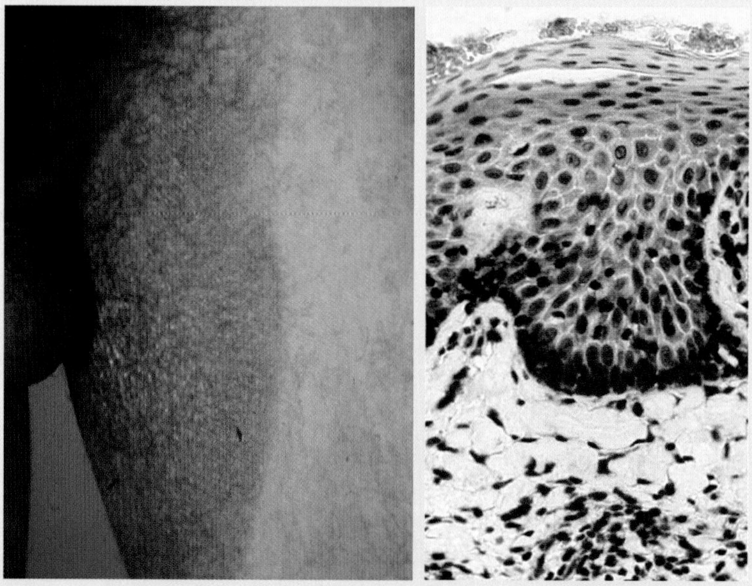

CD8

Epidermotropic infiltrate

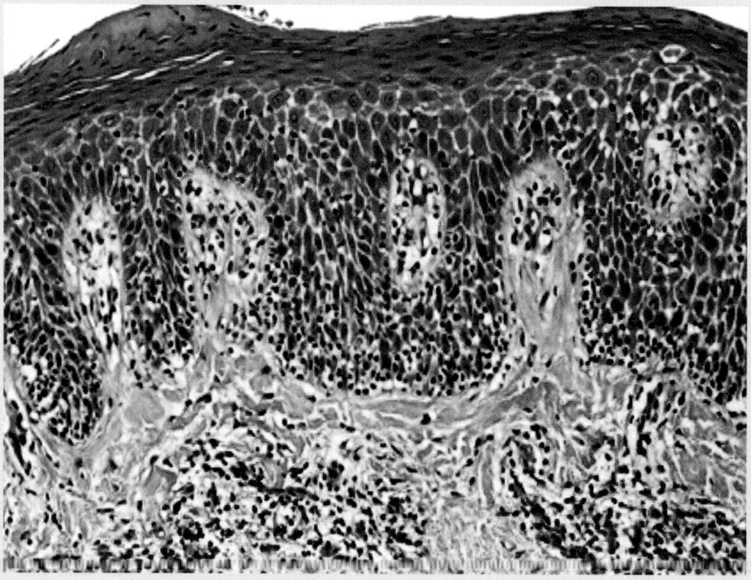

PRIMARY CUTANEOUS PERIPHERAL LYMPHOMA (PTL), UNSPECIFIED (NOS)

Cl: Disseminated patches and plaques, sometimes with blisters, erosions, necrosis, and ulceration. Rapid progression with poor prognosis.

Hi:

- Epidermotropic infiltrate with pagetoid pattern
- Small to medium-sized pleomorphic lymphoid cells
- Necrotic keratinocytes

Immunophenotype: CD3+, CD4−, CD8+, TIA-1+, CD30−, CD45RA+, CD56−.

Genotype : Clonal T-cell receptor rearrangement.

DD: Febrile ulceronecrotic Mucha–Habermann disease.

References

Berti, E., Tomasini, D., Vermeer, M.H., Meijer, C.J., Alessi, E., and Willemze, R. (1999) Primary cutaneous CD8-positive epidermotropic cytotoxic T cell lymphomas. A distinct clinicopathological entity with an aggressive clinical behavior. *Am J Pathol* **155**(2): 483–92.

Kamarashev, J., Burg, G., Mingari, M.C., Kempf, W., Hofbauer, G., and Dummer, R. (2001) Differential expression of cytotoxic molecules and killer cell inhibitory receptors in CD8+ and CD56+ cutaneous lymphomas. *Am J Pathol* **158**(5): 1593–8.

Robson, A., Assaf, C., Bagot, M., et al. (2015) Aggressive epidermotropic cutaneous CD8+ lymphoma: a cutaneous lymphoma with distinct clinical and pathological features. Report of an EORTC Cutaneous Lymphoma Task Force Workshop. *Histopathology* **67**(4): 425–41.

Differential Diagnosis: Febrile Ulceronecrotic PLEVA (Mucha–Habermann Disease)

Ulceronecrotic plaques

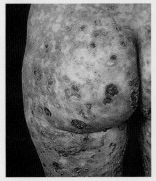
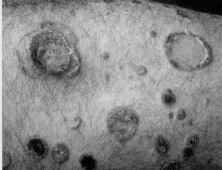

Band-like epidermotropic infiltrate in the upper dermis

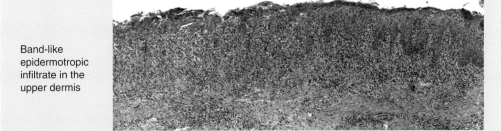

PRIMARY CUTANEOUS PERIPHERAL LYMPHOMA (PTL), UNSPECIFIED (NOS)

Differential Diagnosis: Febrile Ulceronecrotic PLEVA (Mucha–Habermann Disease)

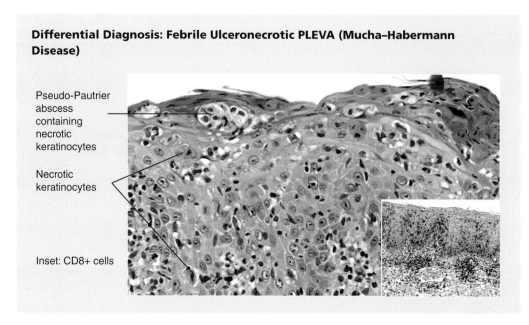

Pseudo-Pautrier abscess containing necrotic keratinocytes

Necrotic keratinocytes

Inset: CD8+ cells

Cl: Generalized necrotic plaques, which may merge into large erosions and ulcerations. In addition, there are general symptoms like fever, nausea, diarrhea, and involvement of the central nervous system. The differentiation from aggressive CD8+ epidermotropic T-cell lymphoma (Berti) is obscure.

Hi:

- Epidermotropic lymphoid infiltrate in the upper dermis
- Necrotic keratinocytes

Immunophenotype: CD3+, CD4+, CD8+, CD30−, CD56−, CD57−.

DD: Aggressive CD8+ epidermotropic T-cell lymphoma; pityriasis lichenoides et varioliformis acuta (PLEVA).

References

Arellano Lorca, J., Yanez Silva, I., Soto Vilches, F., Luna Heine, A., and Corredoira Salum, Y. (2016) [Febrile ulceronecrotic Mucha–Habermann disease] *Rev Med Chil* **144**(9): 1214–17.

Aytekin, S., Balci, G., and Duzgun, O.Y. (2005) Febrile ulceronecrotic Mucha–Habermann disease: a case report and a review of the literature. *Dermatol Online J* **11**(3): 31.

Degos, R., Duperrat, B., and Daniel, F. (1966) [Hyperthermic ulcero-necrotic parapsoriasis. Subacute form of parapsoriasis guttata] *Ann Dermatol Syphiligr (Paris)* **93**(5): 401–96.

Fink-Puches, R., Soyer, H.P., and Kerl, H. (1994) Febrile ulceronecrotic pityriasis lichenoides et varioliformis acuta. *J Am Acad Dermatol* **30**(2 Pt 1): 261–3.

Helmbold, P., Gaisbauer, G., Fiedler, E., Stucker, M., Wolter, M., and Marsch, W. (2006) Self-limited variant of febrile ulceronecrotic Mucha-Habermann disease with polyclonal T-cell receptor rearrangement. *J Am Acad Dermatol* **54**(6): 1113–15.

Herron, M.D., Bohnsack, J.F., and Vanderhooft, S.L. (2005) Septic, CD-30 positive febrile ulceronecrotic pityriasis lichenoides et varioliformis acuta. *Pediatr Dermatol* **22**(4): 360–5.

Kaufman, W.S., McNamara, E.K., Curtis, A.R., Kosari, P., Jorizzo, J.L., and Krowchuk, D.P. (2012) Febrile ulceronecrotic Mucha–Habermann disease (pityriasis lichenoides et varioliformis acuta fulminans) presenting as Stevens–Johnson syndrome. *Pediatr Dermatol* **29**(2): 135–40.

Lopez-Estebaranz, J.L., Vanaclocha, F., Gil, R., Garcia, B., and Iglesias, L. (1993) Febrile ulceronecrotic Mucha–Habermann disease. *J Am Acad Dermatol* **29**(5 Pt 2): 903–6.

Nanda, A., Alshalfan, F., Al-Otaibi, M., Al-Sabah, H., and Rajy, J.M. (2013) Febrile ulceronecrotic Mucha–Habermann disease (pityriasis lichenoides et varioliformis acuta fulminans) associated with parvovirus infection. *Am J Dermatopathol* **35**(4): 503–6.

Sotiriou, E., Patsatsi, A., Tsorova, C., Lazaridou, E., and Sotiriadis, D. (2008) Febrile ulceronecrotic Mucha–Habermann disease: a case report and review of the literature. *Acta Derm Venereol* **88**(4): 350–5.

Yang, C.C., Lee, J.Y., and Chen, W. (2003) Febrile ulceronecrotic Mucha–Habermann disease with extensive skin necrosis in intertriginous areas. *Eur J Dermatol* **13**(5): 493–6.

EXTRANODAL NK/T-CELL LYMPHOMA

Extranodal NK/T-Cell Lymphoma, Nasal Type (Subcutaneous)

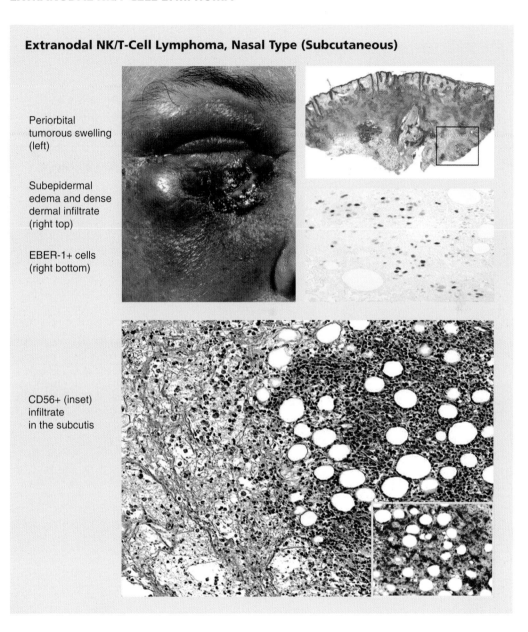

Periorbital
tumorous swelling
(left)

Subepidermal
edema and dense
dermal infiltrate
(right top)

EBER-1+ cells
(right bottom)

CD56+ (inset)
infiltrate
in the subcutis

Cl: Ulcerated plaque or nodule.

Hi: Dermal and subcutaneous infiltrate, composed of small to medium-sized pleomorphic lymphoid cells with angioinvasive growth.

Immunophenotype: CD2+, CD3ε+, CD56+, TIA-1+, granzyme B+, perforin+, EBV+ (EBER).

EXTRANODAL NK/T-CELL LYMPHOMA

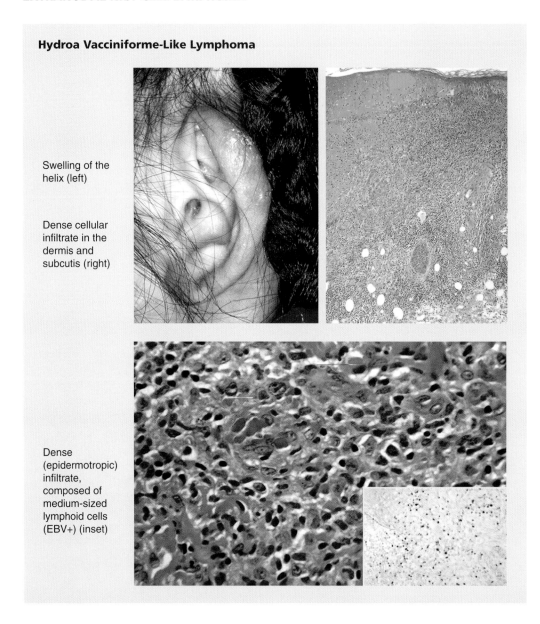

Hydroa Vacciniforme-Like Lymphoma

Swelling of the helix (left)

Dense cellular infiltrate in the dermis and subcutis (right)

Dense (epidermotropic) infiltrate, composed of medium-sized lymphoid cells (EBV+) (inset)

Hydroa-like lymphoma encompasses a group of rare lymphoproliferative disorders of the skin, associated with chronic EBV infection. The oral mucosa may be involved.

CI: Edema, vesiculopapular eruptions, small blisters, crusts, necrotic areas, and scars occur mainly on the nose, ears, and limbs of children and young adults. The lesions are not induced or exacerbated by UV radiation. There is often high fever, malaise, weight loss, failure to thrive, lymphadenopathy, hepatosplenomegaly, and hypersensitivity to insect bites. Antibodies to EBV can be detected in the serum. Progression to visceral and lymph node involvement.

ANGIOIMMUNOBLASTIC T-CELL LYMPHOMA

Hi:
- Epidermal degeneration and necrosis
- Dense perivascular/periadnexal nodular infiltrate in the dermis and subcutis, with some epidermotropism
- Medium-sized lymphocytes with irregular, hyperchromatic nuclei
- Angiocentric/angiodestructive pattern may be seen in some cases

Immunohistochemistry: CD3+, CD8+, TIA-1+, granzyme B+, CD4−, CD45RO+, CD2+, CD43+, CD5−, CD7−; CD56 is variably expressed; CD30 reactivity can be seen.

Genotype: Clonal rearrangement of the T-cell receptor gene. EBV DNA or RNA sequences are detected by PCR or *in situ* hybridization.

DD: Hydroa vacciniforme; lupus erythematosus.

References

Chen, H.H., Hsiao, C.H., and Chiu, H.C. (2002) Hydroa vacciniforme-like primary cutaneous CD8-positive T-cell lymphoma. *Br J Dermatol* **147**(3): 587–91.

Doeden, K., Molina-Kirsch, H., Perez, E., Warnke, R., and Sundram, U. (2008) Hydroa-like lymphoma with CD56 expression. *J Cutan Pathol* **35**(5): 488–94.

Iwatsuki, K., Xu, Z., Takata, M., et al. (1999) The association of latent Epstein–Barr virus infection with hydroa vacciniforme. *Br J Dermatol* **140**(4): 715–21.

Kim, T.H., Lee, J.H., Kim, Y.C., and Lee, S.E. (2015) Hydroa vacciniforme-like lymphoma misdiagnosed as cutaneous lupus erythematosus. *J Cutan Pathol* **42**(3): 229–31.

Magana, M., Massone, C., Magana, P., and Cerroni, L. (2016) Clinicopathologic features of hydroa vacciniforme-like lymphoma: a series of 9 patients. *Am J Dermatopathol* **38**(1): 20–5.

Plaza, J.A. and Sangueza, M. (2015) Hydroa vacciniforme-like lymphoma with primarily periorbital swelling: 7 cases of an atypical clinical manifestation of this rare cutaneous T-cell lymphoma. *Am J Dermatopathol* **37**(1): 20–5.

Zhang, G., Bai, H.X., Yang, L., et al. (2013) NK-/T-cell lymphoma resembling hydroa vacciniforme with positive CD4 marker expression: a diagnostic difficulty. *Am J Dermatopathol* **35**(1): 94–7.

Angioimmunoblastic T-Cell Lymphoma

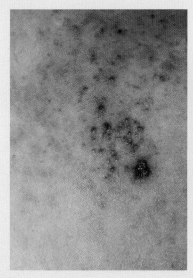
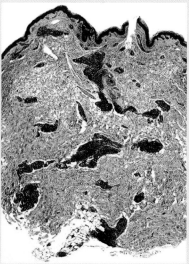

Maculopapular eruption on the trunk (left)

Dense perivascular infiltrates in the dermis (right)

ANGIOIMMUNOBLASTIC T-CELL LYMPHOMA

Angioimmunoblastic T-Cell Lymphoma

Vascular hyperplasia and pleomorphic lymphoid infiltrate

This systemic malignant lymphoproliferative disorder shows clonal growth of atypical lymphoid cells accompanied by the proliferation of high endothelial venules and follicular dendritic cells.

Cl: Skin involvement occurs in up to 50% of cases, usually in the form of a generalized maculopapular eruption with a predilection for the trunk, mimicking a viral exanthema, drug eruption or erythroderma of any cause. General symptoms include fever, weight loss, night sweats, lymphadenopathy, hepato- and splenomegaly, and polyclonal hypergammaglobulinemia.

Hi: Various types have been differentiated.

- Prominent vascular hyperplasia with epithelioid endothelial cells
- Dense perivascular infiltrates of pleomorphic cells involving superficial and deep dermis
- Reactive infiltrate of mature B-cells, plasma cells, and histiocytes

Immunophenotype: Mature T-helper cells: CD3+, CD4+, CD8+/−, PD-1+, ICOS+, bcl-6+, CD10+, CXCL-13+. Increased number of dermal dendritic cells (factor XIIIa).

Genotype: Clonal TCR gamma gene rearrangement was found in some cases.

DD: Drug reaction; viral exanthema; dermatomyositis; chronic urticaria; purpura fulminans.

References

Botros, N., Cerroni, L., Shawwa, A., et al. (2015) Cutaneous manifestations of angioimmunoblastic T-cell lymphoma: clinical and pathological characteristics. *Am J Dermatopathol* **37**(4): 274–83.

Brown, H.A., Macon, W.R., Kurtin, P.J., and Gibson, L.E. (2001) Cutaneous involvement by angioimmunoblastic T-cell lymphoma with remarkable heterogeneous Epstein–Barr virus expression. *J Cutan Pathol* **28**(8): 432–8.

Ferran, M., Gallardo, F., Baena, V., Ferrer, A., Florensa, L., and Pujol, R.M. (2006) The 'deck chair sign' in specific cutaneous involvement by angioimmunoblastic T cell lymphoma. *Dermatology* **213**(1): 50–2.

Frizzera, G., Moran, E.M., and Rappaport, H. (1975) Angio-immunoblastic lymphadenopathy. Diagnosis and clinical course. *Am J Med* **59**(6): 803–18.

Jayaraman, A.G., Cassarino, D., Advani, R., Kim, Y.H., Tsai, E., and Kohler, S. (2006) Cutaneous involvement by angioimmunoblastic T-cell lymphoma: a unique histologic presentation, mimicking an infectious etiology. *J Cutan Pathol* **33**(Suppl 2): 6–11.

Kaffenberger, B., Haverkos, B., Tyler, K., Wong, H.K., Porcu, P., and Gru, A.A. (2015) Extranodal marginal zone lymphoma-like presentations of angioimmunoblastic T-cell lymphoma: a T-cell lymphoma masquerading as a B-cell lymphoproliferative disorder. *Am J Dermatopathol* **37**(8): 604–13.

Kang, M., Bhatia, N., Sauder, A., and Feurdean, M. (2016) Angioimmunoblastic T cell lymphoma mimicking chronic urticaria. *Case Rep Med* **2016**: 8753235.

Mahendran, R., Grant, J.W., Hoggarth, C.E., and Burrows, N.P. (2001) Angioimmunoblastic T-cell lymphoma with cutaneous involvement. *J Eur Acad Dermatol Venereol* **15**(6): 589–90.

Mangana, J., Guenova, E., Kerl, K., et al. (2017) Angioimmunoblastic T-cell lymphoma mimicking drug reaction with eosinophilia and systemic symptoms (DRESS syndrome). *Case Rep Dermatol* **9**(1): 74–9.

Martel, P., Laroche, L., Courville, P., et al. (2000) Cutaneous involvement in patients with angioimmunoblastic lymphadenopathy with dysproteinemia: a clinical, immunohistological, and molecular analysis. *Arch Dermatol* **136**(7): 881–6.

Miladi, A., Thomas, B.C., Beasley, K., and Meyerle, J. (2015) Angioimmunoblastic t-cell lymphoma presenting as purpura fulminans. *Cutis* **95**(2): 113–15.

Murakami, T., Ohtsuki, M., and Nakagawa, H. (2001) Angioimmunoblastic lymphadenopathy-type peripheral T-cell lymphoma with cutaneous infiltration: report of a case and its gene expression profile. *Br J Dermatol* **144**(4): 878–84.

Saito, K., Okiyama, N., Shibao, K., Maruyama, H., and Fujimoto, M. (2016) Angioimmunoblastic T-cell lymphoma mimicking dermatomyositis. *J Dermatol* **43**(7): 837–9.

Smithberger, E.S., Rezania, D., Chavan, R.N., Lien, M.H., Cualing, H.D., and Messina, J.L. (2010) Primary cutaneous angioimmunoblastic T-cell lymphoma histologically mimicking an inflammatory dermatosis. *J Drugs Dermatol* **9**(7): 851–5.

Suarez, A.E., Artiga, M.J., Santonja, C., et al. (2016) Angioimmunoblastic T-cell lymphoma with a clonal plasma cell proliferation that underwent immunoglobulin isotype switch in the skin, coinciding with cutaneous disease progression. *J Cutan Pathol* **43**(12): 1203–10.

Yoon, G.S., Choi, Y.K., Bak, H., et al. (2009) Angioimmunoblastic T cell lymphomas: frequent cutaneous skin lesions and absence of human herpes viruses. *Ann Dermatol* **21**(1): 1–5.

Cutaneous Mature B-Cell Lymphoid Neoplasms (CBCL)

For the characteristic growth pattern of B-cell infiltrates in the skin, see above.

The skin is a secondary lymphoid organ, to which lymphoid cells home and may organize in a pattern corresponding to the various structures of the reactive lymph follicle: germinal center, mantle zone, marginal zone, and interfollicular area (Table 12.1).

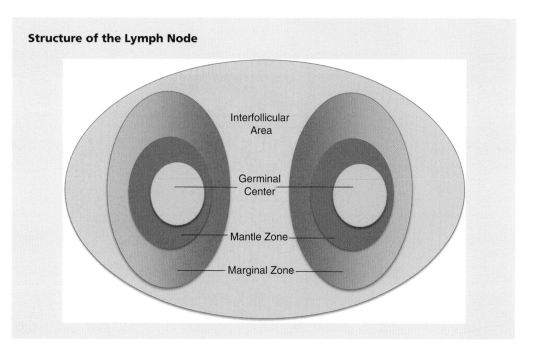

Structure of the Lymph Node

Interfollicular Area

Germinal Center

Mantle Zone

Marginal Zone

MARGINAL ZONE LYMPHOMA

Table 12.1 Immunophenotypical profiles of some cutaneous B-cell lymphomas.

	Bcl-2	Bcl-6	CD 10	t(14;18)	MUM-1 IRF-4	CD 21
MZL/ICY	+	-	-	-	-	+
FCL	-	+	+	-	-	-
DLBCL	+	+	-	+/-	+	-

DLBCL, diffuse large B-cell lymphoma; FCL, follicle center cell lymphoma; MZL/ICY, marginal zone lymphoma/immunocytoma. Red squares indicate diagnostic hallmarks.

Cutaneous Marginal Zone B-Cell Lymphoma (MZL; MALT Type)

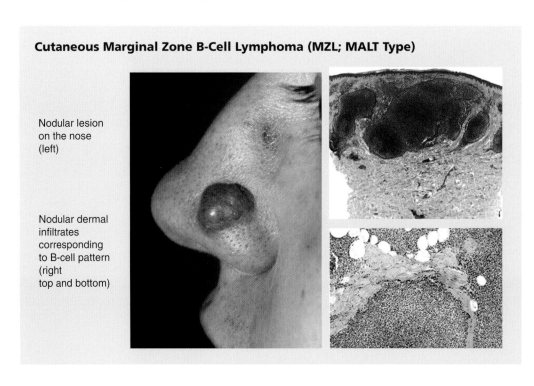

Nodular lesion on the nose (left)

Nodular dermal infiltrates corresponding to B-cell pattern (right top and bottom)

MARGINAL ZONE LYMPHOMA

Cutaneous Marginal Zone B-Cell Lymphoma (MZL; MALT Type)

Small
monomorphic
B-cells (left)

Monocytoid
marginal
zone cells (right)

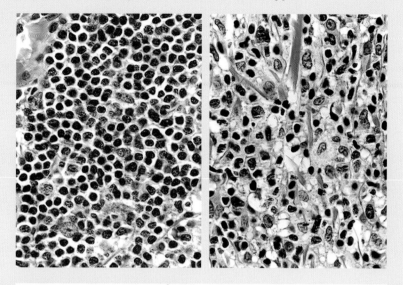

B-cell marker
CD20

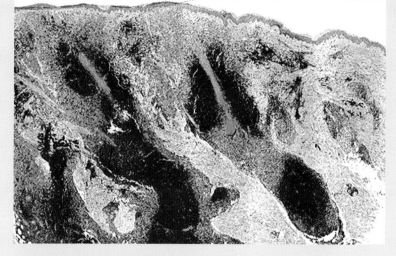

Bcl-2+ marginal
zone cells
(left)

Colonisation of
reactive
germinal centers
by bcl-2+
tumor cells
(right)

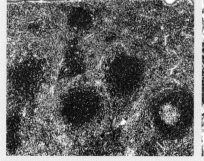
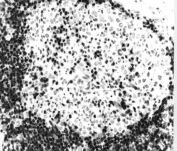

MARGINAL ZONE LYMPHOMA

Cutaneous Marginal Zone B-Cell Lymphoma (MZL; MALT Type)

Lambda positive monotypic plasma cells (left)

CD123+ plasmacytoid dendritic cells at the border of the Infiltrates (right)

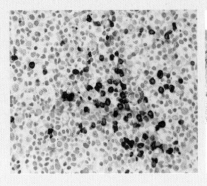
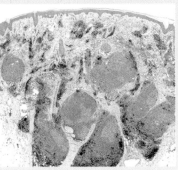

Cl: Red to violaceous infiltrated plaques or firm nodules on an erythematous background. In contrast to follicle center cell lymphoma, which is preferentially located on the head and neck, the sites of predilection of MZL are the trunk and arms.

Hi:

- Nodular well-circumscribed infiltrates in the dermis (B-cell pattern)
- Sometimes "inverse pattern" on scanning magnification: darker centers surrounded by brighter zones of pale-staining cells
- Marginal zone cells with reniform nuclei and monocytoid appearance or plasma cell differentiation in the periphery
- Reactive germinal centers
- The cellular population in the interfollicular areas is represented by small lymphocytes, lymphoplasmacytoid cells, and aggregations of plasma cells
- Occasionally, the infiltrate is arranged around adnexal structures analogous to lymphoepithelioid lesions of MALT lymphoma of the gastrointestinal tract

Immunophenotype: Neoplastic cells: CD20+, bcl-2+, bcl-6-, MUM1-; aggregates of monotypic plasma cells; numerous reactive CD3+ T-cells.

DD: Follicle center cell lymphoma; immunocytoma; B-cell pseudolymphoma.

References

Baldassano, M.F., Bailey, E.M., Ferry, J.A., Harris, N.L., and Duncan, L.M. (1999) Cutaneous lymphoid hyperplasia and cutaneous marginal zone lymphoma: comparison of morphologic and immunophenotypic features. *Am J Surg Pathol* **23**(1): 88–96.

Cerroni, L., Signoretti, S., Hofler, G., et al. (1997) Primary cutaneous marginal zone B-cell lymphoma: a recently described entity of low-grade malignant cutaneous B-cell lymphoma. *Am J Surg Pathol* **21**(11): 1307–15.

de la Fouchardiere, A., Balme, B., Chouvet, B., et al. (1999) Primary cutaneous marginal zone B-cell lymphoma: a report of 9 cases. *J Am Acad Dermatol* **41**(2 Pt 1): 181–8.

de Leval, L., Harris, N.L., Longtine, J., Ferry, J.A., and Duncan, L.M. (2001) Cutaneous b-cell lymphomas of follicular and marginal zone types: use of Bcl-6, CD10, Bcl-2, and CD21 in differential diagnosis and classification. *Am J Surg Pathol* **25**(6): 732–41.

Kempf, W., Kerl, H., and Kutzner, H. (2010) CD123-positive plasmacytoid dendritic cells in primary cutaneous marginal zone B-cell lymphoma: a crucial role and a new lymphoma paradigm. *Am J Dermatopathol* **32**(2): 194–6.

Kutzner, H., Kerl, H., Pfaltz, M. C., and Kempf, W. (2009). CD123-positive plasmacytoid dendritic cells in primary cutaneous marginal zone B-cell lymphoma: diagnostic and pathogenetic implications. *Am J Surg Pathol* **33**(9), 1307–131

Servitje, O., Gallardo, F., Estrach, T., et al. (2002) Primary cutaneous marginal zone B-cell lymphoma: a clinical, histopathological, immunophenotypic and molecular genetic study of 22 cases. *Br J Dermatol* **147**(6): 1147–58.

Spencer, J., Perry, M.E., and Dunn-Walters, D.K. (1998) Human marginal-zone B cells. *Immunol Today* **19**(9): 421–6.

Tomaszewski, M.M., Abbondanzo, S.L., and Lupton, G.P. (2000) Extranodal marginal zone B-cell lymphoma of the skin: a morphologic and immunophenotypic study of 11 cases. *Am J Dermatopathol* **22**(3): 205–11.

MARGINAL ZONE LYMPHOMA

Variant: Immunocytoma

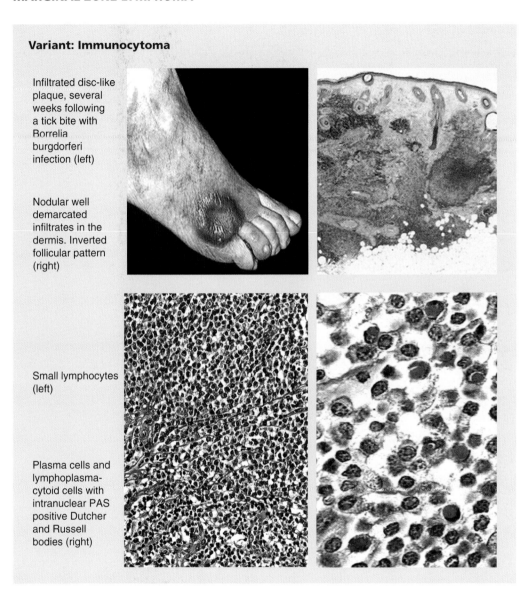

Infiltrated disc-like plaque, several weeks following a tick bite with Borrelia burgdorferi infection (left)

Nodular well demarcated infiltrates in the dermis. Inverted follicular pattern (right)

Small lymphocytes (left)

Plasma cells and lymphoplasma-cytoid cells with intranuclear PAS positive Dutcher and Russell bodies (right)

Similar to the pathogenetic role of *Helicobacter pylori* in mucosa-associated lymphoid tumor (MALT), *Borrelia burgdorferi* infection can induce immunocytoma, which is a variant of marginal zone lymphoma, rich in plasma cells.

Cl: Mostly solitary infiltrated plaque or tumor. History may reveal infection with *Borrelia burgdorferi*.

Hi:

• Nodular well-demarcated dermal infiltrates (B-cell pattern)

• Predominantly composed of plasma cells and lymphoplasmacytoid cells

• Globular intranuclear inclusions of immuno-globulin in plasma cells and plasmacytoid cells (Dutcher bodies). The number is varia-ble, sometimes very few, and one has to search for them, predominantly in the upper dermis

• Intracytoplasmic inclusions (Russell bodies)

DD: Other cutaneous B-cell lymphomas or pseudolymphomas.

MARGINAL ZONE LYMPHOMA

References

Braun-Falco, O., Guggenberger, K., Burg, G., and Fateh-Moghadam, A. (1978) Immunozytom unter dem Bild einer Acrodermatitis chronica atrophicans. *Hautarzt* **29**: 644–7.

Cerroni, L., Zochling, N., Putz, B., and Kerl, H. (1997) Infection by Borrelia burgdorferi and cutaneous B-cell lymphoma. *J Cutan Pathol* **24**(8): 457–61.

Demirkesen, C., Tuzuner, N., Su, O., Eskazan, A.E., Soysal, T., and Onsun, N. (2004) Primary cutaneous immunocytoma/marginal zone B-cell lymphoma: a case with unusual course. *Am J Dermatopathol* **26**(2): 119–22.

Duncan, L.M. and LeBoit, P.E. (1997) Are primary cutaneous immunocytoma and marginal zone lymphoma the same disease? *Am J Surg Pathol* **21**(11): 1368–72.

Goodlad, J.R., Davidson, M.M., Hollowood, K., et al. (2000) Primary cutaneous B-cell lymphoma and Borrelia burgdorferi infection in patients from the Highlands of Scotland. *Am J Surg Pathol* **24**(9): 1279–85.

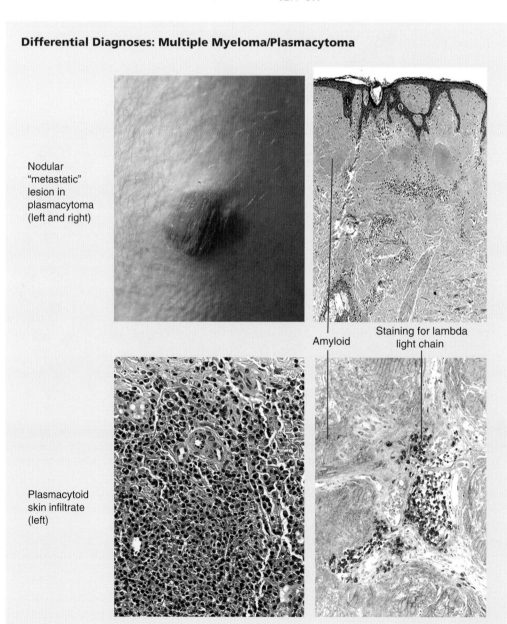

Differential Diagnoses: Multiple Myeloma/Plasmacytoma

Nodular "metastatic" lesion in plasmacytoma (left and right)

Amyloid

Staining for lambda light chain

Plasmacytoid skin infiltrate (left)

FOLLICLE CENTER LYMPHOMA

Cl: Nodular secondary skin involvement.

Hi: Dermal infiltrates with plasma cells showing light chain restriction. Deposits of AL amyloid may be found.

DD: Other cutaneous B-cell lymphomas; B-pseudolymphomas.

Reference

Becker, M.R., Rompel, R., Plum, J., and Gaiser, T. (2008) Light chain multiple myeloma with cutaneous AL amyloidosis. *J Dtsch Dermatol Ges* **6**(9): 744–5.

Primary Cutaneous Follicle Center Lymphoma (FCL)

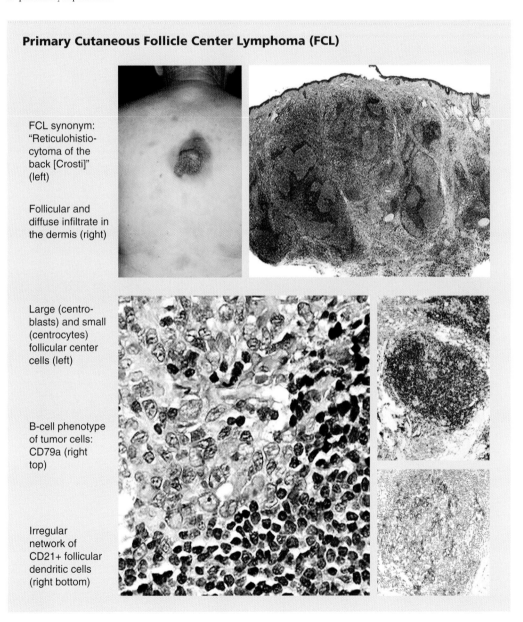

FCL synonym: "Reticulohistiocytoma of the back [Crosti]" (left)

Follicular and diffuse infiltrate in the dermis (right)

Large (centroblasts) and small (centrocytes) follicular center cells (left)

B-cell phenotype of tumor cells: CD79a (right top)

Irregular network of CD21+ follicular dendritic cells (right bottom)

A primary cutaneous B-cell lymphoma with predominance of centrocyte-like tumor cells, which may show a (1) follicular, (2) follicular and diffuse, or (3) diffuse growth pattern. The clinical course is slowly progressive.

Cl: Solitary, rarely multiple, red-brown nodular lesions or thick plaques with smooth surface on the trunk, head, and neck. Hard consistency is very typical.

FOLLICLE CENTER LYMPHOMA

Primary Cutaneous Follicle Center Lymphoma (FCL)

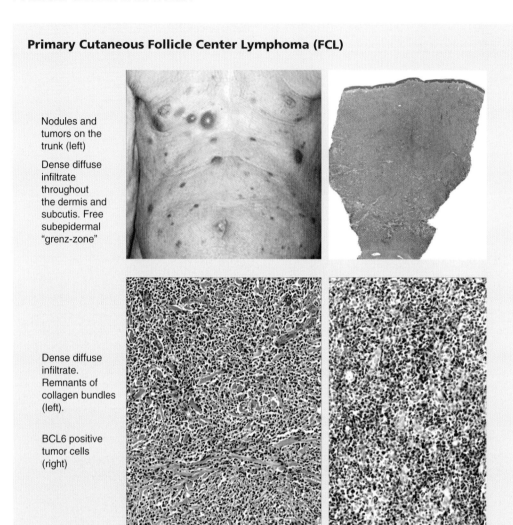

Nodules and tumors on the trunk (left)

Dense diffuse infiltrate throughout the dermis and subcutis. Free subepidermal "grenz-zone"

Dense diffuse infiltrate. Remnants of collagen bundles (left).

BCL6 positive tumor cells (right)

Hi:

- Dermal infiltrate (B-cell pattern: no epidermotropism)
- Growth pattern depending on the subtype:
  - Follicular
  - Follicular and diffuse
  - Diffuse
- Lack of polarization, reduced mantle zone
- Mixed large (centroblasts) and small (centrocytes) follicular center cells
- In contrast to marginal zone lymphoma and pseudolymphoma, tingible body macrophages are usually absent
- Irregular networks of follicular dendritic cells (CD21)

Immunophenotype: CD20+, CD79a+, CD10+, bcl-6 +, bcl-2− (90%), MUM-1−; networks of CD21+ follicular dendritic cells.

Genotype: Monoclonal rearrangement of Ig heavy chain genes (80% of cases).

DD: Other cutaneous B-cell lymphomas; B-pseudolymphomas.

References

Berti, E., Alessi, E., and Caputo, R. (1991) Reticulohistiocytoma of the dorsum (Crosti's disease) and other B-cell lymphomas. *Semin Diagn Pathol* **8**(2): 82–90.

Berti, E., Alessi, E., Caputo, R., Gianotti, R., Delia, D., and Vezzoni, P. (1988) Reticulohistiocytoma of the dorsum. *J Am Acad Dermatol* **19**: 259–72.

DIFFUSE LARGE B-CELL LYMPHOMA (DLBCL)

Caro, M.S.F. (1952) Reticulohistiocytoma of the skin. *Arch Dermatol* **65**: 701–13.

Cerutti, P. and Santoianni, P. (1973) A relatively benign reticulosis: Crosti's "reticulohistiocytoma of the back". *Int J Dermatol* **12**(1): 35–40.

Crosti, A. (1951) Micosi fungoid e reticulo-istiocitomi cutanei maligni. *Minerva Dermatol* **26**: 3–11.

Dilly, M., Ben-Rejeb, H., Vergier, B., ct al. (2014) Primary cutaneous follicle center lymphoma with Hodgkin and Reed-Sternberg-like cells: a new histopathologic variant. *J Cutan Pathol* **41**(10): 797–801.

Diffuse Large B-Cell Lymphoma (DLBCL)

These lymphomas are composed of large B-cells (centroblasts and immunoblasts) and show an aggressive course. DLBCL includes a variety of different entities, formerly referred to as centroblastic lymphoma, immunoblastic lymphoma, "reticulohistiocytoma" or "reticulosarcoma." Two forms of primary cutaneous DLBCL are distinguished in the WHO-EORTC Consensus Classification: DLBCL leg type and DLBCL others. The new WHO classification (2018) has changed "DLBCL, others" to "DLBCL, NOS."

Variant: Cutaneous Diffuse Large B-Cell Lymphoma (Leg Type)

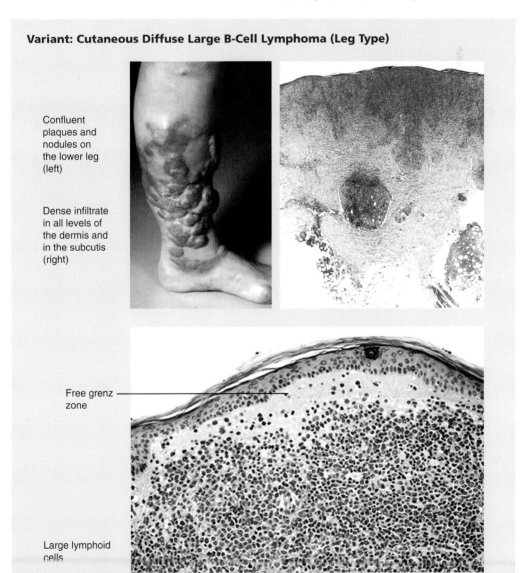

Confluent plaques and nodules on the lower leg (left)

Dense infiltrate in all levels of the dermis and in the subcutis (right)

Free grenz zone

Large lymphoid cells

DIFFUSE LARGE B-CELL LYMPHOMA (DLBCL)

Diffuse Large B-Cell Lymphoma (DLBCL)

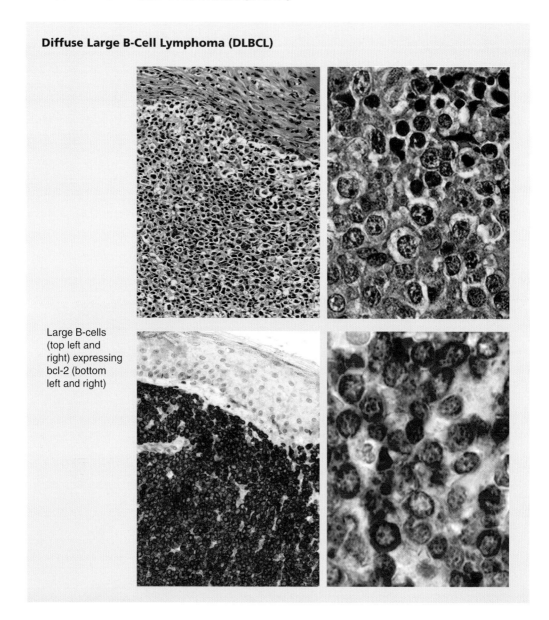

Large B-cells (top left and right) expressing bcl-2 (bottom left and right)

Cl: Most commonly seen on the lower legs. Rapidly growing solitary or multiple confluent infiltrated plaques or tumors. Smooth surface, sometimes ulcerated.

DIFFUSE LARGE B-CELL LYMPHOMA (DLBCL)

Diffuse Large B-Cell Lymphoma (DLBCL), Non-Leg Type

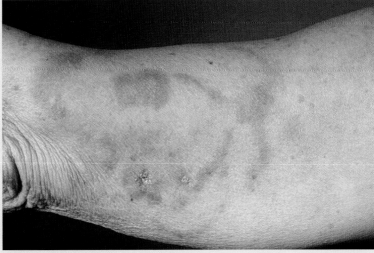

Arciform infiltrates on the arm

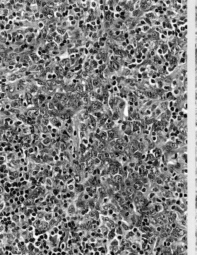
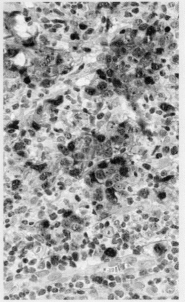

Diffuse large cell infiltrate (left), MUM-1+ (right)

Other localisation (non-leg type) can be involved and basically show the same clinical and histological features.

Hi:

- Diffuse dermal infiltrate, sparing a subepidermal grenz zone
- Large B-cells with abundant cytoplasm:
  - Centroblast: large non-cleaved follicular center cells, showing large vesicular nuclei with small nucleoli attached to the nuclear membrane
  - Immunoblasts: large cells with round nuclei and prominent central nucleoli
  - Occasionally multilobated, anaplastic or large cleaved cells

Immunophenotype: CD20+ or CD79a+, CD10−/+, bcl-2+++, bcl-6+/−, MUM-1/IRF-4++, IgM+.

Genotype: Monoclonal rearrangement of Ig heavy chain genes.

DIFFUSE LARGE B-CELL LYMPHOMA (DLBCL)

References

Kodama, K., Massone, C., Chott, A., Metze, D., Kerl, H., and Cerroni, L. (2005) Primary cutaneous large B-cell lymphomas: clinicopathologic features, classification, and prognostic factors in a large series of patients. *Blood* **106**(7): 2491–7.

Hallermann, C., Kaune, K.M., Gesk, S., et al. (2004) Molecular cytogenetic analysis of chromosomal breakpoints in the IGH, MYC, BCL6, and MALT1 gene loci in primary cutaneous B-cell lymphomas. *J Invest Dermatol* **123**(1): 213–19.

Senff, N.J., Zoutman, W.H., Vermeer, M.H., et al. (2009) Fine-mapping chromosomal loss at 9p21: correlation with prognosis in primary cutaneous diffuse large B-cell lymphoma, leg type. *J Invest Dermatol* **129**(5): 1149–55.

Variant: T-Cell-Rich B-Cell Lymphoma (DLBCL)

Preauricular infiltrate with superficial ulceration and scarring (left)

Dense infiltrate of T-lymphocytes (top right) with scattered large B-cells (bottom left), expressing CD20 (bottom right)

CD20

This extremely rare variant of a primary cutaneous diffuse large B-cell lymphoma is defined by the predominance (75–90%) of non-neoplastic T-cells admixed with *scattered* tumoral cells expressing B-cell pheno- and genotype.

Cl: Solitary nodule or deep subcutaneous tumor. Multiple lesions are rare. The most frequent site of involvement is the head and neck area. Association with Gardner's syndrome and with Epstein–Barr virus infection has been reported.

Hi:
- Background of diffuse infiltrate of small lymphocytes expressing T-cell phenotype

- Scattered large pleomorphic tumor cells with clear cytoplasm and multilobular nuclei (starry sky appearance), resembling Hodgkin or Reed–Sternberg cells
- Centroblasts and immunoblasts can be observed
- Marked vascular proliferation is found in some cases

Immunophenotype: Tumor cells bear B-cell markers.

Genotype: Clonal rearrangement of Ig heavy chain genes.

DD: Burkitt's lymphoma; lymphocyte-predominant Hodgkin's lymphoma; small to medium-sized T-cell lymphoma; lymphomatoid granulomatosis.

References

Arai, E., Sakurai, M., Nakayama, H., Morinaga, S., and Katayama, I. (1993) Primary cutaneous T-cell-rich B-cell lymphoma. *Br J Dermatol* **129**(2): 196–200.

Dommann, S.N., Dommann-Scherrer, C.C., Zimmerman, D., Dours-Zimmermann, M.T., Hassam, S., and Burg, G. (1995) Primary cutaneous T-cell-rich B-cell lymphoma. A case report with a 13-year follow-up. *Am J Dermatopathol* **17**(6): 618–24.

Kamarashev, J., Dummer, R., Schmidt, M.H., Kempf, W., Kurrer, M.O., and Burg, G. (2000) Primary cutaneous T-cell-rich B-cell lymphoma and Hodgkin's disease in a patient with Gardner's syndrome. *Dermatology* **201**(4): 362–5.

Li, S., Griffin, C.A., Mann, R.B., and Borowitz, M.J. (2001) Primary cutaneous T-cell-rich B-cell lymphoma: clinically distinct from its nodal counterpart? *Mod Pathol* **14**(1): 10–13.

Sander, C.A., Kaudewitz, P., Kutzner, H., et al. (1996) T-cell-rich B-cell lymphoma presenting in skin. A clinicopathologic analysis of six cases. *J Cutan Pathol* **23**(2): 101–8.

Take, H., Kubota, K., Fukuda, T., Shinonome, S., Ishikawa, O., and Shirakura, T. (1996) An indolent type of Epstein–Barr virus-associated T-cell-rich B-cell lymphoma of the skin: report of a case. *Am J Hematol* **52**(3): 221–3.

Cutaneous Spindle B-Cell Lymphoma

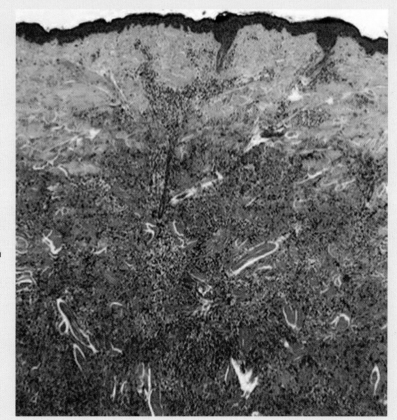

Diffuse dermal infiltrate without epidermotropism

Cutaneous Spindle B-Cell Lymphoma

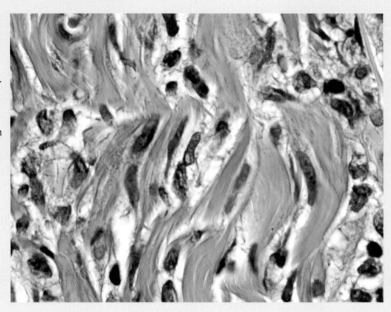

Indian filing pattern of spindle-shaped lymphoid cells (expressing B-lymphocyte markers) between collagen bundles

Spindle cell morphology is not a distinct pathognomonic feature designating a specific nosological entity. It is seen as a variant of diffuse large B-cell lymphoma by some authors, but recent molecular studies indicate that it rather represents a form of peripheral cutaneous follicle center lymphoma (PCFCL).

Cl: Inconspicuous plaques or nodular lesions.

Hi:

- Diffuse dense infiltrate in a fascicular pattern
- Spindle-shaped lymphoid cells spreading between collagen bundles

Immunophenotype: CD20+, CD79a+, Bcl-6+, CD10+, CD21+.

Genotype: Clonal rearrangement of Ig heavy chain genes.

DD: Various mesenchymal or epithelial spindle cell tumors.

References

Cerroni, L., El-Shabrawi-Caelen, L., Fink-Puches, R., LeBoit, P.E., and Kerl, H. (2000) Cutaneous spindle-cell B-cell lymphoma: a morphologic variant of cutaneous large B-cell lymphoma. *Am J Dermatopathol* **22**(4): 299–304.

Charli-Joseph, Y., Cerroni, L., and LeBoit, P.E. (2015) Cutaneous spindle-cell B-cell lymphomas: most are neoplasms of follicular center cell origin. *Am J Surg Pathol* **39**(6): 737–43.

Forcucci, J., Ralston, J., and Lazarchick, J. (2016) Diagnosing spindle cell variant of primary cutaneous B-cell lymphoma: potential pitfalls and solutions. *Ann Clin Lab Sci* **46**(2): 209–12.

Garrido, M.C., Rios, J.J., Riveiro-Falkenbach, E., Escamez, P.J., Ronco, M.A., and Rodriguez-Peralto, J.L. (2015) Primary cutaneous spindle cell B-cell lymphoma of follicle origin mimicking acne rosacea. *Am J Dermatopathol* **37**(6): e64–7.

Goodlad, J.R. (2001) Spindle-cell B-cell lymphoma presenting in the skin. *Br J Dermatol* **145**(2): 313–17.

Jghaimi, F., Hocar, O., Akhdari, N., Amal, S., and Belaabidia, B. (2013) Primary cutaneous spindle-cell B-cell lymphoma of follicle center cell origin. *Am J Dermatopathol* **35**(8): 871–3.

Kimura, Y., Arakawa, F., Kiyasu, J., et al. (2012) A spindle cell variant of diffuse large B-cell lymphoma is characterized by T-cell/myofibrohistio-rich stromal alterations: analysis of 10 cases and a review of the literature. *Eur J Haematol* **89**(4): 302–10.

Nozawa, Y., Wang, J., Weiss, L. M., Kikuchi, S., Hakozaki, H., and Abe, M. (2001) Diffuse large B-cell lymphoma with spindle cell features. *Histopathology* **38**(2): 177–8.

Ries, S., Barr, R., LeBoit, P., McCalmont, T., and Waldman, J. (2007) Cutaneous sarcomatoid B-cell lymphoma. *Am J Dermatopathol* **29**(1): 96–8.

Wang, L., Lv, Y., Wang, X., Wei, K., and Zhang, Y. (2010) Giant primary cutaneous spindle cell B-cell lymphoma of follicle center cell origin. *Am J Dermatopathol* **32**(6): 620–32.

EXTRACUTANEOUS B-CELL LYMPHOMA (BCL) WITH FREQUENT SKIN INVOLVEMENT

Yun, S.J., Lee, K.H., Yang, D.W., et al. (2009) Primary cutaneous spindle cell B-cell lymphoma with multiple figurate erythema-like manifestation. *J Cutan Pathol* **36**(1): 49–52.

Extracutaneous B-Cell Lymphoma (BCL) with Frequent Skin Involvement

Mantle Cell Lymphoma

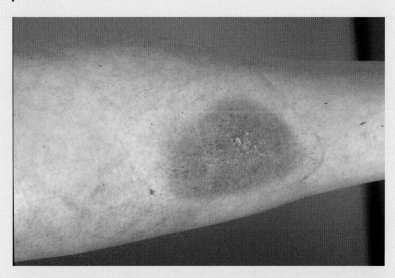

Circumscribed infiltrate on the lower leg

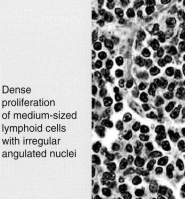

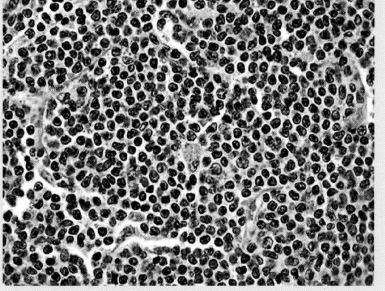

Dense proliferation of medium-sized lymphoid cells with irregular angulated nuclei

Lymphomatous proliferation of mantle zone cells in the lymphoid follicles may secondarily involve the skin. However, cases with primary (blastoid) mantle cell lymphoma have been reported.

Cl: Inconspicuous plaques and nodules.

Hi:
- Nodular dermal infiltrate
- Grenz zone
- Monotonous proliferation of small to medium-sized lymphoid cells, slightly larger than normal lymphocytes

EXTRACUTANEOUS B-CELL LYMPHOMA (BCL) WITH FREQUENT SKIN INVOLVEMENT

- Irregular angulated or cleaved nuclei, scant pale cytoplasm, dispersed chromatin
- Lymphoblasts may be present in blastic forms of mantle cell lymphoma
- Indian file spreading of tumor cells between collagen bundles

Cytochemistry: Alkaline phophatase-positive cell membrane.

Immunophenotype: CD20+, bcl-2+, bcl-6−, cyclin D1+.

Genotype: Clonal rearrangement of Ig heavy chain genes; t(11;14).

DD: Other B-cell lymphomas.

References

Bertero, M., Novelli, M., Fierro, M.T., and Bernengo, M.G. (1994) Mantle zone lymphoma: an immunohistologic study of skin lesions. *J Am Acad Dermatol* **30**(1): 23–30.

Cao, Q., Li, Y., Lin, H., Ke, Z., Liu, Y., and Ye, Z. (2013) Mantle cell lymphoma of blastoid variant with skin lesion and rapid progression: a case report and literature review. *Am J Dermatopathol* **35**(8): 851–5.

Cesinaro, A.M., Bettelli, S., Maccio, L., and Milani, M. (2014) Primary cutaneous mantle cell lymphoma of the leg with blastoid morphology and aberrant immunophenotype: a diagnostic challenge. *Am J Dermatopathol* **36**(2): e16–18.

Estrozi, B., Sanches, J.A. Jr, Varela, P.C., and Bacchi, C.E. (2009) Primary cutaneous blastoid mantle cell lymphoma-case report. *Am J Dermatopathol* **31**(4): 398–400.

Geerts, M.L. and Busschots, A.M. (1994) Mantle-cell lymphomas of the skin. *Dermatol Clin* **12**(2): 409–17.

Geerts, M.L., Burg, G., Schmoeckel, C., and Braun, F.O. (1984) Alkaline phosphatase positive lymphoma. *Dermatologica* **169**(6): 342–7.

Geerts, M.L., Burg, G., Schmoeckel, C., and Braun, F.O. (1984) Alkaline phosphatase activity in non-Hodgkin's lymphomas and pseudolymphomas of the skin. *J Dermatol Surg Oncol* **10**(4): 306–12.

Gru, A.A., Hurley, M.Y., Salavaggione, A.L., et al. (2016) Cutaneous mantle cell lymphoma: a clinicopathologic review of 10 cases. *J Cutan Pathol* **43**(12): 1112–20.

Lynch, D.W., Verma, R., Larson, E., Geis, M.C., and Jassim, A.D. (2012) Primary cutaneous mantle cell lymphoma with blastic features: report of a rare case with special reference to staging and effectiveness of chemotherapy. *J Cutan Pathol* **39**(4): 449–53.

Moody, B.R., Bartlett, N.L., George, D.W., et al. (2001) Cyclin D1 as an aid in the diagnosis of mantle cell lymphoma in skin biopsies: a case report. *Am J Dermatopathol* **23**(5): 470–6.

Sen, F., Medeiros, L.J., Lu, D., et al. (2002) Mantle cell lymphoma involving skin: cutaneous lesions may be the first manifestation of disease and tumors often have blastoid cytologic features. *Am J Surg Pathol* **26**(10): 1312–18.

Burkitt's Lymphoma (BL)

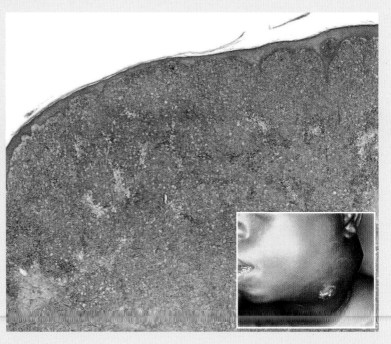

Cohesive dense dermal infiltrate, per continuitatem from lymph nodes of the neck (inset)

EXTRACUTANEOUS B-CELL LYMPHOMA (BCL) WITH FREQUENT SKIN INVOLVEMENT

Burkitt's Lymphoma (BL)

Monomorphous infiltrate with scattered macrophages, featuring a starry sky pattern (left)

Smear preparation of tumor cells with scant cytoplasm and small vacuoles (right)

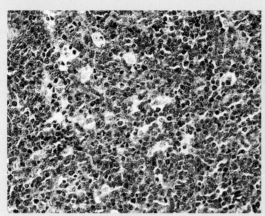
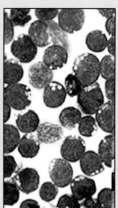

Burkitt's lymphoma (BL) is an aggressive B-cell lymphoma, associated with Epstein–Barr virus (EBV) infection in most cases and featuring translocation of the c-myc gene. HIV-induced immunodeficiency may be a predisposing factor.

Cl: The jaws of children in equatorial Africa and sporadically children and young adults in other countries are most commonly affected. Skin may be affected by secondary invasion from regional lymph nodes.

Hi:

- Diffuse cohesive monomorphous non-epidermotropic infiltrate
- Medium-sized lymphoid cells with large nuclei and narrow basophilic cytoplasmatic rim showing small lipid vacuoles
- Many mitotic figures and spontaneous cell death
- Scattered pale macrophages (starry sky pattern), containing ingested remnants of apoptotic tumor cells

Immunophenotype: The tumor cells express B-cell-associated antigens (CD19, CD20, CD22), are positive for CD10 and Bcl-6 (pointing to a germinal center origin), and are negative for CD5, CD23, Bcl-2, and TdT.

Genotype: t(8;14) translocation of the myc gene.

DD: Other B-cell lymphomas and pseudolymphomas; T-cell-rich B-cell lymphoma; lymphocyte-rich Hodgkin's lymphoma.

References

Burkitt, D. (1958) A sarcoma involving the jaws in African children. *Br J Surg* **46**: 218–23.

Mann, R.B., Jaffe, E.S., Braylan, R.C., et al. (1976) Nonendemic Burkitts's lymphoma. A B-cell tumor related to germinal centers. *N Engl J Med* **295**(13): 685–91.

Rogers, A., Graves, M., Toscano, M., and Davis, L. (2014) A unique cutaneous presentation of Burkitt lymphoma. *Am J Dermatopathol* **36**(12): 997–1001.

Rogge, T. (1975) [Burkitt's lymphoma with skin infiltrates] *Hautarzt* **26**(7): 379–82.

EXTRACUTANEOUS B-CELL LYMPHOMA (BCL) WITH FREQUENT SKIN INVOLVEMENT

Lymphomatoid Granulomatosis (Liebow) (LYG)

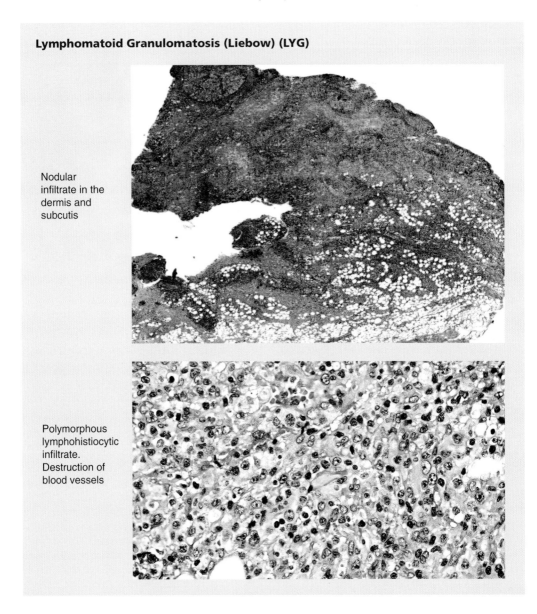

Nodular infiltrate in the dermis and subcutis

Polymorphous lymphohistiocytic infiltrate. Destruction of blood vessels

Lymphomatoid granulomatosis (LYG), originally described by Liebow et al., is a rare multisystemic angiocentric and angiodestructive lymphoproliferative disease involving extranodal sites, especially the lungs, skin (in more than 50% of patients), kidneys, and brain. It is EBV positive in most cases and may progress to diffuse large B-cell lymphoma. Although the predominant infiltrating cells are T-cells, the T-cell receptor genes are not clonally rearranged. These findings indicate that LYG is an angiocentric T-cell-rich B-cell lymphoproliferative disorder.

Cl: The clinical features of cutaneous LYG are diverse, transient and manifest as scattered nodules, eroded and crusted lesions, recurrent skin ulcerations, facial edema, papules or folliculitis-like eruptions. EBV infection is an important etiological factor.

Hi:
- Nodular polymorphous lymphohistiocytic infiltrate involving the dermis and subcutis
- Angiocentric and angiodestructive features, inducing necrosis
- No epidermal involvement

INTRAVASCULAR LYMPHOMAS

Immunophenotype: EBV+ in CD20+ B-cells; reactive T-cell infiltrate CD2+, CD3+, CD4+, CD5+, CD7+, CD45RO+.

Genotype: Clonal rearrangement of Ig heavy chain genes.

DD: Vasculitis; other lymphomas.

References

Beaty, M.W., Toro, J., Sorbara, L., et al. (2001) Cutaneous lymphomatoid granulomatosis: correlation of clinical and biologic features. *Am J Surg Pathol* **25**(9): 1111–20.

Brodell, R.T., Miller, C.W., and Eisen, A.Z. (1986) Cutaneous lesions of lymphomatoid granulomatosis. *Arch Dermatol* **122**(3): 303–6.

James, W.D., Odom, R.B., and Katzenstein, A.L. (1981) Cutaneous manifestations of lymphomatoid granulomatosis. Report of 44 cases and a review of the literature. *Arch Dermatol* **117**(4): 196–202.

Katzenstein, A.L., Carrington, C.B., and Liebow, A.A. (1979) Lymphomatoid granulomatosis: a clinico-pathologic study of 152 cases. *Cancer* **43**(1): 360–73.

Liebow, A.A., Carrington, C.R., and Friedman, P.J. (1972) Lymphomatoid granulomatosis. *Hum Pathol* **3**(4): 457–8.

McNiff, J.M., Cooper, D., Howe, G., et al. (1996) Lymphomatoid granulomatosis of the skin and lung. An angiocentric T-cell-rich B-cell lymphoproliferative disorder. *Arch Dermatol* **132**(12): 1464–70.

Intravascular Lymphomas

Intravascular Large B-Cell Lymphoma (IV-LBCL) (Systemic Angioendotheliomatosis)

Violet erythemas on the leg (left)

Vessels filled with infiltrating cells (right)

Intravascular pleomorphic cells (left and right)*

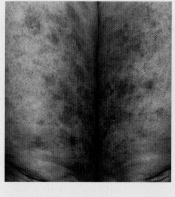
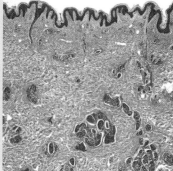
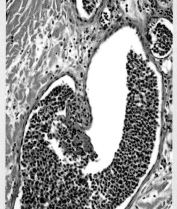
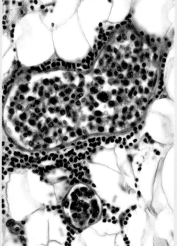

Courtesy of Omar P Sangueza, Winston-Salem/USA

INTRAVASCULAR LYMPHOMAS

Intravascular large B-cell lymphoma is a systemic, diffuse large B-cell lymphoma. Some cases are EBV-associated.

Cl: Erythematous or violaceous plaques or nodules on the face, trunk or lower extremities resembling livedo racemosa.

Hi: Large atypical cells in the lumina of capillaries and venules.

Immunophenotype: B-cell markers.

DD: Reactive angioendotheliomatosis; erythema nodosum; livedo reticularis.

References

Barnett, C.R., Seo, S., Husain, S., and Grossman, M.E. (2008) Intravascular B-cell lymphoma: the role of skin biopsy. *Am J Dermatopathol* **30**(3): 295–9.

Berger, T.G. and Dawson, N.A. (1988) Angioendotheliomatosis. *J Am Acad Dermatol* **18**(2 Pt 2): 407–12.

Kiyohara, T., Kumakiri, M., Kobayashi, H., Shimizu, T., Ohkawara, A., and Ohnuki, M. (2000) A case of intravascular large B-cell lymphoma mimicking erythema nodosum: the importance of multiple skin biopsies. *J Cutan Pathol* **27**(8): 413–18.

Kong, Y.Y., Dai, B., Sheng, W.Q., et al. (2009) Intravascular large B-cell lymphoma with cutaneous manifestations: a clinicopathologic, immunophenotypic and molecular study of three cases. *J Cutan Pathol* **36**(8): 865–70.

Lazova, R., Slater, C., and Scott, G. (1996) Reactive angioendotheliomatosis. Case report and review of the literature. *Am J Dermatopathol* **18**(1): 63–9.

Perniciaro, C., Winkelmann, R.K., Daoud, M.S., and Su, W.P. (1995) Malignant angioendotheliomatosis is an angiotropic intravascular lymphoma. Immunohistochemical, ultrastructural, and molecular genetics studies. *Am J Dermatopathol* **17**(3): 242–8.

Pfleger, L. and Tappeiner, J. (1959) Zur Kenntnis der systemisierten Endotheliomatose der cutanen Blutgefaesse (Reticuloendotheliomatose?). *Hautarzt* **10**: 359–63.

Sitthinamsuwan, P., Chinthammitr, Y., Pattanaprichakul, P., and Sukpanichnant, S. (2017) Random skin biopsy in the diagnosis of intravascular lymphoma. *J Cutan Pathol* **44**(9): 729–33.

Wang, L., Li, C., and Gao, T. (2011) Cutaneous intravascular anaplastic large cell lymphoma. *J Cutan Pathol* **38**(2): 221–6.

Wick, M.R. and Rocamora, A. (1988) Reactive and malignant "angioendotheliomatosis": a discriminant clinicopathological study. *J Cutan Pathol* **15**(5): 260–71.

Intravascular T Cell Lymphoma

Clinical and histological features correspond to the more frequent B-cell variant.

Some cases are EBER positive.

DD: Benign atypical intravascular CD30(+) T-cell proliferation.

References

Au, W.Y., Shek, W.H., Nicholls, J., Tse, K.M., Todd, D., and Kwong, Y.L. (1997) T-cell intravascular lymphomatosis (angiotropic large cell lymphoma): association with Epstein–Barr viral infection. *Histopathology* **31**(6): 563–7.

Deetz, C.O., Gilbertson, K.G. 2nd, Anadkat, M.J., Dehner, L.P., and Lu, D. (2011) A rare case of intravascular large T-cell lymphoma with an unusual T helper phenotype. *Am J Dermatopathol* **33**(8): e99–102.

Gebauer, N., Nissen, E.J., Driesch, P., Feller, A.C., and Merz, H. (2014) Intravascular natural killer cell lymphoma mimicking mycosis fungoides: a case report and review of the literature. *Am J Dermatopathol* **36**(5): e100–4.

Iacobelli, J., Spagnolo, D.V., Tesfai, Y., et al. (2012) Cutaneous intravascular anaplastic large T-cell lymphoma: a case report and review of the literature. *Am J Dermatopathol* **34**(8): e133–8.

Kempf, W., Keller, K., John, H., and Dommann-Scherrer, C. (2014) Benign atypical intravascular CD30+ T-cell proliferation: a recently described reactive lymphoproliferative process and simulator of intravascular lymphoma: report of a case associated with lichen sclerosus and review of the literature. *Am J Clin Pathol* **142**(5): 694–9.

Martinez-Escala, M.E., Guggina, L.M., Cotliar, J., Winter, J.N., and Guitart, J. (2016) Cutaneous involvement in a case of intravascular T-cell lymphoma with a gammadelta phenotype. *Am J Dermatopathol* **38**(2): e27–9.

Perniciaro, C., Winkelmann, R.K., Daoud, M.S., and Su, W.P. (1995) Malignant angioendotheliomatosis is an angiotropic intravascular lymphoma. Immunohistochemical, ultrastructural, and molecular genetics studies. *Am J Dermatopathol* **17**(3): 242–8.

Riveiro-Falkenbach, E., Fernandez-Figueras, M.T., and Rodriguez-Peralto, J.L. (2013) Benign atypical intravascular CD30(+) T-cell proliferation: a reactive condition mimicking intravascular lymphoma. *Am J Dermatopathol* **35**(2): 143–50.

Sepp, N., Schuler, G., Romani, N., et al. (1990) "Intravascular lymphomatosis" (angioendotheliomatosis): evidence for a T-cell origin in two cases. *Hum Pathol* **21**(10): 1051–8.

Wang, L., Chen, S., Ma, H., et al. (2015) Intravascular NK/T-cell lymphoma: a report of five cases with cutaneous manifestation from China. *J Cutan Pathol* **42**(9): 610–17.

Wang, L., Li, C., and Gao, T. (2011) Cutaneous intravascular anaplastic large cell lymphoma. *J Cutan Pathol* **38**(2): 221–6.

Secondary Skin Involvement in Leukemias/Lymphomas

Chronic Lymphocytic Leukemia (CLL)

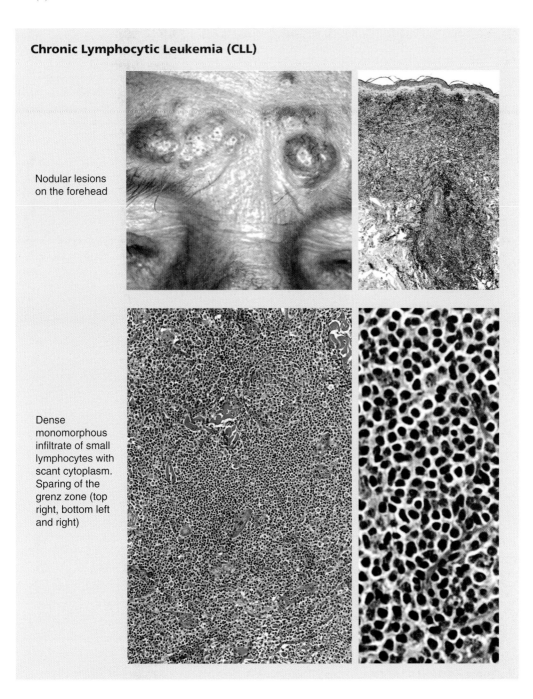

Nodular lesions on the forehead

Dense monomorphous infiltrate of small lymphocytes with scant cytoplasm. Sparing of the grenz zone (top right, bottom left and right)

B-CLL is an accumulative disease of long-lived, mature, monoclonal CD5+ B-cells that express high levels of the antiapoptotic protein bcl-2. Specific skin lesions occur in approximately 8% of patients with B-CLL. Many more patients suffer from non-specific symptoms including purpura, ecchymoses, and maculopapular eruptions.

Cl: Specific lesions present as red or violaceous macules, papules or nodules with smooth surface, preferentially on the face and the ears. Specific infiltrates may be seen at the site of herpes zoster and herpes simplex scars and in association with *Borrelia burgdorferi* infection.

Hi: Dense monomorphous infiltrates of small lymphocytes with chromatin-dense nuclei, small nucleoli, and scant cytoplasm. Variable numbers of eosinophils, neutrophils, and plasma cells may be present.

Immunophenotype: CD19+, CD20+, CD79a+, CD5+, CD23+; monoclonal expression of Ig light chains, sIgM or sIgD.

DD: Cutaneous B-cell lymphomas and pseudolymphomas.

References

Cerroni, L., Zenahlik, P., Hofler, G., Kaddu, S., Smolle, J., and Kerl, H. (1996) Specific cutaneous infiltrates of B-cell chronic lymphocytic leukemia: a clinicopathologic and prognostic study of 42 patients. *Am J Surg Pathol* **20**(8): 1000–10.

Cerroni, L., Zenahlik, P., and Kerl, H. (1995) Specific cutaneous infiltrates of B-cell chronic lymphocytic leukemia arising at the site of herpes zoster and herpes simplex scars. *Cancer* **76**(1): 26–31.

Kash, N., Fink-Puches, R., and Cerroni, L. (2011) Cutaneous manifestations of B-cell chronic lymphocytic leukemia associated with Borrelia burgdorferi infection showing a marginal zone B-cell lymphoma-like infiltrate. *Am J Dermatopathol* **33**(7): 712–15.

Tapia, G., Mate, J.L., Fuente, M.J. (2013) Cutaneous presentation of chronic lymphocytic leukemia as unique extramedullar involvement in a patient with normal peripheral blood lymphocyte count (monoclonal B-cell lymphocytosis). *J Cutan Pathol* **40**(8): 740–4.

Myeloid and Monocytic Leukemias

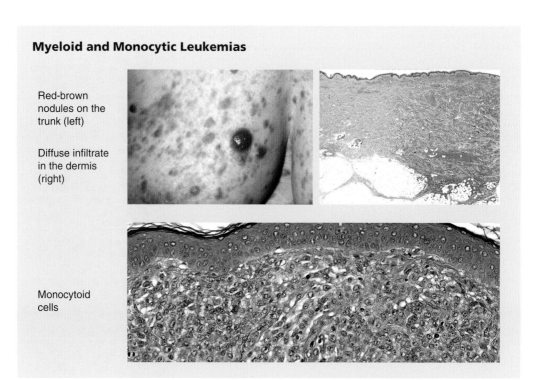

Red-brown nodules on the trunk (left)

Diffuse infiltrate in the dermis (right)

Monocytoid cells

Myeloid and Monocytic Leukemias

Indian filing pattern of tumor cells between collagen bundles (left)

Chloroacetates-terase (Leder) stain of myeloid cells (right)

Cl: In acute myelomonocytic leukemia, mucocutaneous lesions are found in up to 30% of patients. On the skin, they present in a very typical fashion as disseminated red to violaceous thin plaques and papules.

Hi:

- Dense nodular and diffuse pleomorphic infiltrate in the dermis, extending into the subcutis
- Mature and immature cells of the granulocytic series, including atypical myelocytes, eosinophilic metamyelocytes, and neutrophils
- Indian file formation of tumor cells between collagen bundles is very typical

Cytochemistry: Most cells are positive for naphthol-ASD-chloroacetatesterase (Leder stain), lysozyme, and myeloid peroxidase.

Immunophenotype: CD68+, CD14+, MPO+, CD13+, CD33+, CD34+, ERG+, MNDA+, myeloid dendritic cell antigens (BDCA3).

References

Burg, G., Schmoeckel, C., Braun-Falco, O., and Wolff, H.H. (1978) Monocytic leukemia. Clinically appearing as 'malignant reticulosis of the skin'. *Arch Dermatol* **114**(3): 418–20.

Ferran, M., Gallardo, F., Ferrer, A.M., et al. (2008) Acute myeloid dendritic cell leukaemia with specific cutaneous involvement: a diagnostic challenge. *Br J Dermatol* **158**(5): 1129–33.

Kaddu, S., Zenahlik, P., Beham-Schmid, C., Kerl, H., and Cerroni, L. (1999) Specific cutaneous infiltrates in patients with myelogenous leukemia: a clinicopathologic study of 26 patients with assessment of diagnostic criteria. *J Am Acad Dermatol* **40**(6 Pt 1): 966–78.

T-Zone Lymphoma

Papulomacular rash on the abdomen. Swelling of inguinal lymph nodes (left)

Dense dermal infiltrate (mid)

Lymph node: proliferation of interfollicular tumor cells between reactive lymph follicles (right)

Pleomorphic "interfollicular" haloed tumor cells with abundant cytoplasm (left)

CD45+ tumor cells (right top). CD20+ B-cells (right mid). Factor XIIIa+ dendritic cells (right buttom)

T-zone lymphoma (TZL) is a rare subtype of nodal peripheral T-cell lymphoma characterized by a clonal expansion of T-zone lymphocytes accompanied by a proliferation of other T-zone constituents.

Cl: Non-specific symptoms are frequent but specific lesions are rarely found and may present as widespread papulonodular rash. Peripheral lymph nodes are enlarged.

Hi:

- Diffuse and perivascularly arranged lymphocytic infiltrate in the dermis and subcutis
- Tightly packed, medium-sized pleomorphic lymphocytes with abundant clear haloed cytoplasm

Lymph node: Effaced architecture; interfollicular proliferation of medium-sized lymphocytes with abundant clear cytoplasm. Increased number of factor XIIIa + dermal dendritic cells and postcapillary venules.

Immunophenotype: CD3+, CD43+, CD45RO+; negative for CD20, CD21, and CD30.

References

Bernengo, M.G. and Massobrio, R. (1990) Cutaneous manifestations in T-zone lymphoma. *Curr Probl Dermatol* **19**: 161–6.

Helbron, D., Brittinger, G., and Lennert, K. (1979) [T-zone lymphoma – clinical symptoms, therapy, and prognosis (author's transl)] *Blut* **39**(2): 117–31.

Kazakov, D.V., Kempf, W., Michaelis, S., et al. (2002) T-zone lymphoma with cutaneous involvement: a case report and review of the literature. *Br J Dermatol* **146**(6): 1096–100.

Lennert, K. (1978) Malignant lymphoma, lymphocytic, T-zone type (T-zone lymphoma). In: Lennert, K. (ed.) Malignant Lymphomas other than Hodgkin's Disease. Berlin: Springer-Verlag.

Adult T-Cell Leukemia/Lymphoma (ATLL)

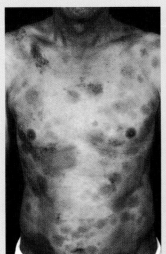

Disseminated erythematous plaques (left)

Medium to large pleomorphic cells (right)

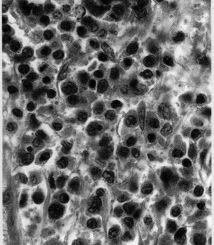

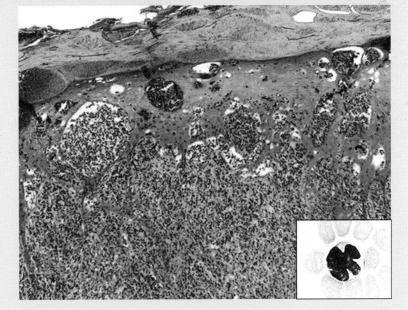

Epidermotropic dermal infiltrate

"Flower cell" in the peripheral blood (inset)

Adult T-cell leukemia/lymphoma is a peripheral T-cell lymphoma, etiologically associated with human T-cell leukemia virus-1 (HTLV-1), which is endemic in south-western Japan and the Caribbean. **Cl**: Various subtypes can be differentiated: acute, chronic, lymphomatous, and smoldering. Skin involvement occurs in about 50% of cases, presenting as purpuric papules, nodules or tumors, or as erythroderma. Peripheral blood smears show atypical lymphoid cells with polylobulated, convoluted nuclei (so-called flower cells) and leukocytosis, sometimes in conjunction with anemia. Additional findings are hypoalbuminemia, hypergammaglobulinemia, and hypercalcemia.

Hi: Histologically, ATLL shares some features with MF.

- Perivascular or diffuse infiltrate in the upper dermis
- Medium to large pleomorphic cells
- Prominent epidermotropism with formation of large Pautrier microabscesses
- Plasma cells and eosinophils are less frequent than in MF

DD: Mycosis fungoides; anaplastic large cell lymphoma CD30+.

References

Chan, H.L., Su, I.J., Kuo, T.T., et al. (1985) Cutaneous manifestations of adult T cell leukemia/lymphoma. Report of three different forms. *J Am Acad Dermatol* **13**(2 Pt 1): 213–19.

Wang, C., Yao, Z., Liao, J., et al. (1999) Clinicopathologic, immunophenotypic and ultrastructrual analyses of ATLL patients with cutaneous involvement. *Chin Med J (Engl)* **112**(5): 461–5.

Immature Hematopoietic Malignancies

Blastic Plasmacytoid Dendritic Cell Neoplasm

Contusiform hemorrhagic plaques (left)

Dermal infiltrate extending to the subcutis (right)

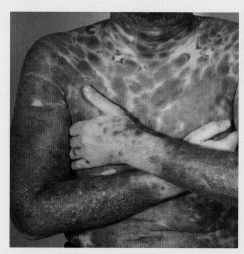
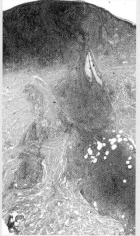

Blastic Plasmacytoid Dendritic Cell Neoplasm

Densely packed
blastic tumor
cells with
irregular nuclei.
Erythrocyte
extravasation
(left)

CD56+ tumor
cells (right)

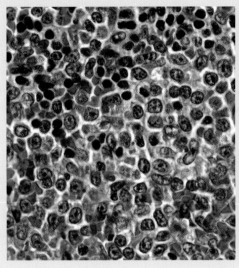
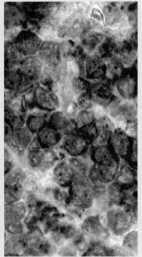

This neoplasm, formerly referred to as CD4+/ CD56+ hematodermic blastic NK-cell lymphoma, blastoid NK-cell leukemia/lymphoma or agranular CD4+ CD56+ hematodermic neoplasm, is a tumor of plasmacytoid dendritic cells (CD123+).

Cl: Skin involvement occurs in 87% of cases and manifests with very typical, rapidly growing and expanding contusiform, brownish infiltrated confluent plaques or nodules. The oral mucosa is commonly involved.

Hi:

- Diffuse dermal infiltrates without epidermotropism
- Densely packed, medium-sized and blast-like "lymphoid" tumor cells
- Scant cytoplasm, no granulation
- Irregular nuclei with one or several nucleoli
- Erythrocyte extravasation
- Mitoses are rare
- Few concomitant small T-lymphocytes, no eosinophils or plasma cells

Immunophenotype: CD4+, CD56+, CD123+, BDCA2+, TCL-1+, CD3−, CD8−, TIA-1−, CD34−, CD68−, MPO−, CD1a−, EBV−

Genotype: No clonal rearrangement of T-cell receptor genes or immunoglobulin heavy or light chain genes.

DD: Unique clinical feature: contusiform confluent plaques.

References

Cota, C., Vale, E., Viana, I., et al. (2010) Cutaneous manifestations of blastic plasmacytoid dendritic cell neoplasm-morphologic and phenotypic variability in a series of 33 patients. *Am J Surg Pathol* **34**(1): 75–87.

Garnache-Ottou, F., Feuillard, J., and Saas, P. (2007) Plasmacytoid dendritic cell leukaemia/lymphoma: towards a well defined entity? *Br J Haematol* **136**(4): 539–48.

Giagounidis, A.A., Heinsch, M., Haase, S., and Aul, C. (2004) Early plasmacytoid dendritic cell leukemia/ lymphoma coexpressing myeloid antigens. *Ann Hematol* **83**(11): 716–21.

Kazakov, D.V., Mentzel, T., Burg, G., Dummer, R., and Kempf, W. (2003) Blastic natural killer-cell lymphoma of the skin associated with myelodysplastic syndrome or myelogenous leukaemia: a coincidence or more? *Br J Dermatol* **149**(4): 869–876.

Petrella, T., Bagot, M., Willemze, R., (2005) Blastic NK-cell lymphomas (agranular CD4+CD56+ hematodermic neoplasms): a review. *Am J Clin Pathol* **123**(5): 662–75.

Petrella, T., Comeau, M.R., Maynadie, M., et al. (2002) 'Agranular CD4+ CD56+ hematodermic neoplasm' (blastic NK-cell lymphoma) originates from a population of CD56+ precursor cells related to plasmacytoid monocytes. *Am J Surg Pathol* **26**(7): 852–62.

Petrella, T., Dalac, S., Maynadie, M., et al. (1999) CD4+ CD56+ cutaneous neoplasms: a distinct hematological entity? Groupe Francais d'Etude des Lymphomes Cutanes (GFELC). *Am J Surg Pathol* **23**(2): 137–46.

Precursor Lymphoblastic Leukemia/Lymphoma

The skin is not the primary site of manifestation and the diagnosis is based on findings in the lymph nodes, peripheral blood, and bone marrow. B- and T-lymphoblastic leukemia/ lymphoma has to be differentiated pheno-or genotypically. "Metastatic" nodules in the skin show monomorphous sheets of atypical imma- ture blast cells with finely dispersed chromatin.

Reference

Sander, C.A., Medeiros, L.J., Abruzzo, L.V., Horak, I.D., and Jaffe, E.S. (1991) Lymphoblastic lymphoma presenting in cutaneous sites. A clinicopathologic analysis of six cases. *J Am Acad Dermatol* **25**(6 Pt 1): 1023–31.

CHAPTER 13

Cutaneous Cysts

Atlas of Dermatopathology: Tumors, Nevi, and Cysts, First Edition. Günter Burg, Heinz Kutzner,
Werner Kempf, Josef Feit, and Bruce R. Smoller.
© 2019 John Wiley & Sons Ltd. Published 2019 by John Wiley & Sons Ltd.

STRATIFIED SQUAMOUS EPITHELIUM

Cutaneous cysts are benign encapsulated firm or fluctuant lesions, containing material of various types. Pseudocysts clinically are similar to cysts but do not have a capsule. Overviews on the various types of cysts and pseudocysts are given in the following papers.

References

Grosshans, E. and Cribier, B. (1994) [Cutaneous cysts and pseudocysts. I] *Ann Dermatol Venereol* **121**(8): 594–9.

Grosshans, E. and Cribier, B. (1994) [Cutaneous cysts and pseudocysts. II] *Ann Dermatol Venereol* **121**(9): 647–53.

Massa, M.C. and Medenica, M. (1985) Cutaneous adnexal tumors and cysts: a review. Part I. Tumors with hair follicular and sebaceous glandular differentiation and cysts related to different parts of the hair follicle. *Pathol Annu* **20**(Pt 2): 189–233.

Massa, M.C. and Medenica, M. (1987) Cutaneous adnexal tumors and cysts: a review. Part II Tumors with apocrine and eccrine glandular differentiation and miscellaneous cutaneous cysts. *Pathol Annu* **22**(Pt 1): 225–76.

Raff, M. (1979) [Cutaneous cysts and cystic skin tumors] *Hautarzt* **30**(5): 229–35.

Thaller, S.R. and Bauer, B.S. (1987) Cysts and cyst-like lesions of the skin and subcutaneous tissue. *Clin Plast Surg* **14**(2): 327–40.

Cysts with Epithelial Lining

Stratified Squamous Epithelium

Epidermal (Infundibular) Cysts

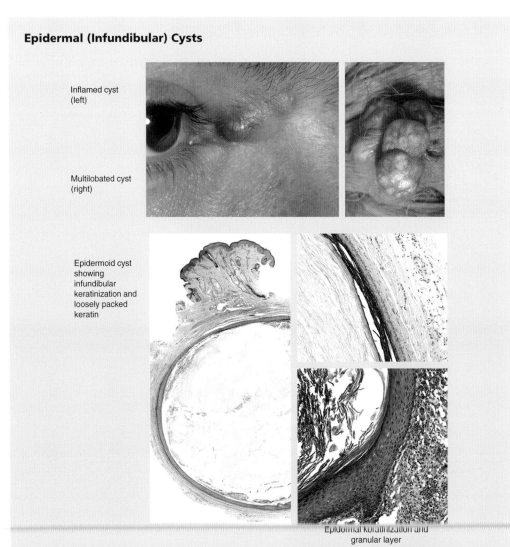

Inflamed cyst (left)

Multilobated cyst (right)

Epidermoid cyst showing infundibular keratinization and loosely packed keratin

Epidermal keratinization and granular layer

STRATIFIED SQUAMOUS EPITHELIUM

This most common cyst is filled with isolated hair shafts and keratinous material (squames) derived from the cornified mural layer. Epidermal cyst is not an "atheroma" but rather a genuine infundibular follicular cyst.

Cl: Round, slowly growing nodule, showing a central pore in some cases. Fixed or slightly movable beyond the overlying erythematous smooth skin surface. Preferred localisations are face, neck, and back. Frequent rupture of the epithelial cyst wall with subsequent bacterial infection leading to abscess formation, bursting, and draining.

Hi:

- Cyst wall shows flattened epithelium with infundibular-type epidermal keratinization and granular layer
- Basket-weave hyperkeratosis filling the cystic cavity
- Ruptured cysts show suppurative inflammation with granulomatous reaction, followed by fibrosis
- Little or no proliferative activity of the cyst wall epithelium
- Trichilemmal-type focal mural epithelium may be encountered in hybrid cysts

DD: Trichilemmal cyst; cystic adnexal tumor; cystic basal cell carcinoma; cutaneous metastasis.

Variant: Epidermal Proliferating Cyst

Epidermal cyst with proliferation of squamous epithelium on the bottom of the cyst wall

Hi: Proliferation of squamous epithelium on the bottom of the cyst wall is an unusual feature.

Variant: Epidermal Cyst with Pigment and Vellus Hairs

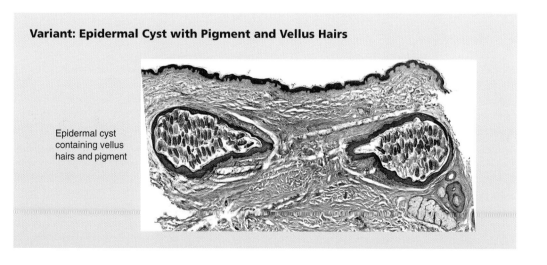

Epidermal cyst containing vellus hairs and pigment

STRATIFIED SQUAMOUS EPITHELIUM

Hi: Vellus hairs and pigment in the cyst cavity.

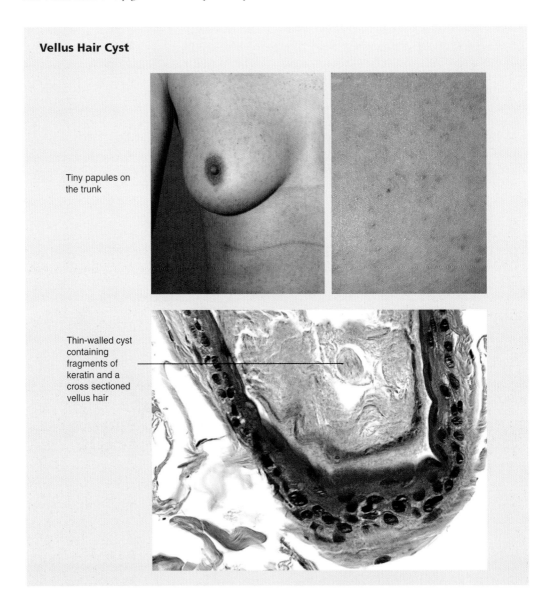

Vellus Hair Cyst

Tiny papules on the trunk

Thin-walled cyst containing fragments of keratin and a cross sectioned vellus hair

Similar to epidermal cysts, vellus hair cysts arise from the infundibular portion of the hair follicle and contain multiple small vellus hair shafts.
Cl: Multiple tiny papules preferentially on the chest and back, present since birth as part of an autosomal dominant disease (eruptive vellus hair cysts), and manifesting in puberty.
Hi:
• Small thin-walled cyst with stratified squamous epithelium, filled with densely packed keratinous masses (squames)

• Multiple small vellus hair shafts within the cyst
DD: Steatocystoma; adnexal tumors.

References

Ahn, S.K., Chung, J., Lee, W.S., Lee, S.H., and Choi, E.H. (1996) Hybrid cysts showing alternate combination of eruptive vellus hair cyst, steatocystoma multiplex, and epidermoid cyst, and an association among the three conditions. *Am J Dermatopathol* **18**(6): 645–9.

STRATIFIED SQUAMOUS EPITHELIUM

Plewig, G. (1990) Eruptive vellus hair cysts. A follicular cyst of the sebaceous duct (sometimes). *Am J Dermatopathol* **12**(5): 538–9.

Sanchez Yus, E. and Requena, L. (1990) Eruptive vellus hair cyst and steatocystoma multiplex. *Am J Dermatopathol* **12**(5): 536–7.

Trichilemmal (Isthmus-Catagen) Cyst

Firm nodule on the scalp

Trichilemmal keratinization. No granular layer. Abrupt transition to densely packed keratin

Granulomatous inflammation and cholesterol clefts

Arising mostly from the isthmus of anagen hair.
Cl: Solitary or multiple mobile firm, sometimes calcifying nodule(s) preferentially on the scalp (90%), face, back, and anogenital region.
Hi:
- Cyst wall consisting of pale stratified squamous epithelial layer
- No granular layer
- Abrupt transition between epithelial cells and homogeneous pale eosinophilic keratinous masses, filling the lumen of the cyst
- Dystrophic calcification, inflammatory granulomatous reaction, cholesterol cristals (clefts), and foamy macrophages are sometimes found

STRATIFIED SQUAMOUS EPITHELIUM

Immunohistochemistry: Epithelial layer showing strong positivity for CK17 and calretinin.

DD: Epidermal cyst; adnexal tumors; proliferating trichilemmal tumor.

References

Ivan, D., Bengana, C., Lazar, A.J., Diwan, A.H., and Prieto, V.G. (2007) Merkel cell tumor in a trichilemmal cyst: collision or association? *Am J Dermatopathol* **29**(2): 180–3.

Nakamura, T. (2011) Comparative immunohistochemical analyses on the modes of cell death/keratinization in epidermal cyst, trichilemmal cyst, and pilomatricoma. *Am J Dermatopathol* **33**(1): 78–83.

Su, W., Kheir, S.M., Berberian, B., and Cockerell, C.J. (2008) Merkel cell carcinoma in situ arising in a trichilemmal cyst: a case report and literature review. *Am J Dermatopathol* **30**(5): 458–61.

Milia

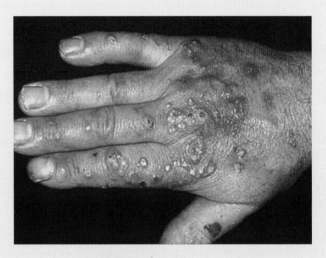

Multiple milia following blister formation in a patient with porphyria cutanea tarda

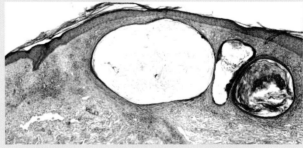

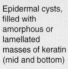

Epidermal cysts, filled with amorphous or lamellated masses of keratin (mid and bottom)

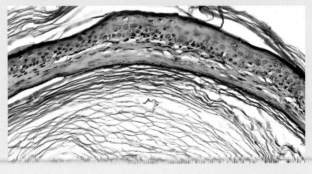

STRATIFIED SQUAMOUS EPITHELIUM

Milia are tiny epidermal cysts arising from the infundibular portion of vellus hairs or dermal sweat ducts, without connection to the overlying epidermis.

Cl: Primary milia temporarily present as yellowish tiny papules in the face of infants. They usually disappear within a few weeks. Secondary milia occur in the aftermath of blistering dermatoses (e.g. porphyria cutanea tarda, dystrophic epidermolysis) or after superficial wounds.

Hi:

- Cyst wall with stratified squamous epithelium
- Cyst lumen filled with keratinous material
- Often connected to a vellus hair follicle

DD: Tiny adnexal tumors; steatocystoma; vellus hair cyst.

References

Cho, S.H., Cho, B.K., and Kim, C.W. (1997) Milia en plaque associated with pseudoxanthoma elasticum. *J Cutan Pathol* **24**(1): 61–3.

Terui, H., Hashimoto, A., Yamasaki, K., and Aiba, S. (2016) Milia en plaque as a distinct follicular hamartoma with cystic trichoepitheliomatous features. *Am J Dermatopathol* **38**(3): 212–17.

Follicular Hybrid Cyst

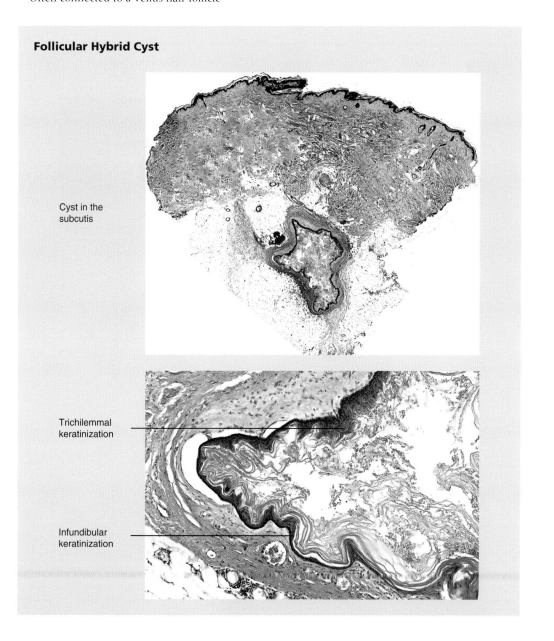

Cyst in the subcutis

Trichilemmal keratinization

Infundibular keratinization

STRATIFIED SQUAMOUS EPITHELIUM WITH SWEAT GLAND COMPONENTS: HIDROCYSTOMA

Follicular hybrid cyst shows combined features of both infundibular and trichilemmal keratinization in different portions of the cyst.

Cl: Cystic lesions, preferentially localized on the face.

Hi:
- Infundibular keratinization in one portion of the cyst
- Trichilemmal keratinization in another portion of the cyst
- Abrupt transition from infundibular to trichilemmal keratinization

DD: Pilar cyst; epidermal cyst.

References

Dargent, J.L., Aupaix, F., and Herin, M. (2013) Follicular hybrid cyst with isthmic-catagen, pilomatrical, and syringocystadenoma papilliferum components. *Am J Dermatopathol* **35**(3): 399–400.

Miyake, H., Hara, H., Shimojima, H., and Suzuki, H. (2004) Follicular hybrid cyst (trichilemmal cyst and pilomatricoma) arising within a nevus sebaceus. *Am J Dermatopathol* **26**(5): 390–3.

Requena, L. and Sanchez Yus, E. (1991) Follicular hybrid cysts. An expanded spectrum. *Am J Dermatopathol* **13**(3): 228–33.

Hidrocystoma (Cystadenoma)

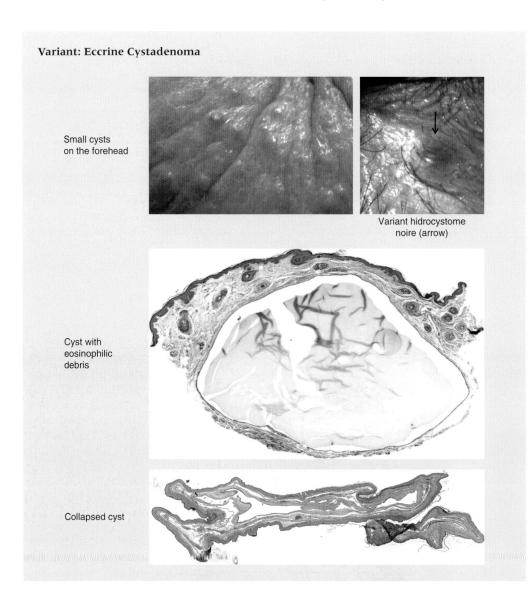

Variant: Eccrine Cystadenoma

Small cysts on the forehead

Variant hidrocystome noire (arrow)

Cyst with eosinophilic debris

Collapsed cyst

STRATIFIED SQUAMOUS EPITHELIUM WITH SWEAT GLAND COMPONENTS: HIDROCYSTOMA

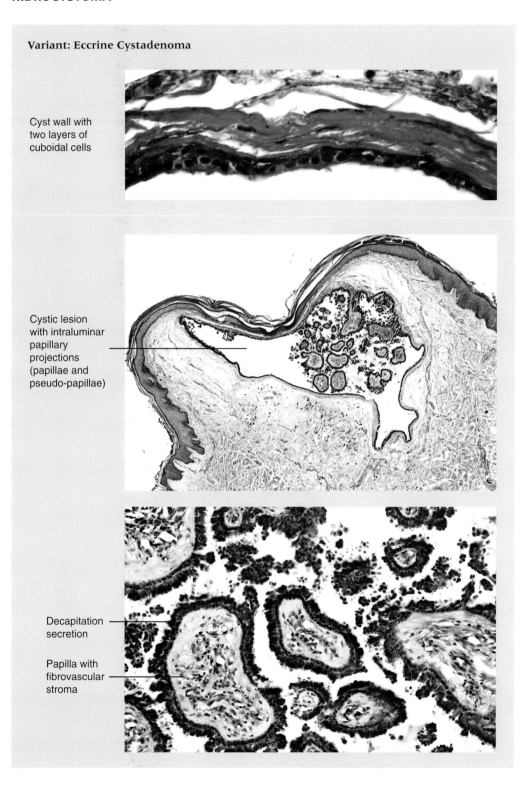

Variant: Eccrine Cystadenoma

Cyst wall with two layers of cuboidal cells

Cystic lesion with intraluminar papillary projections (papillae and pseudo-papillae)

Decapitation secretion

Papilla with fibrovascular stroma

STRATIFIED SQUAMOUS EPITHELIUM WITH SWEAT GLAND COMPONENTS: HIDROCYSTOMA

Hidrocystomas may contain eccrine or apocrine components or both in the cystic wall of stratified squamous epithelium.

Cl: Solitary or multiple intradermal cystic lesions. Location: face or scalp. Lipofuscin-filled "hidrocystome noire" may simulate nodular malignant melanoma due to the blue-black color of intracystic pigment (Tyndall effect).

Hi:
- Cystic cavity may be dilated or collapsed
- Cyst wall lined with secreting epithelium with double layer of cuboidal cells
- Eccrine or apocrine secretion
- Intraluminar papillary projections
- Cyst cavity empty or filled with amorphous eosinophilic masses or dark lipofuscin pigment

Variant: Apocrine Cystadenoma

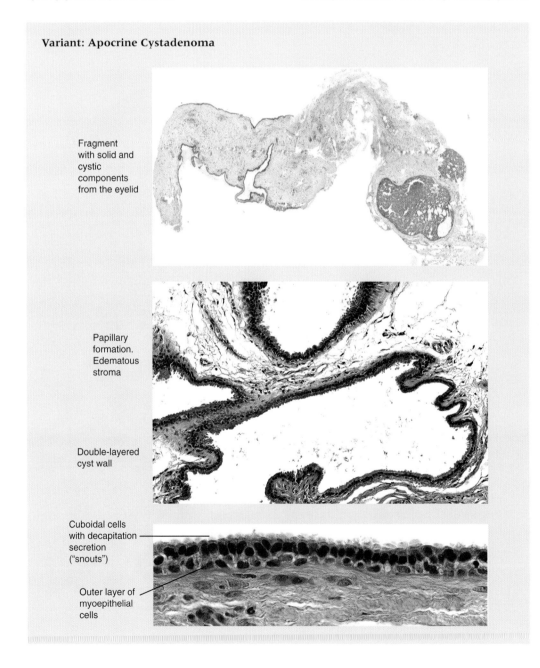

Fragment with solid and cystic components from the eyelid

Papillary formation. Edematous stroma

Double-layered cyst wall

Cuboidal cells with decapitation secretion ("snouts")

Outer layer of myoepithelial cells

STRATIFIED SQUAMOUS EPITHELIUM

Cl: This small solitary translucent cystic lesion is typically located in the periorbital area (eyelid). Lesions on the penis with similar morphological features are known as median raphe cysts.

Hi:

- Dilated cyst, sometimes with intracystic papillary formations
- Combination of papilla (with stroma) and pseudopapillae (epithelial mounts without stroma)
- Epithelial cyst wall consists of:
  - inner layer of cuboidal cells with decapitation secretion
  - outer layer, consisting of myoepithelial cells
- Edematous or compact stroma

DD: Digital papillary adenocarcinoma (aggressive digital papillary adenocarcinoma) is an invasive adnexal carcinoma on palms and soles simulating a benign apocrine cystadenoma. Hallmarks are cystic structures with a double layer of apocrine epithelia on the inside and a contiguous outer layer of myoepithelia ("*in situ*" type of adenocarcinoma). There is a marked combination of solid and cystic parts, with papillae and pseudopapillae in the latter. Pleomorphism may be moderate. Proliferative activity and mitoses are conspicuous features. Pathologists should be aware that a proliferative apocrine hidrocystoma or cystadenoma on palms and soles in most cases represents a digital papillary adenocarcinoma.

References

Molina-Ruiz, A.M., Llamas-Velasco, M., Rutten, A., Cerroni, L., and Requena, L. (2016) "Apocrine hidrocystoma and cystadenoma"-like tumor of the digits or toes: a potential diagnostic pitfall of digital papillary adenocarcinoma. *Am J Surg Pathol* **40**(3): 410–18.

Sugiyama, A., Sugiura, M., Piris, A., Tomita, Y., and Mihm, M.C. (2007) Apocrine cystadenoma and apocrine hidrocystoma: examination of 21 cases with emphasis on nomenclature according to proliferative features. *J Cutan Pathol* **34**(12): 912–17.

Yanagi, T., Sawamura, D., Nishie, W., Abe, M., Shibaki, A., and Shimizu, H. (2006) Multiple apocrine hidrocystoma showing plane pigmented macules. *J Am Acad Dermatol* **54**(2 Suppl): S53–4.

Steatocystoma, Multiplex and Simplex

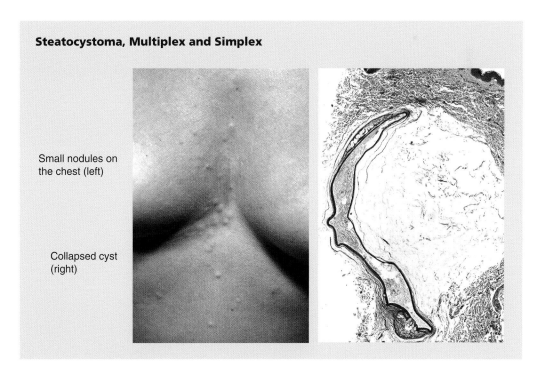

Small nodules on the chest (left)

Collapsed cyst (right)

STRATIFIED SQUAMOUS EPITHELIUM

Steatocystoma, Multiplex and Simplex

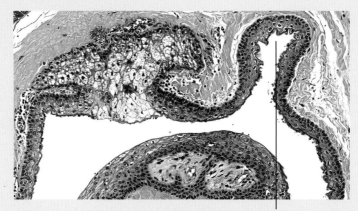

Sebaceous gland in cyst-wall

Typical crenellated inner layer of epithelial cyst wall

While steatocystoma multiplex is an autosomal dominant inherited disease, steatocystoma simplex is not. Lesions manifest in puberty. They are considered to be hamartomas of the pilar-sebaceous structure.

Cl: Yellowish or skin-colored round nodules, preferentially located in the sternal region, axilla, arms or genital area.

Hi:

- The cyst wall shows a characteristically wavy (crenellated) luminal surface
- Flat sebaceous glands within the cyst wall
- The cyst may be collapsed, and contain lipids and keratinous material

Immunohistochemistry: Marked expression of calretinin in the upper crenelated epithelial layer.

DD: Epidermoid cysts; vellus hair cysts; milia; adnexal tumors; acne.

References

Ahn, S.K., Chung, J., Lee, W.S., Lee, S.H., and Choi, E.H. (1996) Hybrid cysts showing alternate combination of eruptive vellus hair cyst, steatocystoma multiplex, and epidermoid cyst, and an association among the three conditions. *Am J Dermatopathol* **18**(6): 645–9.

Fernandez-Flores, A. (2015) On steatocystoma, sebaceous duct cyst, isthmic-anagenic cyst, and CK19. *Am J Dermatopathol* **37**(9): 733–4.

Sabater-Marco, V. and Perez-Ferriols, A. (1996) Steatocystoma multiplex with smooth muscle. A hamartoma of the pilosebaceous apparatus. *Am J Dermatopathol* **18**(5): 548–50.

Sanchez Yus, E. and Requena, L. (1990) Eruptive vellus hair cyst and steatocystoma multiplex. *Am J Dermatopathol* **12**(5): 536–7.

Tomkova, H., Fujimoto, W., and Arata, J. (1997) Expression of keratins (K10 and K17) in steatocystoma multiplex, eruptive vellus hair cysts, and epidermoid and trichilemmal cysts. *Am J Dermatopathol* **19**(3): 250–3.

Dermoid Cyst

Cyst with stratified epithelium

STRATIFIED SQUAMOUS EPITHELIUM

Dermoid Cyst

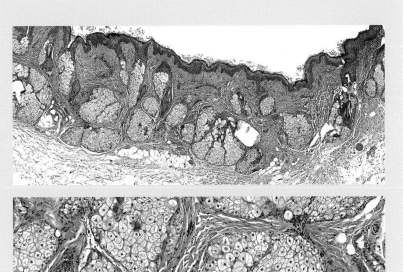

Mature epidermal appendages attached to the cyst (top and below)

This cyst develops in embryological fusion lines and contains ectodermal and mesenchymal elements. It is present from birth.

Cl: Well-defined, hard, yellow or skin-colored nodule, sometimes with vellus hairs. Preferential localisations are the periorbital and midline areas of the face.

Hi:

- Cyst wall consists of stratified squamous epithelium
- Various mature epidermal appendages such as hairs with sebaceous glands and sweat glands are attached to the cyst
- Smooth muscle may be apparent in the cyst wall

DD: Epidermal cyst; steatocystoma.

Reference

Kudo, Y., Katagiri, K., Ishii, Y., et al. (1997) Conjunctival dermoid cyst in an infant. *J Am Acad Dermatol* **36**(5 Pt 1): 784–5.

STRATIFIED SQUAMOUS EPITHELIUM

Pilonidal Sinus (Pilonidal Cyst)

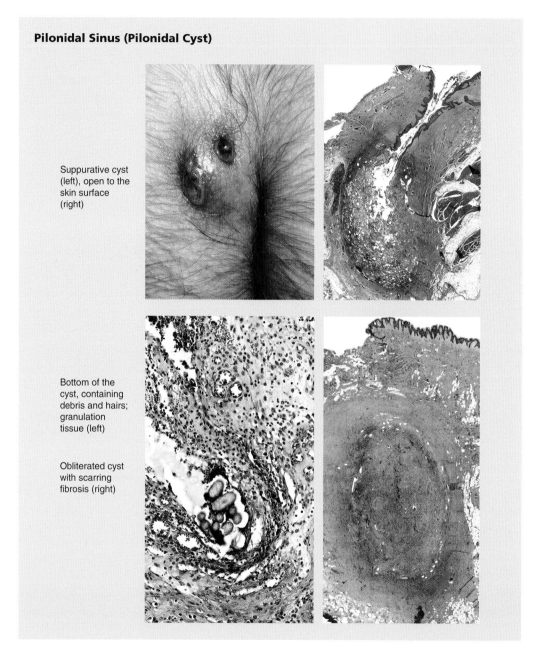

Suppurative cyst (left), open to the skin surface (right)

Bottom of the cyst, containing debris and hairs; granulation tissue (left)

Obliterated cyst with scarring fibrosis (right)

Pilonidal sinus is part of the acne tetrad and may result from local infection and inflammation in the sacral area, corresponding to granulomatous reaction following ingrown hair of the beard. In rare cases, squamous cell carcinoma may develop within the chronic inflammatory process.

Cl: The hair-bearing area in the gluteal fold is the typical localisation, where a fluctuant inflamed cystic lesion with draining to the surface develops.

Hi:
- Remnants of a ruptured epithelial cyst with stratified squamous epithelium
- Granulomatous inflammation containing multiple hair shafts without epithelial lining
- Scarring fibrosis as late-stage manifestation

DD: Other inflamed cysts; acneiform lesions.

NON-STRATIFIED SQUAMOUS EPITHELIUM

References

Kim, Y.A. and Thomas, I. (1993) Metastatic squamous cell carcinoma arising in a pilonidal sinus. *J Am Acad Dermatol* **29**(2 Pt 1): 272–4.

Val-Bernal, J.F., Azcarretazabal, T., and Garijo, M.F. (1999) Pilonidal sinus of the penis. A report of two cases, one of them associated with actinomycosis. *J Cutan Pathol* **26**(3): 155–8.

Non-Stratified Squamous Epithelium

Some adnexal tumors, delineated in the respective chapter, and other cysts of non-stratified squamous epithelium are not further discussed here.

- Eccrine hidrocystoma
- Apocrine hidrocystoma
- Papillary apocrine cystadenoma
- Bronchiogenic cyst
- Branchial cleft cyst
- Thyroglossal duct cyst
- Ciliated cyst of the vulva
- Omphalomesenteric cyst
- Gartner's duct cyst
- Endometriosis

Reference

Kurban, R.S. and Bhawan, J. (1991) Cutaneous cysts lined by nonsquamous epithelium. *Am J Dermatopathol* **13**(5): 509–17.

Cutaneous Ciliated Cyst of the Lower Limb

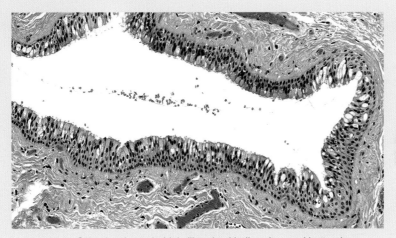

Cyst showing cuboidal ciliated epithelium (top and bottom)

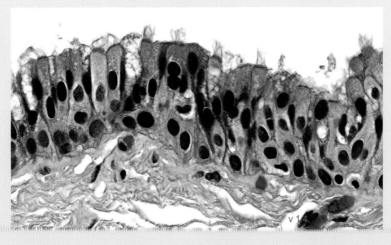

NON-STRATIFIED SQUAMOUS EPITHELIUM

Develops almost exclusively in women, originating from heterotopic tissue of the Müllerian duct and manifesting on the lower extremities. However, other locations and presentation in men also occur.

Cl: Solitary lesion presenting as subcutaneous swelling on the back or lower extremities.

Hi:

* Deep dermis or subcutis
* The cyst wall consists of cylindrical or cuboidal epithelium, lined by ciliated cells
* Cavity microscopically empty or filled with oily fluid

DD: Various cysts; apocrine hidrocystoma.

References

Ashton, M.A. (1995) Cutaneous ciliated cyst of the lower limb in a male. *Histopathology* **26**(5): 467–9.

Bivin, W.W. Jr, Heath, J.E., Drachenberg, C.B., Strauch, E.D., and Papadimitriou, J.C. (2010) Cutaneous ciliated cyst: a case report with focus on mullerian heterotopia and comparison with eccrine sweat glands. *Am J Dermatopathol* **32**(7): 731–4.

Fontaine, D.G., Lau, H., Murray, S.K., Fraser, R.B., and Wright, J.R. (2002) Cutaneous ciliated cyst of the abdominal wall: a case report with a review of the literature and discussion of pathogenesis. *Am J Dermatopathol* **24**(1): 63–6.

Hung, T., Yang, A., Binder, S.W., and Barnhill, R.L. (2012) Cutaneous ciliated cyst on the finger: a cutaneous mullerian cyst. *Am J Dermatopathol* **34**(3): 335–8.

Reserva, J.L., Carrigg, A.B., Schnebelen, A.M., Hiatt, K.M., and Cheung, W.L. (2014) Cutaneous ciliated cyst of the scalp: a case report of a cutaneous ciliated eccrine cyst and a brief review of the literature. *Am J Dermatopathol* **36**(8): 679–82.

Sickel, J.Z. (1994) Cutaneous ciliated cyst of the scalp. A case report with immunohistochemical evidence for estrogen and progesterone receptors. *Am J Dermatopathol* **16**(1): 76–9.

Tachibana, T., Sakamoto, F., Ito, M., Ito, K., Kaneko, Y., and Takenouchi, T. (1995) Cutaneous ciliated cyst: a case report and histochemical, immunohistochemical, and ultrastructural study. *J Cutan Pathol* **22**(1): 33–7.

Median Raphe Cyst

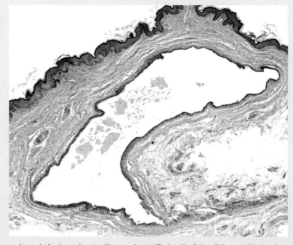

Irregularly shaped cyst with pseudostratified epithelial wall (top and bottom)

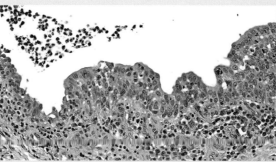

This cyst is a result of defects in embryological development of the median raphe, which extends from the urethra to the anus and normally is closed before birth.

Cl: Small translucent papules on the penis or perineum.

Hi:

- Irregularly shaped hidrocystoma-like cyst in the mid dermis
- Cyst wall lined by pseudostratified columnar epithelium
- No connection with the epidermis
- Occasionally mucin-secreting cyst wall or pigmented or ciliated

DD: Apocrine cystadenoma.

References

Dini, M., Baroni, G., and Colafranceschi, M. (2001) Median raphe cyst of the penis: a report of two cases with immunohistochemical investigation. *Am J Dermatopathol* **23**(4): 320–4.

Nishida, H., Kashima, K., Daa, T., et al. (2012) Pigmented median raphe cyst of the penis. *J Cutan Pathol* **39**(8): 808–10.

Romani, J., Barnadas, M.A., Miralles, J., Curell, R., and de Moragas, J.M. (1995) Median raphe cyst of the penis with ciliated cells. *J Cutan Pathol* **22**(4): 378–81.

Cysts without Epithelial Lining (Pseudocysts)

Oral Mucous Cyst and Superficial Mucocele of the Lip

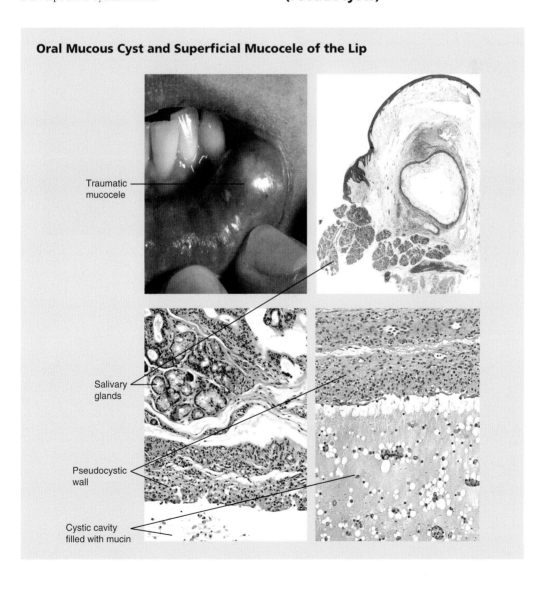

Traumatic mucocele

Salivary glands

Pseudocystic wall

Cystic cavity filled with mucin

Cl: Translucent submucosal node developing on lip, tongue or buccal mucosa in the vicinity of salivary glands, following minor injury.

Hi:

*   Deposit of sialomucin (PAS, alcian blue), produced by salivary glands in the vicinity
*   Fibrous and inflammatory reactions provide a pseudocystic wall
*   Remnants of ruptured salivary duct

Reference

Henry, C.R., Nace, M., and Helm, K.F. (2008) Collagenous spherulosis in an oral mucous cyst. *J Cutan Pathol* **35**(4): 428–30.

Digital Myxoid Cyst

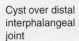 Cyst over distal interphalangeal joint

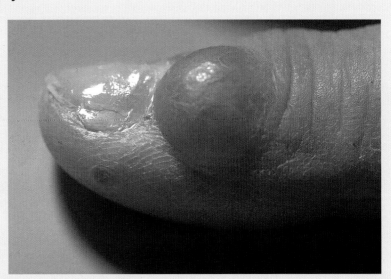

Mucin deposits (HE, alcian blue)

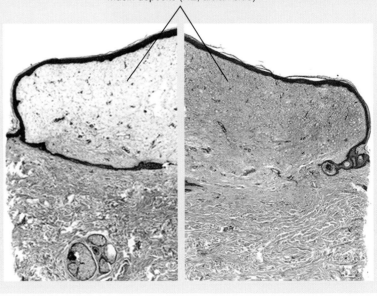

This cyst is considered to be either a variant of a ganglion connected with an interphalangeal joint or resulting from independent proliferation of fibroblasts, producing glucosaminoglycans.

DD of Digital Myxoid Cyst: Cutaneous Myxoma

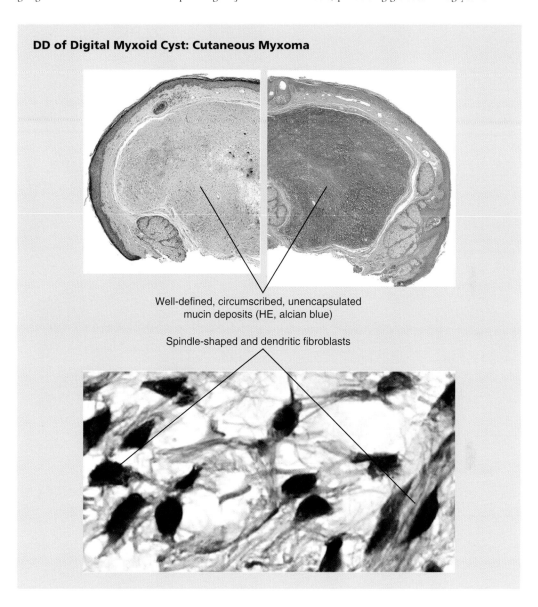

Well-defined, circumscribed, unencapsulated mucin deposits (HE, alcian blue)

Spindle-shaped and dendritic fibroblasts

Cl: Translucent small cysts over the dorsal aspects of interphalangeal joints, preferentially of the fingers.

Hi:
- Very thin ("membranous") overlying epidermis
- No cyst wall
- Mucinous deposits within the dermis
- Lack of vessels within mucinous zones
- Occasionally, histiocytic or granulomatous inflammatory response along with a fibrous pseudocapsule

DD: Cutaneous myxoma; wart; digital fibrokeratoma; digital synovial cyst (ganglion).

Reference

Radice, F. and Gianotti, R. (1993) Cutaneous ganglion cell tumor of the skin. Case report and review of the literature. *Am J Dermatopathol* **15**(5): 488–91.

Synovial Cyst (Ganglion)

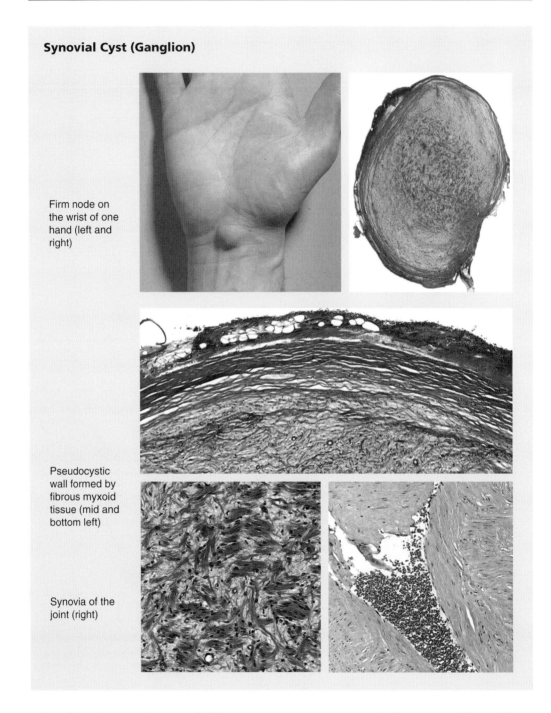

Firm node on the wrist of one hand (left and right)

Pseudocystic wall formed by fibrous myxoid tissue (mid and bottom left)

Synovia of the joint (right)

Cl: Small pseudocyst, often proceeded by trauma. Location: extremities, near joints.

Hi:
• Wall formed by fibrous tissue

• Connection with the synovia of the underlying joint
• Amorphous myxoid material in the cystic cavity
• Fibrous scar formation

Index

A

ABCD (A:asymmetry; B:border; C:colour; D:diameter)
         rule 189
Abrikossoff granular cell tumor 354
acantholytic acanthoma 26–7
acantholytic (angiosarcoma-like) squamous cell
         carcinoma 316–17
acantholytic SCC (epithelioma spinocellulare segregans of
         Delacretaz) 74–6
acantholytic solar keratosis 16
acanthomas
    non-viral 19–31
        acantholytic acanthoma 26–7
        callus, factitial acanthoma 20–1
        knuckle pads (chewing pads) 21–2
        large cell acanthoma 23–4
        pale (clear) cell acanthoma 22
        porokeratoma (porokeratosis Mibelli) 30–1
        solar lentigo 19–20
        warty dyskeratoma 27
    viral 31–9
        acrokeratosis verruciformis (Hopf) 37
        bowenoid papulosis 35–6
        molluscum contagiosum 38–9
        verruca vulgaris/variants 31–4
acanthosis nigricans 14–15
acanthotic seborrheic keratosis 4
accessory nipple 218
accessory tragus 217
acquired fibrokeratoma 216
acquired immunodeficiency syndrome/human
         immunodeficiency virus (AIDS/HIV) 273,
         299, 303
acquired melanocytic nevi, common 155–71
    compound nevus 157–8
    dermal nevus, with maturation 158–60
        "activated" acral (lentiginous) melanocytic nevus 162–3
        ancient nevus 170–1
        balloon cell nevus 161
        combined nevus 167
        eczematoid melanocytic (Meyerson's) nevus 165–6
        genital melanocytic nevus 162–3
        halo nevus (leukoderma centrifugum acquisitum;
                 Sutton nevus) 163–4
        Miescher's nevus (dermal nevus) 160
        nevus in pregnancy 168–9
        osteo-nevus of Nanta 166
        recurrent (persistent) melanocytic nevus
                 (pseudomelanoma) 167–8
    junctional nevus 156
    melanosis neviformis (pigmented hairy
                 epidermal nevus) 155

acral arteriovenous hemangioma (cirsoid aneurysm) 256–7
acral lentiginous melanoma (ALM) 189, 194–6
acral pseudolymphomatous angiokeratoma of children
         (APACHE) 269
acroangiodermatitis Mali (pseudo-Kaposi's sarcoma) 276–7
acroasphyctic digitorum angiokeratoma (Mibelli) 267, 269
acrochordon 209–10
acrokeratosis verruciformis (Hopf) 37–8
acrolentiginous melanoma 206
acrospiroma, "eccrine" (misnomer) 97–8
actinic solar keratoses 15–18
"activated" acral (lentiginous) melanocytic nevus 161–2
activated (irritated) seborrheic keratosis 7
adenoid-cystic basal cell carcinoma 62–3
adenoma sebaceum associated with Pringle–Bourneville
         disease 319–21
adipophilin 117
adnexal structures 85–144
    hair follicle differentiation 119–43
        benign neoplasms 121–40
            pilar sheath acanthoma 121–2
            pilomatricoma (calcifying epithelioma
                     Malherbe) 137–8
            proliferating trichilemmal (pilar) tumor (PTT)
                     (proliferating trichilemmal cyst) 138–40
            trichadenoma (Nikolowski) 136–7
            trichilemmoma (tricholemmoma) 122–3
            trichoblastoma (trichoblastic fibroma; immature
                     trichoepithelioma) 127–31
            trichoepithelioma (sclerosing epithelial
                     hamartoma) 131–3
            trichoepithelioma (superficial
                     trichoblastoma) 125–6
            trichofolliculoma (folliculosebaceous cystic
                     hamartoma) 133–5
            tumor of the follicular infundibulum
                     (infundibuloma) 124–5
        malignant neoplasms 140–3
            malignant pilomatricoma (pilomatrical
                     carcinoma) 140–1
            trichilemmal carcinoma 141–2
            trichoblastic carcinoma 142–3
        nevi, hyperplasia, and hamartomas 119–21
            conical infundibular acanthoma (giant dilated pore
                     of Winer) 120–1
    pilosebaceous mesenchyme, benign neoplasms,
                 trichodiscoma (follicular fibroma;
                 fibrofolliculoma; perifollicular
                 fibroma) 143
    sebaceous differentiation 110–19
        benign neoplasms 114–18
            Muir–Torre syndrome 115–16

Atlas of Dermatopathology: Tumors, Nevi, and Cysts, First Edition. Günter Burg, Heinz Kutzner,
Werner Kempf, Josef Feit, and Bruce R. Smoller.
© 2019 John Wiley & Sons Ltd. Published 2019 by John Wiley & Sons Ltd.